EMOT

Founded by C. K. Ogden

The International Library of Psychology

GENERAL PSYCHOLOGY
In 38 Volumes

EMOTION

A Comprehensive Phenomenology of Theories and their Meanings for Therapy

JAMES HILLMAN

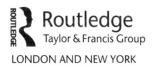

Routledge
Taylor & Francis Group

LONDON AND NEW YORK

First published in 1960 by
Routledge
2 Park Square, Milton Park, Abingdon, Oxfordshire OX14 4RN
711 Third Avenue, New York, NY 10017

First issued in paperback 2014

Routledge is an imprint of the Taylor and Francis Group, an informa business

© 1960 James Hillman

British Library Cataloguing in Publication Data
A CIP catalogue record for this book
is available from the British Library

Emotion
ISBN 0415-21026-7
General Psychology: 38 Volumes
ISBN 0415-21129-8
The International Library of Psychology: 204 Volumes
ISBN 0415-19132-7

ISBN 13: 978-1-138-88247-8 (pbk)
ISBN 13: 978-0-415-21026-3 (hbk)

To

the spirits of my grandfathers

JOEL HILLMAN AND JOSEPH KRAUSKOPF

CONTENTS

Contents

PART III. INTEGRATION

PREFATORY NOTE

THIS BOOK is a slightly revised version of my Doctor's Dissertation submitted in the Spring of 1958 to the Faculty of Arts of the University of Zurich, and my first debt is due to Professor Wilhelm Keller under whom I studied. He generously believed in and warmly encouraged my work throughout. His range of knowledge, his critical acuity and the thoroughness with which he went through the work provided the example of the master without which this book would not have been possible. Although the phenomenological method and philosophical approach to the problems of psychology reflect his attitudes, we sometimes came to different conclusions. But wherever we disagreed, his was always the larger spirit graciously allowing me, his student, the right of way; and I wish to thank him here for all he did for me and for this book.

Dr. K. W. Bash gave freely of his valuable time to read the entire typescript and he brought many corrections and raised many questions which led me deeper into the work. Dr. C. A. Meier and Dr. Marvin Spiegelman read through parts of the work in its early stages and made useful suggestions. I am further indebted to Dr. Meier for his sustained interest in the progress of the work from 1955 onward, and also for the seed idea of the problem of emotion theory which fell in my mind during one of his lectures at the C. G. Jung Institute, Zurich. Mr. Morris Philipson helped me to think more clearly in Part One and Dr. Robert Stein encouraged me towards some of my conclusions in Part Three. To these five gentlemen I am very grateful indeed because without their kind interest my shortcomings would be even more obvious.

I turned over to Mr. A. K. Donoghue the task of checking the quotations in my text against the originals. I wish to thank him here for his tireless effort and help with many fine points, especially with my shaky Latin. Although this task of preparing the book for the press was largely in his hands, I must assume the ultimate responsibility for any error which might appear.

In particular, I am responsible for rendering into English those quotations from foreign languages which were not available to me in authorized translations.

Frau Dr. Katja Liepmann translated the bulk of the typescript into German in order to comply with University requirements. I owe her much for her loyal and sympathetic sharing of the problems of the work when it was in thesis form.

I am grateful to Mme Danielle Rhally-Python for her work on the bibliography. I should also like to thank the many people who so kindly assisted me in the libraries where I worked: the Zurich Zentralbibliothek, the Library of the Burghölzli Clinic, the University Library in Cambridge, the Library of the Department of Psychology there, and the Library of Trinity College, Dublin.

I owe thanks to many others too: my former teachers—especially Prof. E. J. Furlong—at Trinity College, Dublin; Dr. C. G. Jung for a conversation about emotion; all the workers in the field whose writings I have made use of; Miss Una Thomas, Mrs. Virginia Coleman and Mrs. Alice Maurer for their secretarial work; Mr. Norman Franklin, Mr. C. A. Thurley; friends and colleagues in Zurich; and my wife, Catharina.

J. H.

Zurich,
  August 15, 1959.

PART I

Introduction

'As there is no man so temperate but that he sometimes experienceth the violence of Passions, and that the disorder thereof is a fate from which very few can fence themselves; so it is the Subject whereupon Philosophers have most exercised their brains, and is the part of Moral Philosophy which hath oftest been examined; But if I may speak my sense with freedom, and if I may be permitted to censure my Masters, I am of opinion, that there is no point in the whole body of Philosophy, that hath been treated of with more ostentation and less of profit . . .'—*The Use of the Passions*, J. F. Senault (transl. by Henry, Earl of Monmouth), London, 1649.

A. THE PROBLEM

FROM all the evidence at hand the concept of emotion has become central to the issues of our time. Wherever we turn in the various fields and sciences of contemporary life we come up against this concept which is used to refer to a crucial problem in each area.

In psychotherapy, the concept of emotion plays a significant role: the abreaction and catharsis of repressed emotions in the method of Freud, the emotionally-toned complex in Jung, the emotional basic needs in Horney, are concepts essential to the theory and practice of these therapies. Writers from all the various schools of psychotherapy make much of 'emotional insight' [1] and of the 'affective contact' [2] in the transference phenomenon, etc. Case histories, technical papers and the theoretical literature all show that emotion is the centre theme of every analysis and of every transformation in every analysis.

Emotion is also the key concept in psychosomatic medicine.[3] Research into the history of this field[4] shows that emotion has long been recognized as playing the crucial role in the body-mind relation, but it is in the twentieth century that this has been particularly stressed.[5] Psycho-surgery also turns on the concept of emotion. Allison and Allison write:

> Freeman and Watts have emphasized the point that '... emotional tension is the prime requisite for success in Prefrontal Lobotomy'. It appears that as yet there is no psychiatric diagnosis that causes one to think immediately of psycho-surgery. Rather, there is a constellation of symptoms described by Arnot as, 'a fixed state of tortured self-concern'. Inner emotional tension is implied in this description, and Robinson states the following in this regard: 'Psycho-surgery, then, not only relieves emotional tension; it prevents the development of future tensions. ...' [6]

In psychiatry, not only does diagnosis and classification make use of the concept of emotion and of emotional categories, but in

---

[1] Zilboorg, G., 'The Emotional Problem and the Therapeutic Role of Insight', *Yearbook of Psychoanalysis*, Vol. IX, N.Y., 1953, pp. 199–219.

[2] Carp (ed.), *The Affective Contact* (Report from International Congress for Psychotherapeutics), Amsterdam, 1952.

[3] EBC, p. vii.

[4] Margetts, E. L., 'Historical Notes on Psychosomatic Medicine', RDPM 54, pp. 41–68.

[5] De Crinis, M., *Der Affekt und seine körperlichen Grundlagen*, Leipzig, 1944, p. 14; EBC, p. vii.

[6] Allison, H. W., and Allison, S. G., 'Personality Changes Following Transorbital Lobotomy', *J. Abn. Soc. Psychol.*, 1954, pp. 219–23.

3

particular the indications for the various, physically violent, methods of treatment often depend upon the generic concept of emotion or upon specific concepts of emotion such as 'excitement', 'depression', 'indifference', etc. In point here, Anton-Stephens, reporting on the use of chlorpromazine, says:

> *Psychic Indifference.* This is perhaps the characteristic psychiatric response to chlorpromazine. Patients responding well to the drug have developed an attitude of indifference both to their surroundings and their symptoms best summarized by the current phrase 'couldn't care less'.[1]

In addition to the important role the concept of emotion plays in the spurt of interest in chemical therapies of mental disorders and in the new 'wonder-drugs' now habitually employed to change emotional states, the concept of emotion stands out importantly in the regions where psychiatry and sociology meet, e.g. the world-wide burdens of alcoholism and juvenile delinquency.

If we turn to the literature of psycho-diagnostics and clinical testing (with its influential ramifications in modern society), we find again the concept of emotion is crucial. The subject tested and/or diagnosed is assessed in accordance with various concepts such as 'emotional maturity', 'emotional attachments', 'emotional instability', 'emotional insecurity', and the like. In the field of developmental psychology, research occupies itself more and more with the emotional aspects of earliest childhood and the emotions in the mother-child relationship, and seeks therein causes and cures for many later psychological disorders.

In short, one is led to conclude that much, if not all, of the judgments concerning aetiology, diagnosis, treatment and cure in these several related fields of psychology depend to a great extent upon the concept of emotion in the mind of the practitioner.

In a wider field, wherever we turn to examine contemporary problems we find 'emotion' playing a leading part. Sociologists make use of the concept in many areas of their work: political phenomena, propaganda and mass psychology, the sociology of the family and community, and also in their publications on the shadowy aspects of society, e.g. prostitution, sexual perversions, delinquency, etc. In economics, concepts of emotion have recently come to the fore in studies of motivational research, or the emotional aspects of purchasing. The role of the concept of emotion in ethics, in education and in aesthetics is traditional and so central to those fields that it does not need pointing out here. The concept appears in theological debate whenever 'faith' or 'belief' is discussed, and especially in

---

[1] Anton-Stephens, D., 'Preliminary Observations on the Psychiatric Uses of Chlorpromazine', *J. Ment. Sci.*, 1954, pp. 543–57.

regard to questions of 'enthusiasm', 'mysticism' and, of course, in the recent crusades of 'revivalism'. In semantics and modern linguistic analysis, the 'emotive' meaning of words and statements has become one of the main topics to exercise the minds of those whose writings are found in the professional journals. Parapsychology too gives importance to emotional factors.[1]

In particular, there are many authors who make of the concept of emotion a basis for their respective fields of inquiry: Shand[2] on character; Denison[3] on civilization; Collingwood[4] on art; Grimberg[5] on delinquency; Bleuler[6] on psychopathology, to name but a few. We might mention, as well, the use of specific concepts of emotion such as 'dread', 'disgust', 'fear', etc., which are fundamental to existential philosophy.

Yet when we come home to systematic (academic or theoretical) psychology to inquire quite naïvely: 'What is emotion; how is it defined; what is its origin, nature, purpose; what are its properties and laws; everyone uses this concept "emotion"—what are we speaking about?', we find a curious and overwhelming confusion. Stout writes:

> If we ask the question, What is an emotion? The first answer that occurs to common sense is a list of specific emotions—fear, anger, hope, suspense, jealousy, and the like. When we push the inquiry further, and ask what character these states have in common which leads us to apply the same name 'emotion' to all of them, we find psychologists giving various and inconsistent answers.[7]

In the same vein Claparède writes:

> The psychology of affective processes is the most confused chapter in all psychology. Here it is that the greatest differences appear from one psychologist to another. They are in agreement neither on the facts nor on the words.[8]

The *Encyclopedia Britannica* (1955), states:

> Our knowledge of the topic emotion is much less complete than our knowledge of the other topics in the field of psychology.

The introduction to a modern dictionary of psychology says:

> In preparing our definitions we have been struck by the extreme

---

[1] Mangan, G., 'A Review of Published Research on the Relationship of some Personality Variables to ESP Scoring Level', *Parapsychol. Mono.* 1, N.Y., 1958.
[2] Shand, A. F., *The Foundations of Character*, London, 2nd edn., 1920.
[3] Denison, J. H., *Emotion as the Basis of Civilization*, N.Y. and London, 1928.
[4] Collingwood, R. G., *The Principles of Art*, Oxford, 1938.
[5] Grimberg, L., *Emotion and Delinquency*, London, 1928.
[6] Bleuler, E., *Lehrbuch der Psychiatrie*, Berlin, 1916 (Chapters I and II).
[7] Stout, G. F., *A Manual of Psychology*, 5th ed., London, 1938, p. 362.
[8] Claparède, E., FE 28, p. 124.

difficulty of finding a good technical meaning for many of the terms in common psychological use. This is particularly true in the field of emotion.[1]

A recent theoretical paper on emotion begins:

> . . . no genuine order can be discerned within this field. Instead, examination of current treatments of emotion reveals a discouraging state of confusion and uncertainty. Substantial advances have been made in recent years with respect to theories of learning and motivation, but the phenomena of emotion have not, as a rule, been considered in these formulations and remain a tangle of unrelated facts.[2]

A review of a recent volume of some six hundred pages written by many hands and devoted entirely to the subject, 'feelings and emotions', concludes:

> The total impression of the book is that we are still far from a solution;—we do not even have a consensual definition of feelings and emotions.[3]

The latest psychological dictionary available (1958) complains: 'Emotion is virtually impossible to define . . . except in terms of conflicting theories'.[4]

To present the problem more sharply, we can find four different kinds of theories of emotion in the *Encyclopedia Britannica* and four principal kinds of theories in Helsen's textbook.[5] Marston[6] offers five, as does Grossart,[7] and Masserman gives thirteen different conceptual connotations.[8]

Furthermore, those workers who are at grips with the phenomena of emotion take great pains to avoid conceptual or theoretical discussion, while some try to get rid of the problem altogether. Wittkower,[9] in a masterly paper on the influence of emotion on body functions, writes: 'Thus the philosophical side of the problem—the nature of emotions, the nature of affective-somatic relations—has

[1] Warren, H. C., *Dictionary of Psychology and Cognate Sciences*, 1934 (quoted by C. A. Ruckmick, *The Psychology of Feeling and Emotion*, 1936, p. 112).
[2] Brown, J. S. and Farber, I. E., 'Emotions Conceptualized as Intervening Variables', *Psychol. Bull.*, 1951, pp. 465–95.
[3] Zinkin, J., Book Review in *J. Nerv. Ment. Dis.*, 1954, p. 91.
[4] English, H. B., and English, A. C., *A Comprehensive Dictionary of Psychological and Psychoanalytical Terms*, N.Y., 1958.
[5] Helsen, H., ed., *Theoretical Foundations of Psychology* (Chapter VI, 'Feeling and Emotion', by J. C. Beebe-Center), N.Y., 1951.
[6] Marston, W. M., 'Analysis of Emotions', *Encyclopedia Britannica*, 14th edn., 1929.
[7] Grossart, Fr., 'Zur Kritik der herrschenden Gefühlstheorien', *Arch. f. d. Gesamte Psychol.*, 74, 1930, p. 402 f.
[8] Masserman, J. H., 'A Biodynamic Psychoanalytic Approach to the Problems of Feeling and Emotion', FE 50, p. 40–1.
[9] Wittkower, E., 'Studies on the influence of emotions on the functions of the organs', *J. Ment. Sci.*, 1935, p. 534.

been purposely disregarded.' Grimberg,[1] too, 'does not intend to discuss the psychology of emotions'; while Whately Smith's[2] book on the measurement of emotion begins: 'It is no part of the intended scope of this book to deal fully with the general theory of Emotion.' Abély[3] finds that emotion 'does not enter within the frames of his work', even though the work is an explanatory account of affective phenomena. Karnosh reports:

> In all this setting of desire on the part of both physicians and laymen for knowledge about how man emotes and about what structures in the brain and what physiological devices therein produce emotions, practically every standard text on neurology says nothing. Out of ten textbooks on basic and clinical neurology, the word 'emotion' was found in the index in only two of them, and the references were single ones. . . .

> In other words, if one is to be guided by modern texts in neurology and neurophysiology, one is justified in concluding that the emotions have no major representation in the central nervous system and, what is more puzzling, that organic diseases of emotions do not exist.[4]

Bond,[5] in his paper called 'The Avoidance of "Emotion" in Medical Literature', asks the question: Why is medical literature full of detours and euphemisms instead of using the word 'emotion'?

This in turn leads to a kind of scepticism about the possibility of theorizing about emotion. Bentley[6] says: 'But whether emotion is to-day more than a heading of a chapter, I am still doubtful.' Elmgren[7] writes: 'No real model, so to speak, of affective phenomena exists at the present time.' For him this is due largely to the fact that 'no psychological phenomena are organized on such different levels of complexity as are affective reactions'. Cobb[8] draws a conclusion for us: 'The moral of all this is, of course, that no person with only one point of view can explain the whole phenomenon of emotion.'

Dissatisfaction, avoidance, confusion and scepticism meet us at every turn, and it is impressive to find Descartes stating:

> There is nothing in which the defective nature of the sciences which we have received from the ancients appears more clearly than in what they have written on the passions; . . .[9]

[1] Grimberg, L., *Emotion and Delinquency*, p. 114 fn.
[2] Smith, W. Whately, *The Measurement of Emotion*, London, 1922, p. 17.
[3] Abély, P., 'Etude Clinique', *Les Facteurs vasculaires et endocriniens de l'affectivité* (A. M. P. Abély, A. Assailly et B. Lainé), Paris, 1948, p. 47.
[4] Karnosh, L., 'Neurology and Human Emotions', *J. Am. Med. Assoc.*, 147, 1951, p. 289.
[5] Bond, E. D., 'The Avoidance of "Emotion" in Medical Literature', *J. Nerv. Ment. Dis.*, 1947, pp. 260–1.
[6] Bentley, M., 'Is "Emotion" More than a Chapter Heading?', FE 28, p. 23.
[7] Elmgren, J., 'Emotions and Sentiments in Recent Psychology', FE 50, p. 142.
[8] Cobb, S., *Emotions and Clinical Medicine*, N.Y., 1950, p. 110.
[9] Descartes, R., 'Les Passions de l'Ame' (Eng. transl. by Haldane and Ross, *The Philosophical Works of Descartes*, Vol. I, Dover Edition, U.S.A., 1955, p. 331).

Evidently, the fundamental problem of the theory of emotion has not changed.

However, there is some light. Drever in his dictionary of psychology makes the useful distinction between what the authorities agree upon and what they disagree upon in regard to emotion. He says:

> *Emotion:* differently described and explained by different psychologists, but all agree that it is a complex state of the organism, involving bodily changes of a widespread character—in breathing, pulse, gland secretion, etc.—and, on the mental side, a state of excitement or perturbation, marked by strong feeling, and usually an impulse towards a definite form of behaviour. If the emotion is intense there is some disturbance of the intellectual functions, a measure of *dissociation*, and a tendency towards action of an ungraded or *protopathic* character. Beyond this description anything else would mean an entrance into the controversial field.[1]

Drever's statement presented schematically looks like this:

    I. There is agreement about the description of emotion as a complex state of the organism of varying intensity involving:
        (*a*) widespread bodily changes,
        (*b*) a mental state of excitement or perturbation;
        (*c*) strong feeling;
        (*d*) an impulse (usually) towards a specific form of behaviour.
    II. There is disagreement about:
        (*a*) a more exact description of this complex state;
        (*b*) any explanation of this complex state.

Or, to put the matter succinctly, there is agreement about the concept[2] of emotion and disagreement about the theory[3] of emotion.

The question, 'What is emotion', has been answered in so far as one accepts the general notion given in I*a*, *b*, *c*, and *d*, above. But the 'How' of emotion (II*a*) and the 'Why' of emotion (II*b*) involve theoretical controversy. It is here our problem begins.

To sum up:

1. The generic concept 'emotion' and concepts of specific emotions are central in many areas of human life and are particularly crucial to analytical psychotherapy, psychosomatic medicine, psychosurgery, and physical methods of psychiatric treatment.

---

[1] Drever, J., *A Dictionary of Psychology* (Penguin Reference Books), London, 1952, pp. 80–1.

[2] By 'concept' we mean, 'an idea of a class of objects; a general notion' (O.E.D.).

[3] By 'theory' we mean, 'A scheme or system of ideas or statements held as an explanation or account of a group of facts or phenomena; a hypothesis that has been confirmed or established by observation or experiment, and is propounded or accepted as accounting for known facts; a statement of what are held to be the general laws, principles, or causes of something known or observed' (O.E.D.).

2. Systematic psychology has failed to present a unified theory of emotion which goes beyond the terms of general description. It is even doubted if such a unified theory is possible.

3. Emotion-therapy (whether psychological or physical) nevertheless proceeds to diagnose, treat and cure on a basis of a general notion of emotion without adequate theory.

4. Can a unified theory of emotion be developed which might provide a basis for psychotherapy and find agreement among systematic psychologists?

B. THE METHOD

THE *problem* has presented itself: to bring order out of the confusion, agreement out of disagreement. The *method* must still be elaborated. How can we develop a theory of emotion so that it might find approval among therapists and systematic psychologists? How can we integrate the many theories into one? Or, perhaps, the investigation may prove something special about 'emotion', something which gives ground to the confusion, revealing that no integration is possible? If other far more competent investigators have failed, what hopes have we of succeeding?

Clearly, the method we choose is of great importance. Advances in thought are due often not so much to new content, but to ways of ordering old content. What are some of the possible ways of setting about this problem?

1. The *phenomenological* method is the most direct. Following Sartre, we might go directly to the emotions themselves and ask them what they are. He says:

> Therefore, the phenomenologist will interrogate emotion *about consciousness* or *about man*. He will ask it not only what it is but what it has to teach us about a being, one of whose characteristics is exactly that he is capable of being moved. And inversely, he will interrogate consciousness, human reality, about emotion: what must a consciousness be for emotion to be possible, perhaps even to be necessary? [1]

Bochenski,[2] in giving an account of Husserl's phenomenological method, writes: 'Man muss *zu den Sachen selbst* vorstossen. Das ist die erste und fundamentale Regel der phänomenologischen Methode.' (One must go right to the thing itself. This is the first and fundamental rule of the phenomenological method.) In its approach to the thing itself, this method 'brackets out' the testimony of natural

---

[1] Sartre, J. P., *Esquisse d'une théorie des Emotions* (3e ed.), Paris, 1948, p. 10. (Eng. transl. by B. Frechtman, *The Emotions: Outline of a Theory*, N.Y., 1948, p. 15.)

[2] Bochenski, I. M., *Europäische Philosophie der Gegenwart*, Bern, 1951, p. 146.

science, of logic, of history—in short, of all other authority but the authority of the phenomenon itself.

Tertullian, long ago, recommended this direct phenomenological approach, this confrontation method of asking the phenomenon questions and letting it give its own witness. He writes:

> If . . . one is bent on gathering testimonies . . . from the writings of the philosophers, or the poets, or other masters of the world's learning and wisdom, he has need of a most inquisitive spirit, and a still greater memory, to carry out the research. Indeed, some of our people . . . have published works . . . in which they relate and attest the nature and origin of their traditions, and the grounds on which opinions rest. . . .
>
> I call in a new testimony, yea, one which is better known than all literature, more discussed than all doctrine, more public than all publications, greater than the whole man—I mean all which is man's. Stand forth, O soul . . . stand forth and give thy witness. But I call thee not as when fashioned in schools, trained in libraries, fed up in academies. . . . [1]

Tertullian, in writing about the soul, 'brackets out' other testimony and turns directly to the soul, asking it to teach us what it knows; just as Sartre says the phenomenologist will interrogate emotion about what it has to teach us.

Now, why do we not use this method? Primarily, because it would not end the controversy. Natural scientists, particularly, would not accept being 'bracketed out' in the manner which Husserl describes:

> Thus *all sciences which relate to this natural world*, though they stand never so firm to me, though they fill me with wondering admiration, though I am far from any thought of objecting to them in the least degree, *I disconnect them all, I make absolutely no use of their standards, I do not appropriate a single one of the propositions that enter into their systems, even though their evidential value is perfect, I take none of them, no one of them serves me for a foundation*—so long, that is, as it is understood, in the way these sciences themselves understand it, as a truth *concerning the realities* of this world. [2]

Not only would this method not end the controversy because of its differences with natural science, but the method itself has controversial presuppositions which Buytendijk states clearly:

> Surely all phenomenological analysis of feelings and emotions . . . presuppose[s] a certain implicit idea about human reality and man's existence in the world. . . .
>
> The phenomenological approach to feelings and emotions starts from the undeniable fact that consciousness is always a being conscious of

[1] Tertullian, Q. S. F., *De Testimonio Animae Liber Adversus Gentes* (Opera . . . Omnia, Paris, 1616, p. 124). 'On the Testimony of the Soul', ANCL, XI, pp. 36-7, condensed.)

[2] Husserl, E., *Ideen zu einer reinen Phänomenologie und phänomenologischen Philosophie.* (Eng. transl. by W. B. Gibson, *Ideas*, London and N.Y., 1931, p. 111.)

something else and that we are conscious of our existing, that means our being physically subjected to a given situation.[1]

Not all the approaches to the theory of emotion start out from this premise. Therefore this method would only add another conceptual connotation, another theory to the long list.

Furthermore, a proper phenomenological investigation of emotion would require an analysis of *one* emotion. A classical example is Seneca's work on anger. Scheler's examination of sympathy is an excellent modern example of this approach. One begins with the phenomenon (sympathy), not with the generic concept (emotion). Scheler says: '. . . this short work may perhaps provide an example of how to conduct investigations into the phenomena of the emotional life.'[2] But the examination of one emotion would not solve our problem.

We can nevertheless follow the phenomenologists—Sartre in particular—in the way in which we approach the theories of emotion, turning to them directly, taking them as they appear, and asking them what witness each bears about emotion, about consciousness and about man.

2. The phenomenological method as defined above and the experimental method cancel each other out. Just as natural scientists would refuse the method of phenomenology, so do phenomenologists refuse the experimental method. Sartre says: '. . . essences and facts are incommensurables, and one who begins his inquiry with facts will never arrive at essences.'[3] Nevertheless, we can 'bracket out' the view of Husserl and Sartre, in order to see for ourselves if one can approach the problem with the experimental method.

This method could be used in two ways. The first would be a direct approach to the facts of emotion from which a new theory could be developed. This has been and is being done by competent experimentalists. The professional journals and textbooks give much space to their observational records and, in spite of the maimed animals expended and a ubiquitous 'scientism',[4] these records are often of considerable interest. This method has yielded facts about the provocation of emotion, the neurological 'seat' of emotion, the recognition of emotion, the physiological changes in emotion, etc. But a curious impression emerges after reading through these reports: very little definite is established. It is as if the facts of emotion did not lend themselves to the experimental method which depends so much upon procedures of measurement, the laboratory situation, verification

[1] Buytendijk, F. J. J., 'The Phenomenological Approach to the Problem of Feelings and Emotions', FE 50, p. 129.

[2] Scheler, M., *Zur Phänomenologie und Theorie der Sympathiegefühle*, Halle, 1913, p. iii. (Eng. transl. by P. Heath, *The Nature of Sympathy*, London, 1954, p. li.)

[3] Sartre, J. P., *op. cit.*, p. 7. (Eng. transl., p. 9.)

[4] Woodger, J. H., *Physics, Psychology and Medicine*, Cambridge, 1956, pp. 20–1.

by repetition, prediction, accumulation of data, etc. As examples here are the well-known difficulties in fixing definite facts of emotion through the psychogalvanic phenomena, the Rorschach test, the various introspectionist techniques, anatomo-neurological investigations, experiments in the recognition of emotion through facial expression, the stimulation of 'pseudo-emotion', the analysis of psychosomatic case histories. In all these various empirical attempts to seize the facts of emotion, little results from one experiment or situation which can be verified in the next. A host of 'variables' intervene. Each situation is different; the facts do not check. So, in spite of the wealth of experiments, few decisive laws are gleaned. It is as if emotion were unique and too personal, too spontaneous, too irrational for the methods which seek to fix it. No doubt the confusion and frustration in the field of theory is in part due to this difficulty with the facts. A shining failure of an excellent experimentalist in trying to establish facts about emotion is shown in this (abbreviated) report from Landis. His paper, 'An Attempt to Measure Emotional Traits in Juvenile Delinquency', 1932, has as its purpose: 'Since no comparative evaluation of various methods of testing or measuring emotion, emotional instability, or emotional psychopathy had been made, it seemed worth while to make such a study.' [1] The conclusions follow:

1. Neither age, race, nor social offense is related in constant fashion to either emotional stability or to the tests which we have employed in this investigation.

2. The degree of intellectual capacity (I.Q.) bears no relationship to emotional factors which are involved in delinquency.

3. Thurstone's Personality Schedule . . . fails to give diagnostic results when revised for use with juvenile delinquents.

4. Heidbreder's Temperament Test . . . is of much less value with juvenile delinquents.

5. Our revision of the text and of the scoring of Allport's Ascendancy Submission Test was not successful as a method of measuring character traits.

6. Tests of the appreciation of humor do not yield satisfactory results . . .

7. The Pressey X-O Test, neither in its original nor in our revised form, gave results of practical diagnostic value.

8. That the type of learning curve obtained in learning a maze offers an objective test of emotional stability, as claimed by Ball, we were unable to confirm.

9. Hull's test of waking suggestion gave clear differentiation between individuals, but this difference bore no relationship to other tests or ratings of character traits.

[1] Landis, C., 'An Attempt to Measure Emotional Traits in Juvenile Delinquency', in *Studies in the Dynamics of Behavior* (ed. by K. Lashley), Univ. of Chic., 1932, p. 267.

10. The frequency of the appearance of the psychogalvanic reflex . . . bears no relation to any other measure or rating of emotionality.

11. Case histories . . . do not really lend themselves to the purpose of close scientific analysis.

12. Various statistical procedures designed to show the correlation existing between the functions tested in this study gave negative results.

13. An analysis of the individual test performances . . . shows that conformity with respect to these tests does not agree with conformity in general life situations.

14. In general, it may be concluded that analytical investigations of the personality traits of emotionality or psychopathy are unsatisfactory and fail to bring out decisive evidence.[1]

These results can be contested in many ways, *e.g.* (*a*) the report is 'out of date'; (*b*) the concept 'emotion' was not clearly defined; (*c*) testing delinquents involves other variables than those accounted for by these tests; etc. However it be argued, we bring this only as witness to our view that recourse to facts will lead to new difficulties, not to new solutions.

And further, when these observational records are raised to the level of explanatory hypotheses, there is no theory which integrates the great variety of such hypotheses, nor is there a theory which is not subject to contradictory hypotheses based upon other—or even the same—experimentally derived facts. No theory has been put forward which finds acceptance among workers in the experimental field—to say nothing of finding agreement among those whose hypotheses are not derived by the experimental method. This is not to deride or punish such methods as far as they go, since the development of a variety of contradictory observations and hypotheses is the very life-blood of science. We want only to make clear that turning to the facts or deriving hypotheses experimentally will not solve the problem.

The second way in which we might try the experimental method would be to apply it not to facts, but to hypotheses. We would attempt to construct an over-all theory by integrating the disparate hypotheses. If we place the experimental method within its contemporary context—*modern scientific method*—such an integration is at least conceivable. What is required is the design of an experiment which would verify the hypotheses coming in from all the fields. These would first have to be reduced to a neutral language, e.g. the signs of symbolic logic, or the mathematical language of the probability curve, or the signals for an electronic data processor, etc. Through this reduction, the hypotheses would become factors of an

---

[1] Landis, C., *Ibid.*, p. 310–14 (all italics in original).

over-all, clearly defined system of operations. The host of hypotheses could thus be tested according to the laws of the system, those which failed to prove could be discarded, leaving us with a verified theory of emotion.

It is obvious that the success of this method depends upon the success in achieving a universe of discourse, or agreed system of operations, within which verification has meaning. This requires an initial agreement about the operational definitions, or neutral language, for such key terms of the hypotheses as: 'emotion', 'energy', 'unconscious', 'disorder', 'situation', etc. The degree of success which the general theory will have depends upon the degree of success in agreement about these terms, because a theory is only meaningful—and this is the kernel of this method—in terms of the conceptual definitions assigned to the terms.

It is just here that the method fails. In the first place, in the field of theory of emotion there is no universe of discourse; there are no agreed conceptual definitions. Therefore, no agreed operational definitions can be assigned and no over-all experiment designed. Is this due to the men working in this area—some being wise and knowing what these terms mean, while others persist in foolishness? Hardly. Rather it is because the concepts themselves are not fixed conventions. They are more like living entities, aspects of which are grasped by different individuals. Or as Cobb[1] says, '. . . no person with only one point of view can explain the whole phenomenon of emotion'. Thus the failure of the method in the first place leads to a more fundamental second reason for rejection of this method.

Such terms as 'emotion', 'energy', 'conflict', etc., cannot be reduced to neutral counters. They have a multitude of shadings; they are paradoxical and ambiguous; and they are full of metaphysical and irrational overtones which Mach, Schlick, Carnap and Neurath[2] insisted must be purged from scientific statements. This position—whether it be called 'operationalism', 'scientific world conception' (*wissenschaftliche Weltauffassung*), or 'logical positivism'—always attempts to limit meaning to that assigned by definition. But such a rule for what is meaningful or meaningless is true only within the very limited realm of a rational consciousness. These concepts (emotion, energy, situation, signification, etc.), however, have not only the values assigned by consciousness; they are also involved in unconscious models. This aspect of the concept cannot be reduced to definitions imposed by consciousness, since this aspect makes the concept a living reality, persisting through time, with historical and

[1] ECM, p. 110.
[2] Frank, P., *Modern Science and Its Philosophy*, Harvard Univ. Press, 1949 (Introduction).

sociological associations, ethical implications and psychological qualities. One comes closer to the 'meaning' of such concepts, not by limitation of them as specific signs, but by amplification of them as general symbols. Such an amplification, by circumscribing the concept from many sides, admits both conscious and rational definitions as well as other levels of meaning. The position we argue is reminiscent of the realism of mediaeval philosophy—with one enormous difference. It is a realism re-interpreted in the light of modern depth psychology which modifies the substantial reality of concepts in terms of psychological reality.[1] We take the ontological nature of such concepts as an *esse in anima*,[2] i.e. as realities of the psyche, not as hypostatized *ante rem* substances. The method we challenge is traditional nominalism in a new dress.[3]

It is principally for this reason that modern scientific method does not suit our problem. As disguised nominalism it neglects to give full value and psychological reality to the question it investigates. Its methods are partial methods because it omits the psychological aspect. Therefore, the suggested approaches to the theory of emotion based on this method (Beebe-Center,[4] Duffy,[5] Plutchik,[6] Brown and Farber,[7] and those who find the issue to be only one of semantics or communication) are also unacceptable, because they do not go beyond the logical or intellectual side of the problem. The attitude

---

[1] Jung, C. G., *Psychologische Typen*, Zürich, 1921. (Eng. transl. by H. Baynes, *Psychological Types*, London, 1923.)

[2] *Ibid.*, Chapter I, Section 4.

[3] This position is brilliantly exposed by George Orwell (*Nineteen Eighty-Four*, London, 1949; Penguin Books, 1954, p. 45). Syme, an expert on the language of the future, Newspeak, describes the aims of this language after accusing the hero, Winston, of preferring Oldspeak 'with all its vagueness and useless shades of meaning'. Syme says: 'Don't you see that the whole aim of Newspeak is to narrow the range of thought? In the end we shall make thoughtcrime literally impossible, because there will be no words in which to express it. Every concept that can ever be needed, will be expressed by exactly *one* word, with its meaning rigidly defined and all its subsidiary meanings rubbed out and forgotten. Already . . . we're not far from that point. . . . Every year fewer and fewer words, and the range of consciousness always a little smaller.' One wonders just where the difference lies between the 'purification' of language demanded by modern scientific method and the 'destruction of words' described by Orwell. (See further Part II, Chapter I, where an attempt is made to get rid of the term 'emotion'.) The place where Orwell's vision of totalitarianism and rational nominalism both have part of their source is in the work of Hobbes who also insisted upon exact definitions. For him a 'name is a word taken at pleasure to serve as a mark' (E. W., I, p. 16). It is an arbitrary convention which can be picked up and laid aside at will. That these definitions can be arbitrarily made by the ruler of the state, Hobbes admits, and Orwell's *1984* brings the *Leviathan* up to date.

[4] Beebe-Center, J. G., 'Feeling and Emotion', in *Theoretical Foundations of Psychology*, ed. H. Helsen, N.Y., 1951.

[5] Duffy, E., 'Emotion: An Example of the Need for Reorientation in Psychology', *Psychol. Rev.*, 1934, pp. 187 ff.

[6] Plutchik, R., 'Some Problems for a Theory of Emotion', *Psychosom. Med.*, 1955, pp. 309 ff.

[7] Brown, J. S., and Farber, I. E., *op. cit.*, p. 465.

of modern nominalism, like its traditional counterpart, seeks to sever the logic of rational intellect from its living connection with the psyche, whether these psychological influences be called 'faith' in the world of Occam, 'metaphysics' by Carnap, or 'emotion' in Reichenbach.[1]

This sterile restriction of science to a game of counters and logic to empty tautologies can of course become deadly, as our times show. It is not our aim to further this game. Nor is it conceivable to us that any problem in psychology can be legitimately approached by a method which has as its fundamental and self-righteous attitude the exclusion of the psyche from its role in the development of explanatory hypotheses. Contrary to Reichenbach's statement: 'The satisfaction of psychological desires, however, is not explanation',[2] we maintain that explanation only fully succeeds when it satisfies a sense of necessity and sufficiency to the psyche asking for explanation.

3. This rejection of 'modern scientific method' for our problem leaves this residue: we need a method which bridges the opposition between the mutually exclusive restrictions of the scientific and the phenomenological methods. Such a bridge is the method of *amplification*. Amplification includes statements of facts and statements of essences. It is empirical and scientific in being open to all sorts of evidence. It is objective in that it does not restrict meaning to a system of private conventions set up by any one school of thought. And it is phenomenological as it allows the phenomenon under scrutiny to have its full say. And because amplification comprehends an event from many sides, it prevents the building of compartments between intellect and other aspects of the psyche, between logic and psychology, which would sever a rational investigation of this kind from the life of psychological reality. But the method of amplification is not in itself enough to yield a theory because it presents no structure. Thus we are forced to look further to find a method of systematizing the amplifications.

4. The simplest method for solving our problem—and opposite to amplification—would be *reduction*. This would mean fitting all the various theories into one. However often this has been tried—and most theories, as we shall see, are of this sort—it has failed. Reduction of the many to one has failed mainly because the many hypotheses are antithetical. They use terms such as mind and body, order and disorder, cause and purpose, action and reaction, subject and object, etc., which are pairs of opposites. They do not allow reductions to one member of the pair without violation of the antithetical member.

---

[1] Reichenbach, H., *The Rise of Scientific Philosophy*, Univ. of Calif., 1951 (Chapters XVI and XVII).
[2] *Ibid.*, p. 9.

Unification through reduction would not give full weight to the great range of hypotheses. It would be one-sided and would hardly find agreement.

Furthermore, reduction is a method which achieves unification through reduction to a common root. This means leaving out the specific differences which, when they are included, lead into irreducible pairs of opposites. The closest we can come to a reductive solution is already given in Drever's definition. This is of course not a theory because the specific explanatory hypotheses are missing. Again, the reductive method will not do the job.

5. The *historical* method provides us with a way of reviewing the phenomenology of theories as they appear through time. But here we can find competent works already.[1] There is little sense in going over this ground once more, especially since the historical method is not intended to solve the problem as we presented it. However, an historical viewpoint to the theories can be useful in exposing their background, those conceptual models and root metaphors which come to expression in many ages and places. Therefore, we shall bring in historical comparisons in order to gain perspective and distance when we confront the welter of hypotheses.

6. We can set about the problem through the method of *survey*. But here, too, predecessors[1] have met with little success. At best they have collected the confusion into one place. There are as many views as there are viewers, and so a survey would only be useful if it were accompanied by a system of correlation, or group of categories by means of which the theories could be organized.

7. Such a set of categories could be provided by a method of *types*. Where the reductive method orders by reduction to simpler and narrower roots leaving out differences, the typing method orders through reference to wider categories and classes. It aims to present differences. Broad, who has used this method in ethics, writes

> It appears to me that the best preparation for original work on any philosophical problem is to study the solutions which have been proposed for it by men of genius whose views differ from each other as much as possible. The clash of opinions may strike a light. . . . [2]

Authorities, rather than being omitted as Tertullian and the phenomenologists suggest, are limned one against the other to make differences vivid. The field is not merely surveyed; it is ordered by means of a number of groupings. The way of grouping the theories is, in part, similar to the way of reducing in the reductive method: a single characteristic or property of the theory is seen to colour the

---

[1] See Bibliography, p. 24 below.
[2] Broad, C. D., *Five Types of Ethical Theory*, 1930, London, p. 1.

17

whole theory and to be the characteristic which sets the theory off from the others. Broad says:

> ... it seems likely that each of these great men will have seen some important aspect of the subject, and that the mistake of each will have been to emphasize this aspect to the exclusion of others which are equally relevant.[1]

The typing method, too, has been used by Marston,[2] by Beebe-Center,[3] and by Grossart.[4] Where it serves to order the confusion into a small number of categories, it does not integrate the order into a whole. If the typing method is to succeed, the types must be more than random eclectic categories which evolve out of the data at hand. They must not only allow full play to the wide range of differences of theory. More important, they must themselves be related in a *coherent* system, which is a whole and which covers all the possibilities within the field—similar, for example, to what Jung maintains for his psychological types.[5] The categories must be more than an aggregate of simple classes; they must be together a complex.

In other words, the typing method following Broad can be used for one half of our task: the grouping of theories in Part II. But these groupings can have no effect on the problem of integration which we aim for in Part III, unless the types are interrelated categories forming a whole. Therefore, for integration we need a *special method of types*.

8. The accrued results of our discussion of method so far have led us to see the value of using the *phenomenological* method but in a new way: turning directly to the theories themselves. We have found that a method of *amplification* permits an unrestricted approach to the problem. We have also seen that the *historical* point of view helps in exposing the models of thinking about emotion. And we have seen that we can organize the material through a wide range of *types*. The method for Part II is thus established. It shall be an amplification of the theory of emotion through the phenomenology of theories, grouped through a wide range of types, with relevant historical background.

For Part III, we find we need a *special method of types*. There seems no method better suited to our conditions, nor one which has stood the test of time and which does not present us with new terminological difficulties than the *system of the four causes of Aristotle*. This is the method we propose to use to solve the problem.

Several objections can be urged against this method: the first is that Aristotle did not use the four causes when dealing with the soul

---

[1] Broad, C. D., *Five Types of Ethical Theory*, 1930, London, p. 1.
[2] *Op. cit.*   [3] *Op. cit.*   [4] *Op. cit.*   [5] *Op. cit.*

and with *orexis*; therefore, is the method appropriate? The second objection is that such an Aristotelian framework may give our whole investigation an Aristotelian or Scholastic cast; therefore, is the method not arbitrary? And finally, does this method fulfil our requirements of a special method of types which can embrace disparate kinds of explanation, integrating them into one because this one forms a coherent system covering all the possibilities in the field?

Concerning the first objection, we can point to the work of Shute who also comes upon this problem, writing:

> The interesting question arises, is the motivating power of appetence something which can be analysed in terms of the four causes, or does Aristotle here deal with causality of a completely different order? [1]

After investigation, he concludes that the method is justifiable and suitable for dealing with psychological events. Moreover, we must remember that our work is not on the psychological events themselves (emotions), but on theories about psychological events. And when it comes to theories, we find Aristotle using just this method in the Metaphysics[2] to integrate by means of the system of the four causes the earlier theories of Being, much as we intend to do here with theories of emotion.

Secondly, we need not assume that by using concepts of such an abstract and generic nature as Formal, Material, Efficient and Final we shall be writing Aristotelian philosophy in attempting to deal with modern psychology. More likely, we shall be taking these concepts out of their original context; but for this violation the history of thought presents many precedents. The use of old concepts and old methods in new ways is a crime sanctioned by tradition.

To answer the third objection it is necessary to go into some detail.

We have seen in our analysis of Dreyer's definition that our problem lies in the theory of emotion which we understand as the 'why' of emotion. Aristotle approaches the problem of the 'why' like this: 'Knowledge is the object of our inquiry, and men do not think they know a thing till they have grasped the "why" of it (which is to grasp its primary cause).[3], [4] He then gives the four ways in which the 'why' can be understood, concluding with the statement: 'This then perhaps exhausts the number of ways in which the term "cause" is used.' [5]

---

[1] Shute, C., *The Psychology of Aristotle*, N.Y., 1941, p. 67.

[2] Aristotle (*Collected Works*, transl. ed. by W. D. Ross, Oxford), *Metaphysica*, Bk. A, 7, 988b.

[3] 'The proximate cause, which is primarily responsible for an event' (footnote, *loc. cit.*).

[4] Aristotle, *Physica*, II, 3, 194b.   [5] *Ibid.*, 3, 195a.

He goes over the ground once again even more clearly:

> It is clear then that there are causes, and that the number of them is what we have stated. The number is the same as that of things comprehended under the question 'why'. The 'why' is referred ultimately either (1), in things which do not involve motion, e.g. mathematics, to the 'what' (to the definition of 'straight line' or 'commensurable', etc.), or (2) to what initiated a motion, e.g. 'why did they go to war?—because there had been a raid'; or (3) we are inquiring 'for the sake of what?'— 'that they may rule'; or (4), in the case of things that come into being, we are looking for the matter. The causes, therefore, are these and so many in number.[1]

These four causes—Formal, Efficient, Final and Material—are irreducible to each other. Thus they are each necessary to satisfy the question 'why'. But perhaps more than these are necessary. In other words, do these four cover all the possibilities within the field? Are they sufficient? Aristotle says: 'Now the modes of causation are many, though when brought under heads they too can be reduced in number.'[2] Other modes of causation, of answering the question 'why', can ultimately be reduced to these four, not only because they exhaust the way in which the 'why' can be understood as stated above; but because he makes it explicit elsewhere[3] that he cannot name any others than these four. Therefore, the four causes offer the model for a complete theory because they satisfy the demands for necessary and sufficient explanation. By being an irreducible number of categories and yet still covering all the possibilities within the field, they provide a special method of types for ordering the various explanatory hypotheses which have been put forward to answer the 'why' of emotion.

Aristotle's idea 'that the modes of causation are many' has a modern ring. One is reminded of Verworn's[4] concept of 'conditionalism': 'A state or process is identical with the totality of its conditions. From this follows: A state or condition is scientifically completely known when the totality of its conditions is determined.' Conditionalism as an expanded form of causality has been used by Jung in accounting for such psychological phenomena as dreams.[5] But the concept of multi-causality is also re-entering psychology through the work of Alexander[6] and others in the field of psychosomatics who are concerned largely with the problem of emotion. However, the many modes of causation, the totality of essential conditions for a state or process, used in the psychosomatic approach have not been

---

[1] Aristotle, *Physica*, II, 7, 198a.   [2] *Ibid.*, 3, 195a.
[3] Aristotle, *Metaphysica*, A, 10, 993a.
[4] Verworn, M., *Kausale und Konditionale Weltanschauung*, 3rd edn., 1928.
[5] Jacobi, J., *The Psychology of Jung*, 5th edn., London, 1951, p. 100.
[6] Alexander, F., *Psychosomatic Medicine: Its Principles and Applications*, N.Y., 1950, p. 51.

reduced to basic categories as with Aristotle. It is possible that a revival of these four fundamental causes as a method is very apt to meet the complex problems in this field.

In this respect, it is useful to note the difference between a method of types derived from the material at hand, such as Broad's types of ethical theory or Empson's[1] types of ambiguity, and the method of types based on the model of the four causes. The former types, as random eclectic categories, merely classify. They can only be useful (as in Part II) for purposes of differentiation. The latter types, however, form a coherent whole. They explain, having fulfilled the conditions of necessity and sufficiency. Aristotle maintains for them a certain fundamentality; they are operative in *all* things, or as Wallace puts it:

> The Aristotelian analysis of existence into *dynamis* and *energeia,* or *hyle* and *eidos,* is expressed with more detail in the doctrine of the four *archai* or *aitiai*—that is, principles which enter into the existence or origination or cognition of any object.[2]

Therefore, the second condition which we laid down for our special method of types—that the categories be more than an aggregate of incidental simples, but that they be together a complex whole—is also met.

It is met not only by our arguments based on Aristotle's arguments. It is met as well from another point of view, the psychological one. These four causes form a whole in so far as they complete each other and together form a totality. They are an expression of the idea of the fourfold root which crops up again and again in the history of thought and which is brought forward as a basis of explanation. (See further, Part III, page 246 f.) The four cases are analogous to the four directions. They complete each other and are mutually interdependent for meaning. Together they form a complex through which each gathers its meaning. Each stands to the whole as an aspect of that whole. Each is a phenomenological appearance of the whole, not a mere part of it. They do not make up a whole as simples form a collection, but rather *each is the whole* seen from one side.

In this way, we shall be approaching both that 'complex state of the organism' (Drever), emotion, and those complex theories about that complex state, because we take the theories as witness to the way emotion has appeared to the consciousness of man. We shall get to the origin, nature and purpose of emotion through the phenomenology of theories of emotion: taking them each as they

---

[1] Empson, W., *Seven Types of Ambiguity,* 2nd edn., London, 1949.
[2] Wallace, E., *Outlines of the Philosophy of Aristotle,* 3rd edn., Cambridge, 1887, p. 71.

appear and asking them what testimony they bear about emotion, about consciousness and about man. Only in this way, by giving full authority and validity to each view, by refusing to take 'sides', can we circumambulate the problem and hope to come to an integrated view. Only then when all four views are elaborated and held in mind together can we try to present the 'why' of emotion.

Since every method is a *way of going about* things and every theory or hypotheses a statement *about* things, we offer this method as the proper one for going about complex phenomena. They cannot be gone into, taken apart, analysed and explained in the sense of 'laid out flat'. A definition of *about* is: 'Around the outside; on or towards every side; all round.' So one must quite literally 'go about', circumambulate, the phenomenon, much as a pilgrim views his shrine from all directions, letting it remain intact in its dignity, letting it speak and have its *Wirkung*.

C. THE SCOPE AND PLAN

JUST as the presentation of the problem led to the methodological question of how to go about the problem, so does the presentation of the method lead to the question: within what limits and in what manner is the method to be applied? What is the scope and plan of the work?

Primarily the scope is limited *by the kind of work* this is—a treatise in psychology. Therefore, the scope of the work shall remain within the area proper to psychology. It shall not deal with concepts of emotion, whether elaborated into theory or not, that appear in sociology, political science, education, aesthetics, etc., except in so far as would be indicated by the considerations which follow. However, an attempt shall be made to cover the field of psychology thoroughly, including theories in English, German, French, Spanish and those which appeared originally in other languages.

The scope is also limited *by the problem*. The problem is one of contemporary controversy and contemporary psycho-therapy and psychology, and so this work shall not bring under survey non-current theories except when they are relevant to current theories. We take 'current theories' to mean those going back to the beginning of this century. The works of the nineteenth century need not be dealt with in much detail since their influence remains in the current theories.

The scope is further limited *by the method*, which is not one that relies exclusively upon fact or experiment, upon introspection or metaphysical speculation, upon logic, linguistic analysis, or authority, upon phenomenological or biological reduction, but which is a method of amplification, that is, enlargement of comprehension. So the scope must encompass testimony from all sides. It must include the widest divergences in explanations of emotion, so that if any integration be achieved it will have had the widest possible basis. Clearly, an integration based on few or complementary hypotheses will not solve the problem. This means that it is necessary to present the theories in order to show the collective disunity and to point up their individual inadequacies. It is just this which is the problem. Otherwise, the problem might just be a phantom problem based on hearsay evidence that some think there is a problem. And then in turn the integration would just be a hat-trick for solving make-believe problems. The full experience of the problem in Part II is therefore intimately linked with the value of the integration in Part III.

When we speak of the theories which must be presented, we mean the explanatory hypotheses. A theory has at least one explanatory hypothesis. In selecting these in accordance with what has been said above, we shall use these additional principles. We shall select:

(*a*) those hypotheses which are representative of a body of thought or school;

(*b*) those which find wide agreement or approval;

(*c*) those which are important, even if not representative, in so far as they are persistent;

(*d*) those which are controversial and extreme.

In this way the scope of the work determines its *plan*. Part II, because it will set out the confusion and differentiation, will be the bulk of the book. Part III will attempt the simplicity and integration. The methods to be used in both parts have been already described and will be touched upon again preliminary to each chapter.

It is also within the scope and plan of this work to draw *conclusions* or otherwise present the reader with what Woodger calls 'bright ideas' [1] and which he considers a basic requirement for the development of science. These will come not only at the end; there will be conclusions within the discussion of the different theories as part of pointing out their inadequacies and exposing their conceptual models. Because the problem is many-sided and the method we have chosen is many-sided, the conclusions must fall in at many points. The fundamental conclusion we can state in advance: an amplification of the problem of emotion in our time as it appears in concept and theory, or, in short, the conclusion is the work itself.

---

[1] Woodger, J. H., *op. cit.*, pp. 15 ff.

BIBLIOGRAPHICAL NOTE TO PART ONE

Works on the history of theory of emotion—other than standard works of reference and encyclopediae:

K. Bernecker, *Kritische Darstellung der Geschichte des Affektbegriffes* (von Descartes bis zur Gegenwart), Berlin, 1915.

C. L. Duprat, 'La Psycho-physiologie des passions dans la philosophie ancienne', *Arch.f. d.Gesch. der Phil.*, XI, 1905.

M. Steinitzer, *Die menschlichen und tierischen Gemütsbewegungen als Gegenstand der Wissenschaft*, Munich, 1889.

H. M. Gardiner, R. C. Metcalf and J. G. Beebe-Center, *Feeling and Emotion: A History of Theories*, N.Y., 1937.

O. Byrne, *The Evolution of the Theory and Research on Emotions*, Columbia Univ. Master's Thesis, 1927. (Experimental research and theory only, by a pupil of Marston.)

Fr. M. Ubeda Purkiss, 'Desarrollo histórico de la doctrina sobre las emociones' (in two parts), *La Ciencia Tomista*, 248, 1953, pp. 432–87; 250, 1954, pp. 35–68.

E. B. Titchener, 'An Historical Note on the James-Lange Theory of Emotion', *Am. J. Psychol.*, 1914, pp. 427–47.

G. S. Brett, 'Historical Development of the Theory of Emotions', FE 28, pp. 388–97.

W. A. Hunt, 'Recent Developments in the Field of Emotion', *Psychol. Bull.*, 1941, pp. 249–76.

E. L. Margetts, 'Historical Notes on Psychosomatic Medicine', RDPM 54.

Also:

G. S. Brett, *A History of Psychology* (the three volume edition), London, 1912–21.

T. Laycock, *A Treatise on the Nervous Diseases of Women*, London, 1840.

C. A. Ruckmick, *The Psychology of Feeling and Emotion*, N.Y. and London (Chapters II, IV, V and VI).

C. Spearman, *Psychology Down the Ages* (Vol. I, Chapter X), London, 1937.

E. Wittkower, 'Studies on the Influence of Emotions on the Functions of the Organs', *J. Ment. Sci.*, 81, 1935, pp. 533–682.

II. Works which survey the field—other than general textbooks of psychology:

Feelings and Emotions—The Wittenberg Symposium (ed. by M. Reymert), Clark Univ., 1928.

Feelings and Emotions—The Mooseheart Symposium (ed. by M. Reymert), N.Y., 1950.

D. Rapaport, *Emotions and Memory*, 2nd edn., N.Y., 1950. (Surveys that aspect of emotion to do with memory; written from the psychoanalytic point of view; omits mention of French works.)

S. Strasser, *Das Gemüt*, Utrecht, Antwerpen, Freiburg, 1956. (Surveys the field from the phenomenological point of view; neglects the psychiatric-pathological; no mention of the 'unconscious' in his index.)

P. T. Young, *Emotion in Man and Animal*, N.Y., 1943.

C. A. Ruckmick, *op. cit. sup.*

W. McDougall, 'Organization of the Affective Life', *Acta Psychologica*, 2, 1937.

F. Dunbar, *Emotions and Bodily Changes* (4th edn.), Columbia Univ., 1954. (Reviews a bibliography of over 5,000 entries; from the point of view of American psychosomatic medicine.)

D. B. Lindsley, 'Emotion', in *Handbook of Experimental Psychology* (ed. by S. Stevens), N.Y. and London, 1951. (From the experimental and physiological point of view.)

PART II
Differentiation

The Phenomenology of the Theories of Emotion

'. . . some people do not listen to a speaker unless he speaks mathematically, others unless he gives instances, while others expect him to cite a poet as witness. And some want to have everything done accurately, while others are annoyed by accuracy. . . . Hence one must be already trained to know how to take each sort of argument. . . .'

'For those who wish to get clear of difficulties it is advantageous to discuss the difficulties well; for the subsequent free play of thought implies the solution of the previous difficulties, and it is not possible to untie a knot of which one does not know. But the difficulty of our thinking points to a 'knot' in the object; . . . Hence one should have surveyed all the difficulties beforehand, . . . because people who inquire without first stating the difficulties are like those who do not know where they have to go; . . . Further, he who has heard all the contending arguments, as if they were parties to a case, must be in a better position for judging.'—Aristotle, *Metaphys.* 995a–b.

'. . . men give different names, to one and the same thing, from the difference of their own passions: as they that approve a private opinion, call it opinion; but they that mislike it, heresy: . . .'—Th. Hobbes—*Leviathan*, I, 11.

PRELIMINARY

IT HAS BEEN shown in the Introduction why it is necessary to present these theories—in order to point up their individual inadequacies as well as their collective disunity and in order to have before us, in utmost differentiation, the material which shall later be integrated by our Aristotelian system of types. We must now ask: What should be presented? How should it be presented?

Turning directly to the theories, we are confronted straight off with difficulties. On the one hand, it is not possible to state everything which each writer on emotion has said. On the other hand, most theories are not stated simply and concisely, lending themselves to easy quotation. Therefore, we are obliged to abstract and condense in order to present in as few of the original words as necessary an adequate statement of each theory. Such manipulations with other people's words and ideas are always a gamble. One runs the risk through the act of selection both of displaying one's own prejudices and of misrepresenting the other's intentions. Yet it is still better to make this selection, present these excerpts in their original language wherever we can, than to try to rephrase, interpret or merely report. Direct quotation, even if torn from context, at least serves the author in his own words. Direct quotation is also necessary to the phenomenological approach. It means taking statements as they appear. It is irrelevant to our method if a statement comes from a Nobel-Prize expert or a private gentleman who philosophizes at leisure; nor does it matter if a theory propounded in 1910 is set down alongside one from 1950. A phenomenological amplification is timeless. It is no more based upon a notion of progressive evolution in which last year is outdated by this year than it is based upon sanctions of collective opinion which only wants to hear from the 'big names' and 'authorities in the field'. The statements must be gone to directly and quoted directly and thus exposed for what they are, bracketing out all pre-conceptions.

Which of these original statements should be presented? What constitutes 'an adequate statement of each theory'? What is necessary to a theory—as we have said in the first chapter—is a hypothesis. Every theory is made up of at least one hypothesis. So it is these fundamental hypotheses which shall be presented. And what do we mean by 'fundamental'? We mean that hypothesis upon which the other hypotheses in the theory depend.

Not all the quotations which follow are theories in the full sense, nor even are they overt declarations of hypotheses. Some writers do not present an explicit theory, yet they do have a view of emotion, or they define it, or describe it, or restrict the use of the concept in some way which begs the support of an implicit theory or of a smuggled hypothesis. This kind of statement must also be included in order to cover the full phenomenology of theory. So much for the first question: What should be presented?

To the second question: How should we present this wide range of basic hypotheses? Setting forth statements from scores of authors in several languages, each using the almost private frame of his own discipline, requires indeed a method. The one used here is that of types as discussed above. The types have emerged from the study of the phenomena. These basic hypotheses exhibit a kind of differential morphology, that is to say, these theories appear in different forms. And our method consists simply in grouping the theories in accordance with demonstrable similarities of these forms, or ways of looking at and speaking about emotion. In each theory there appears, nearly always, a fundamental hypothesis upon which the theory turns and this hypothesis is similar, as we shall show, to other hypotheses in other theories. These similarities then form superordinate conceptual categories (*Oberbegriffen*) or types, such as 'unconscious', 'conflict', 'disorder', and the like, each of which usually involves traditional philosophical problems. It is these typical problems which stand behind and govern, so to speak, the difficulties and muddles in theory-forming in the field of emotion. As we go along we aim to expose the basic hypotheses in the light of these typical viewpoints in order to make clear the classic nature of the problems involved. This kind of presentation may open another perspective in this area, perhaps removing the problems from the level of argument to a level of more fruitful reflection.

Furthermore, more fruitful reflection in the light of tradition serves a very practical end. Calling attention to these governing principles—which we can also understand as psychological attitudes —that are involved in the theory of emotion, means calling attention to their consequences for clinical practice. For example, emotion explained in terms of disorder, or in terms of energy, spirit, or muscular activity results in different diagnostic appraisals and different therapeutic measures in each case. As was pointed out in the first part, the concept of emotion is the currency of clinical practice. Ideas about emotion fill the literature and the consulting-room. We believe it is useful to become aware of the density and complexity of these ideas which, when taken for granted and used without discrimination, become the repositories of prejudice, superstition and

30

illusion. It seems far better to become aware of these prejudicial attitudes—and traditional values—attached to the concept of emotion which come out in the fundamental hypotheses of the theories in order to have them clearly in mind. Ideas which we have, but do not know we have in all their traditional complexity, we do not really have. Rather, they have us. Instead of possessing them as instruments, they possess us as prejudices. Hence our method may serve the practical end of discovering to the clinician his possessions.

In addition, this method, where it tends to agree in part with the groupings of other writers who present theories of emotion in terms of the various schools of psychology, i.e. in terms of fundamental viewpoints, is more differentiated and extensive than any we have found in the literature. And we claim it is adequate to this presentation of all the varied, yet relevant, material in the field. These groupings, in as much as they have no inherent relation to each other, are only 'random eclectic categories' such as we mentioned in Part I. Therefore whatever light they shed on the problem of integration is accidental. (They do, of course, provide rubrics for an anthology of theory which is another way of looking at this collection.) However, integration is not the concern of this part. The aim is an ordered differentiation by means of this method of the pandemonium of theory.

THE VARIOUS DENIALS

SOME THEORISTS present no theory; in the phenomenology of theories there are those which deny the existence of anything to theorize about. This denial can take three forms: (*a*) denying the use of the concept 'emotion', or emotional concepts a place in psychology; (*b*) reducing the concept 'emotion' to other concepts; (*c*) polemicizing against emotions as *things* which call for explanations. The issue is spurious, the concept is not useful; emotion is no different from other more basic events. These theories all try to tell us what emotion is not. Let us look at the examples:

> Why introduce into science an unneeded term, such as emotion, when there are already scientific terms for everything we have to describe? . . . I predict: The 'will' has virtually passed out of our scientific psychology today; the 'emotion' is bound to do the same. In 1950 American psychologists will smile at both these terms as curiosities of the past.—M. F. Meyer, 'That Whale among the Fishes—The Theory of Emotions', *Psychol. Rev.*, 1933, p. 300.

Duffy finds 'the concept is not useful in exact psychological investigation'[1] and attempts 'an explanation of "emotional" phenomena without the use of the concept "emotion" ' in a paper with just that title.[2] The substitute categories which she proposes are 'goal direction' and 'intensity or energy mobilization'[3] Hull's textbook[4] does not mention the terms feeling and emotion; and Masserman, who has made many contributions to the study of emotion from the side of experimental psychology, writes:

[1] Duffy, E., 'Emotion: an Example of the Need for Reorientation in Psychology', *Psychol. Rev.*, 1934, p. 197.
[2] Duffy, E., 'An Explanation of "Emotional" Phenomena Without the Use of the Concept "Emotion" ', *J. General Psychol.*, 1941, p. 283f. R. Arnheim ('Emotion and Feeling in Psychology and Art', *Confin. Psychiat.*, 1958, p. 78) agrees in substance with Duffy.
[3] Duffy, E., 'Leeper's "Motivational Theory of Emotion" ', *Psychol. Rev.*, 1948, p. 328.
[4] Hull, C., *Principles of Behavior*, N.Y., 1943.

I myself have used a more circumspect technique for avoiding what I consider a spurious issue by writing an entire textbook, *Principles of Dynamic Psychiatry* (1946), in which the terms 'feeling' and 'emotion' are used only in a brief special section devoted to indicating how generalized, vague, or protean are their meanings. And yet such attempts to dispose of these concepts leave us with an uneasy feeling that possibly . . . we may even yet be burying them prematurely.—J. Masserman, 'A Biodynamic Psychoanalytic Approach to the Problem of Feeling and Emotion', FE 50, p. 41.

He proposes more 'basic determinants' to which emotion can be reduced, concluding flatly that in his studies '. . . nowhere did an emotion per se become manifest as a distinctive entity or even as a separate vector of conduct.' (*ibid.*, p. 50).

Precker in writing on the problem of emotion in connection with theoretical brain models follows the direction of Meyer and others we shall come to later who conceive emotion as something going on continuously, described either as energy (Chapter VI), as autonomic nervous activity (Chapter X B) or as a quantitative function (Chapter VII). Precker writes:

> Emotion may be approached more profitably in other ways, which do not consider it qualitatively different from other behavior. Spinoza said: 'By emotion I understand the modifications of the body by which the power of action is increased or diminished, aided or restrained, and at the same time, the ideas of these modifications.' In our words, we may say that the process we usually call emotion is tied up with distribution of energy in the system. This distribution and redistribution is always going on. . . .
> The important point is that emotion is *not* different from problem-solving.—J. A. Precker, 'Toward a Theoretical Brain-Model', *J. of Personality*, 1953–4, p. 323.

In Precker's statement there is a quotation from Spinoza and part of that quotation refers to 'the ideas of those modifications'. These ideas we can call the subjective or introspective side of emotion. It is not in keeping with the behaviourist approach to give value to this subjective side, and so Precker's 'problem solving', as well as Masserman's 'basic determinants' neglect or deny that emotion is qualitatively different from other behaviour since, perhaps, this qualitative difference might lie in the subjective side of the event. And in the statements which follow, the denial of emotion as an entity and the denial of emotion as an event in consciousness go hand in hand. Without the subjective qualitative difference, reducing emotion to other categories of behaviour is no great trick, but follows quite freely from the behaviourist approach. As Beebe-Center says '. . . in Behaviour Theory the theory of affective and

33

emotional behaviour may involve neither feeling nor emotion'.[1] Hebb presents this way of going about emotion quite clearly:

> Since it seems that the term emotion does not refer to a special kind of event in consciousness, and since in any case we must not slip into the inconsistency of treating an immaterial awareness as a causal agency, the term is not very useful in its traditional significance. At the same time, we must postulate that the disturbances of emotional behaviour have a neural origin; and the term emotion still can be useful to refer to the neural processes that produce emotional behaviour.
>
> It is important to be clear that in this discussion 'emotion' is a reference to the hypothetical neural processes that produce emotional behaviour; explicitly, it refers neither to an immaterial state of consciousness nor to the observable pattern of emotional behaviour.—D. O. Hebb, *The Organization of Behavior*, N.Y. and London, 1949, pp. 237–8.

He denies explicitly both that emotions are special kinds of events in consciousness and also that we have any subjective 'inner' awareness of an emotional state. The names of emotion are learned, not intuitively known.[2] He holds that it is not the stimulus situation which is the main determinant for recognizing an emotion, i.e. we do *not* recognize and name fear by means of a fearful stimulus situation. It is the 'facts of behaviour' which 'must constitute the ultimate reference of emotional terms' (the same, p. 105). But these facts of behaviour are not intuitively grasped by the 'mind' as the 'body' goes through its pattern of behaviour in an isomorphic sense as other writers whom we shall come to later suppose (e.g. Claparède, p. 50–1). No, we recognize our different emotions because we have *learned* to recognize them (the same, p. 101–2). And finally, he rejects the commonsense view of consciousness and arguments from introspection,[3] which make up the main arguments—as we shall come to later—for the qualitative differentiation of emotion, and for regarding emotions as entities.

> As Ryle has shown very forcefully, the commonsense view of consciousness leads directly to absurdities. The only evidence for it, besides, is the demonstrably unreliable evidence of introspection. For some time, psychologists have had to abandon introspection as a crucial argument. The test of any theory is in what a subject *does*.—'The Problem of Consciousness and Introspection', p. 403, in *Brain Mechanisms and Consciousness, A Symposium*, ed. by J. F. Delafresnaye, Oxford, 1954.

Here we can go back to Masserman who also denies introspection

---

[1] Beebe-Center, J. G., 'Feeling and Emotion' in *Theoretical Foundations of Psychology*, ed. by H. Helsen, N.Y., 1951, p. 277.

[2] Hebb, D. O., 'Emotion in Man and Animal: An Analysis of the Intuitive Processes of Recognition', *Psychol. Rev.*, 1946, p. 98.

[3] Hebb, D. O., 'The Problem of Consciousness and Introspection', p. 403, in *Brain Mechanisms and Consciousness*, ed. by J. F. Delafresnaye, Oxford, 1954.

and concludes like Hebb that 'Over-all actions speak louder than (the special kind of actions called) words' (Masserman, p. 49).

Turning to Ryle, whom Hebb used for support, we find him writing vigorously against the idea of emotions as things and against the idea of emotions as internal or private experiences.

> There are two quite different senses of 'emotion', in which we explain people's behaviour by reference to emotions. In the first sense we are referring to the motives or inclinations from which more or less intelligent actions are done. In the second sense we are referring to moods, including the agitations or perturbations of which some aimless movements are signs. In neither of these senses are we asserting or implying that the overt behaviour is the effect of felt turbulence in the agent's stream of consciousness. In a third sense of 'emotion', pangs and twinges are feelings or emotions, but they are not, save *per accidens*, things by reference to which we explain behaviour. They are things for which diagnoses are required, not things required for the diagnoses of behaviour. Impulses, described as feelings which impel action, are paramechanical myths. . . .
>
> Consequently, though the description of the higher-level behaviour of people certainly requires mention of emotions in the first two senses, this mention does not entail inferences to occult inner states or processes. . . . Motives and moods are not the sorts of things which could be among the direct intimations of consciousness, or among the objects of introspection, as these factitious forms of Privileged Access are ordinarily described. They are not 'experiences', any more than habits or maladies are 'experiences'.—G. Ryle, *The Concept of Mind*, London, 1949, pp. 114–15.

There is a curious pressure in all these writers to do away with the tradition of theory about emotion. This tradition has tended to reify the passions and to conceive of the emotions as mental states, as special little entities which 'cause' behaviour. This is what Ryle calls 'the ghost in the machine'. Dunlap puts it this way:

> The so-called emotions of the psychologist . . . remain, however, in the world of myth. They are, so far as I can understand, neither objects, nor occurrences, nor relations, but mystical entities, concerning which a mass of mystical speculation has grown up. . . . They have the same connection with reality as the hypogriff, the demon, and the entelechy.— K. Dunlap, 'Emotion as a Dynamic Background', FE 28, p. 151.

Koffka writes similarly:

> The theory of emotion has suffered from what could be called the static attitude of psychologists. An emotion was considered a sort of *thing*. . . . But, of course, emotions cannot be treated adequately with the thing category. We cannot take them and cut them to pieces and see what they consist of. Again we are in full agreement with McDougall,

35

who emphasizes 'The obvious fact that there are no such things as "emotions".' . . .—K. Koffka, *Principles of Gestalt Psychology*, London, 1935, p. 401.

Beebe-Center[1] makes clear that emotions are constructs not 'contents'. Landis writes: '*Neither emotion nor emotions exist as discrete entities*'.[2] And Malmo says. 'Whatever else we may say about it emotion is not a thing with tangible properties.' [3] Brown and Farber argue that:

> emotion, if it is to enter usefully into scientific thinking, must be regarded as an *invention* or *inference* on the part of the psychologist. Emotion is not a *thing* in the simple, naïve sense that a chair or table is a thing. Like numerous other terms in common use, it cannot be defined by the simple, fundamental operation of 'pointing at'.—J. S. Brown and I. E. Farber, 'Emotions Conceptualized as Intervening Variables', *Psychol. Bull.* 1951, p. 466.

This kind of argument is not something new—even if made nowadays in the name of Science—but seems to appear whenever reification of psychic functions becomes extreme. For example, the Stoics tended to conceive of the emotions as individual demons and Plutarch took his turn with this kind of polemic:

> For it is very absurd that, making all virtues and vices—and with them all arts, memories, fancies, passions, impulses, and assents—to be bodies, they should affirm that they neither lie nor subsist in any subject, leaving them for a place one only hole, like a prick in the heart, where they crowd the . . . soul, enclosed with so many bodies. . . . Nay, that they should not only make them bodies, but also rational creatures, and even a swarm of such creatures, . . . and should so make of each one of us a park or menagerie or Trojan horse, . . .—Plutarch, *Moralia*, 'Of Common Conceptions, Against the Stoics', Sect. 45, Vol. IV, ed. by W. Goodwin, London, 1870, p. 243.

The 'rational creatures' which Plutarch mentions can be interpreted today as the motivational, purposeful or intentional view of emotion; while the making of each of us into a menagerie or Trojan horse stuffed with substantial bodies called emotions, is just what Ryle calls the ghost in the machine and what Dunlap calls the 'hypogriff, the demon, and the entelechy'.

There are two conclusions which emerge from these views. The first is more evident. We are told that emotion as a term has lost its significance because it is not qualitatively different from other activities of the human organism (or machine) which are going on

[1] Beebe-Center, *op. cit. sup.*, p. 295 f.
[2] Landis, C., 'Emotion' in *Psychology*, Boring, Langfeld and Weld, N.Y., 1935, p. 397.
[3] Malmo, R. B., 'Research: Experimental and Theoretical', RDPM, p. 86.

continuously or which are more basic. These more basic determinants can be called simply problem-solving (Precker) or can be described by a pair of co-ordinate categories (Duffy) or exhaustively elaborated into twenty or more functional factors which enter into the 'intervening variable' called emotion (Brown and Farber).[1] The main point is that the whole issue of emotion in psychology is spurious because emotion can be dissolved into other dynamics. The term 'emotion' has no referent since emotions are neither static substantial bodies, things, distinctive entities, nor events in consciousness, motives, experiences, etc., requiring explanation on these levels. This is the theory of emotion which these denials produce.

This leads to the second conclusion which takes rise in questions unanswered by this theory. Why, for instance, in tradition and today does man conceive emotion in this substantial and mythological way? Why does a denial of introspection as a method go hand in hand with a denial of emotion as an entity, or reality, which can 'cause'? And why is the power to cause allowed only to concepts of a material order? (The argument here has been: since emotions cannot be touched, pointed to, cut up, they are not real, but are immaterial and immaterial events are ghosts which cannot cause.) Introspection, of course, attests to another order of reality which we might call psychic, or psychological, where things might be known without learning, where hippogriffs and demons are real, and where so-called 'occult', 'inner' 'states' are more accessible to immediate apprehension than the atom and the gene. So we might say that this *via negativa* to a theory of emotion yields an intimation that emotion and psychic reality have some significant relation, since a denial of emotion is also a denial of that ghost in the machine which has for quite some time been called the psyche.

[1] Brown, J. S., and Farber, I. E., 'Emotions Conceptualized as Intervening Variables', *Psychol. Bull.*, 1951, p. 492.

II

EMOTION AS A DISTINCT ENTITY

INCLUDED HERE are those views which tend to explain the emotions in terms of units, elements, substances, forces, motives, each with its own nature and way of acting. Also here are those views which see emotion—the generic concept—as a trait, vector, factor, faculty, manifold, field or area which can be charted, measured, described. These theories do not make emotion or the emotions an attribute or property of other psychological functions but take it as a distinct entity. Emotion is not reducible to other more basic determinants but is something substantial, that is, independent and distinct. These are the theories, then, which uphold the 'reality' of emotion and which can tend consequently to make emotion *res*, opposite to those views in the group preceding.

For example, McDougall, whom we have just heard say that there are 'no such things as emotions', also says:

> Sentiments, then, or individually acquired cognitive-affective dispositions, are the material, the substance, the functional units of character.—W. McDougall: 'Organization of the Affective Life', *Acta Psychologica*, 1937, p. 311.

And Shand makes it more explicit:

> The emotions then are forces: they work in certain ways, and in certain directions. They are within us to perform certain functions; though they often exceed their functions, and are imperfect instruments. They need, and in man they acquire, higher systems to control them; but they are essentially organized forces, and as such we shall define them. And if in the course of our inquiry we come upon any so-called 'emotion' which is not such a force, which has neither impulse nor end. . . . we shall for our purpose refuse to accept it as emotion, because it lacks the fundamental character of that class of facts to which we restrict the term.—A. F. Shand, *The Foundations of Character*, London, 2nd edn., 1920, p. 179.

Similar to Shand but in more contemporary language is the view of Saul. What Shand would call character, Saul would call psychodynamics. 'Psychodynamics means "the interplay of emotional forces". . . . Of course the forces themselves are generated by the physiologic activities of the body.' He writes:

> Biologic urges, drives, motivations and emotions are forces. They cannot be dissected out to be seen and handled (at least for the present), but they are none the less real. You know them from experiencing them in yourselves—your loves, hates, ambitions, joys and 'anxious cares and dreads'. They are forces like electricity, which also cannot be seen but must be studied through its effects.—L. J. Saul, *Bases of Human Behavior*, Phila., 1951, p. 19.

It is interesting to note how Saul, in spite of his biophysical approach, falls back on the introspective 'you know them from experiencing them in yourselves' in order to establish the reality of the emotions as distinct entities. He says they are real even though we cannot see them, in the same way that energy is invisible and real. Whether this analogy with energy is necessary in order to establish the reality of an order of events which can be called psychological reality is something we can take up in a later section. It is worth noting again here that certain methods lead to certain results. There appears to be an inherent relation between the method of introspection and conclusions about the 'reality' of emotion; just as there seemed to be an intimate connection in the theories of group one which both denied introspection as a method and the 'reality' of emotion.

Stout[1] holds for 'ultimate qualitative differences' in the emotions, but he does not feel obliged to defend his view, as does Saul, with external justifications from other fields of inquiry since he accepts introspective evidence on face value. He considers the specific quality of each emotion to be a unique and irreducible fact, yet he is not therefore driven to conclude that emotions are substances. The various connotations of independence (irreducibility) can lead to the muddle of substance where physical and psychological reality get confused. Stout keeps clear of this muddle, but it is traditional when we conceive of distinct and unique facts and endow them with 'force', to end up with demons and mannikins. It is not so much an argument whether or not there *are* demons and mannikins, as it is a question of accepting facts as they appear in experience. And if emotional phenomena are *experienced* as demons and mannikins, it is more correct to name them such as was done in the old days and as Jung often does today, or as the 'plain man' does when he speaks of emotion doing this or that to him, and thus make honest and explicit the frame of operations. In this way one avoids the critics in Chapter I who are otherwise justified in holding that 'Vibratory

---

[1] Stout, G. F., *A Manual of Psychology*, 5th edn., London, 1938, p. 371.

motion and electrical units have replaced the movement of fiends as ultimate explanatory principles.' [1]

Taking emotions, now, as specific forces or units of character, then the magnificent panoply of emotional life—1,300 kinds of feelings have been suggested[2]—must either each be unique or must be built out of more basic units. Many opt for the latter view, concocting 'derived' emotions from the mixtures and blendings of more 'elemental' emotions, a habit which particularly infuriates the *anti-res* people of Chapter I. (They too, of course, derive complex behaviour states from more basic determinants, but they are careful to avoid labelling those more simple factors and their synthesized products 'emotions'. Therein only lies the difference; in principle both opponents explain emotion through methods of analysis and synthesis.)

Jorgensen finds each emotion 'to contain a . . . nucleus of specific quality'. He offers that emotions be conceived on the analogy of specific energies of sensation (following Müller's Law), since each has 'its own stamp, its own individuality, its own quality, just as all sensations do. . . .'

> If attention is paid to the phenomena of spontaneous conditions of feeling and emotions, it will be seen that there is a great range of such states, which often appear with such a peculiar stamp that it is easy to describe the condition and name it joy, sorrow, want, shyness, etc. If the physiological basis of emotional life were made up of a series of different specific elements which, in excitement, produce states known as emotions, falling back to a light tone when in a state of repose, as is commonly observed in neurological elements, we would seem to have a simple explanation of most of the phenomena within emotional life.—C. Jorgensen, 'A Theory of the Elements in the Emotions', FE 28, p. 311.

He proposes six basic elements (Fear, Happiness, Sorrow, Want, Anger, Shyness) 'to be considered as the fundamental elements of emotional life'. Descartes, too, found six basic passions: Ribot lists five; Thomas Aquinas eleven; Cobb[3] gives a schema with eight, etc. It would take us too far from the theme to report on all the many lists of 'basic emotions', but the main problem in such lists is the confusion between classification as an order imposed upon phenomena and the order of those phenomena in themselves. The hope in all such views, as we see in the theory of Williams, is to compose variety from simplicity.

---

[1] Ruckmick, C. A., *The Psychology of Feeling and Emotion*, N.Y. and London, 1936, p. 52.

[2] See reference to Orth, FE 28, p. 375. Also W. James writes (*The Principles of Psychology*, Dover edn., 1950, Vol. II, p. 454): '. . . *there is no limit to the number of possible different emotions which may exist.* . . .'

[3] ECM, p. 108.

The units we have are the emotions fear, 'anger-aggression', the mood depression, and the feeling tones pleasure-unpleasure, which vary in intensity and duration, are modified by the evoking subject, and further elaborated by temporal perception and secondary cognition. Thus, as an example, the state of jealousy, which was not encountered as an ictal emotion, is an unpleasant feeling tone with anxiety (mild prolonged fear), that the subject may be (temporal) more fortunate than I (cognition).

It is the prime function of the brain that it is able to create so much with such simple units. An elaborate and flexible visual imagery is based on the function of a rigid receptor organ, the eye; social behaviour is all created from the flexor-extensor relationship. In the affective-emotional sphere all experience results from the integration of equally frugal material.—D. Williams, 'The Structure of Emotions Reflected in Epileptic Experiences', *Brain*, 1956, p. 65.

The 'interplay of emotional forces', to use Saul's phrase, or the way in which the component elements of Jorgensen or the frugal units of Williams combine, that is, *the laws of their relationships*, would be the next step in describing the nature of emotional life. Shand elaborates such laws. This is also what factorial analysis attempts. The factors, the traits, the abilities which are plotted out statistically are conceived as forces with causal properties.

> Just as it is convenient to postulate physical forces in describing the movements of physical objects, so it is also natural to postulate abilities and their absence as primary causes of the successful completion of a task by some individuals and of the failure of other individuals in the same task.—L. L. Thurstone, *The Vectors of the Mind*, Univ. of Chicago, 1935, p. 45.

Burt applies these concepts of traits and factors to the emotions:

> The suggestion I ventured to put forward was that, in the emotional field at any rate, both the observable traits and the underlying factors could be regarded as conative 'forces'. Accordingly, relying on the analogy with physical forces, we may attempt to analyze emotional tendencies into independent 'components' and to recombine the components into composite 'resultants' in accordance with the well-known principles of the 'parallelogram of forces'.—Sir Cyril Burt, 'The Factorial Study of Emotions', FE 50, p. 540.

He further draws the comparison between this way of regarding emotion with Wundt's three-dimensional manifold and its three bi-polar factors.[1]

Burt makes a distinction between observable traits and underlying factors. The latter tend to be conceived as hypothetical index factors

---

[1] J. Elmgren ('Emotions and Sentiments in Recent Psychology', FE 50, pp. 142–6) also works out from Wundt. '. . . the Wundtian emotional theory might serve as a model to our thinking in this field.' His manifold has *six* dimensions, however: Sensitivity; Vividness; Tension; Lability-Stability; Intensity; Integration.

in the manner of Karl Pearson, or as faculties and powers as in the psychologies of the last century which, like Galen's humours, make up types of personality. Whether or not they become hypostatized, a certain idealization sets in if one emphasizes the universals and not the particular observable traits. Allport, well aware of these difficulties, opts for the observable traits and avoids reification in spite of conceiving them boldly as:

> ... biophysical in nature, concrete and personal in their organization, contemporaneous in their effect, capable of functional autonomy, but not structurally independent of one another; ...—G. W. Allport, *Personality*, London, 1951—reprint of 1937, U.S.A. edition—p. 342.

Plutchik, however, suggests that emotion be conceptualized more in keeping with a mathematical norm, rather like Burt's underlying factors against which observable traits can be measured and correlated. He gives a view of emotion which is not concrete, not personal, not biophysical. With his view we have the perfect laboratory emotion: pure, exact, and bloodless. For him there is:

> ... the need for a concept of emotions as idealized states, in somewhat the same way that the physicist conceptualizes the point masses, freely falling bodies and frictionless surfaces to which his laws, strictly speaking, apply. The task of the psychologist, just as it is that of the physicist, is then to show, not why a definition does not approximate reality, but why reality does not approximate the definition.
> 'Pure' emotions in this ideal sense may be defined by various properties which can be approached experimentally only by a series of successive approximations as the different variables which affect the measurement of the emotion are eliminated or kept constant. It is only through a recognition of what these variables are that an effective experimental program can be instituted.—R. Plutchik, 'Some Problems for a Theory of Emotion', *Psychosom. Med.*, 1955, p. 309.

Concluding then with the theories of this group we observe that emotions are said to be functional units of the psyche, forces with a ground and a goal, forces which cause. They can be explained on analogy to the forces of physics. Some say they are biophysical in nature, even generated by the body. They form character, personality, types. They mix with each other in building other emotions, and the way in which they relate can be analysed into laws. If we prefer to see them as traits they are inter-dependent, yet functionally autonomous. If we prefer to see them as elements, they are independent and spontaneous and can be reduced to a few basic units. If we prefer to see them as ideal states they become a background of 'reality' against which we can measure experimentally derived facts. Each has a specific qualitative nucleus which is unique and irreducible. They are discrete, distinct, real entities—but not *things*. In short, emotions are not things but there are such things as emotions.

What we have been given here is a substantial view of qualities. This is particularly explicit in the hypothesis of Jorgensen, but it also comes out for example in the views of Shand[1] and Sullivan[2] for whom emotions are distinct entities and also qualities. These qualities are the stuff of the psyche, a notion of the soul we can find symbolically imaged as a bundle or shimmer of qualities—Pandora's box, the multicoloured robe, the peacock's tail. This idea of quality as impalpable yet independent and irreducible to some other more basic substance we find also in common speech when we say 'he is a man of many qualities', meaning 'virtues' or 'potentialities'. (Virtue, *vir* = man, and *vis* = force all have the common root *uei meaning generally 'active strength'.[3]) Character on this view is composed of emotional qualities called traits, factors, motives the combination of which makes each individual just what he is, his *quale*. As such they are 'forces', not as material substances but as powers, virtues or influences.[4] The notion of quality is active; it is restored to its ancient and potent meaning contrary to the castrated qualities of Cartesian Rationalism, those flimsy, ephemeral, secondary accidents hanging about solid bodies.

This is a view of emotion to be found in the German philosopher Nicolai Hartmann. 'Emotions and everything which belongs to this category are the root of affective life, of psychic strength. They are the stuff of life's inner content and the basis of its richness.'[5]

Through taking emotions as substantial qualities which form character, the problem of emotion therapy becomes one of character refinement. Hartmann points this out, finding the Epicurean ideals of 'refinement, enrichment and education of feeling life, including the heightening of the capacity for enjoyment in the sense of ethical "good taste" (*sapientia*)' to be a method far more conducive to self-mastery (*sophrosyne*) than the 'Stoic blunting and coarsening of feeling life' in order to achieve a kind of negative impassibility.[6] Each emotion—whether it be courage, greed or anxiety—is a quality which can be altered through training. A change in one's emotional life takes place through 'character building', through daily habitual

---

[1] Shand, A. F., 'Character and the Emotions', *Mind*, N.S., V, 1896, pp. 217–18.

[2] Sullivan, H. S., *Clinical Studies in Psychiatry*, N.Y., 1956, pp. 91–127. See further Chapter III below for Sullivan's view.

[3] Walde, A., *Lateinisches Etymologisches Worterbuch*, 3rd edn., Heidelberg, 1940.

[4] See O.E.D., 'force', definition 11a, Newton's use of force as 'influence'.

[5] Hartmann, N., *Ethik* (Chapter XLVII), 3rd edn., Berlin, 1949, pp. 436–7: 'Die Affekte und alles, was dem genus nach zu ihnen gehört, sind die Wurzel des emotionalen Lebens, der seelischen Kraft; sie sind die Materie des inneren Lebensgehalts, der Basis seiner Fülle.

[6] *Ibid.*

practices at courage, greed and anxiety. Although this method of meeting emotion is an aspect of all family and school life as well as a part of all religious disciplines, its efficacy remains questionable. It does not meet head on the problem of the excessive, disordering aspect of emotion. We are still left with questions about the origin of these qualities, their meaning and purpose and, more particularly, the quantitative and physiological aspects of the problem.

III

EMOTION AS AN ACCOMPANIMENT

'*PLEASURE, satisfaction, or emotion are to be looked upon as accompaniments not causes,*' says Pillsbury,[1] and this is the essence of the views of this group. Here emotion is viewed as an aspect, companion, or result of something else, rather like an adjective modifying a static noun, or an adverb modifying a dynamic verb. Emotion is only something secondary (Daly King), an epiphenomenon (Masserman), an after-effect (Malmud). It is in fact so secondary that a special psychology of emotion has no *raison d'être* (Cellérier[2]).

McDougall's theory is well known:

> Emotion was regarded as a mode of experience which accompanies the working within us of instinctive impulses. It was assumed that human nature (our inherited inborn constitution) comprises instincts; that the operation of each instinct, no matter how brought into play, is accompanied by its own peculiar quality of experience which may be called a primary emotion; and that, when two or more instincts are simultaneously at work in us, we experience a confused emotional excitement, in which we can detect something of the qualities of the corresponding primary emotions. The human emotions were then regarded as clues to the instinctive impulses, or indicators of the motives at work in us. . . . I hold fast to the scheme as essentially on the right lines. . . .—W. McDougall, *An Outline of Psychology*, 12th edn., London, 1948, p. 128.

Rivers follows along the same lines as McDougall: 'Each of the emotions can be regarded as an affective aspect of an instinctive reaction. . . .'[3]

[1] Pillsbury W. B. 'The Utility of Emotions', FE 28, p. 120.

[2] Cellérier, L. 'La Vie affective secondaire', *Rev. Phil.*, 104, 1927, p. 357. 'L'émotion n'est ainsi qu'un sentiment secondaire accompagné de réactions internes assez vives pour être perçues. Une psychologie spéciale de l'émotion n'a donc pas raison d'être, ce processes étant, à part le degré d'intensité des réactions, ce qu'est le sentiment secondaire.'

[3] Rivers, W. H. R., *Instinct and the Unconscious*, Cambridge, 1920, p. 37. Elsewhere (*Conflict and Dream*, London, 1923) Rivers holds that in so far as dreams are an attempt to solve conflicts, the emotional character of dreams depends upon the degree

45

Laignel-Lavastine uses the wider term 'tendencies' rather than 'instinct' in describing that which emotions accompany:

> We are essentially tendencies; every creature by the mere fact of his existence, tends to continue in his being, according to Spinoza's principle. These tendencies are varied according to their origin and purpose. . . . Janet divides them essentially into three great categories: the *lower tendencies*, of visceral origin, which have a precise somatic source and give rise to the bodily needs; the *superior tendencies*, whose origin, on the contrary cannot be localized exactly in the body, and whose trend is towards synthetic functions of a superior order, social, religious, aesthetic; and the *intermediate tendencies*, which are characterized, on the one hand by their starting point being still in the organism, and, on the other, by having their end point in the more or less elevated part of the psychic sphere.
>
> There would be, then, emotions in all these varieties of tendencies, these emotions being themselves more or less elevated, more or less idealized, according to whichever tendencies they accompany.—M. Laignel-Lavastine, *The Concentric Method in the Diagnosis of Psychoneurotics*, London, 1931, pp. 16–17.

Although emotions are conceived as accompaniments of *all* tendencies, they would seem to appear only under special circumstances, that is, when there is a 'sudden change in the conditions of adaptation of the affective tone of the tendencies' (p. 16). On the physical side, this sudden change has to do with the imbibition of plain muscle which in turn has to do with variations in the chronaxy (reaction time of tissue to electrical excitation). He calls this a 'physical theory of emotivity' (p. 31) implying that all emotion depends on these basic measurable physiological events. Somehow he slips over the former statement that emotions accompany superior tendencies whose origin cannot be localized in the body.

If we consider these accompaniments as 'indicators of the motives at work in us' (McDougall) they can be experienced as 'feelings'. (Here, feelings would not be considered as substantive events in themselves, but as signs or indicators of something else.[1]) This is how Sullivan[2] understands emotion: the emotion of lust, for example, he calls 'the felt aspect of the genital drive' (p. 295); and the 'uncanny emotions—awe, dread, loathing, horror', he understands as the felt aspects of the dissociated parts of the personality (p. 320; p. 359). Malmud, on the other hand, sees emotion as an accompaniment not

---

of success or failure in the resolution of these conflicts. He does not however elaborate a 'conflict' theory of emotion which such a view implies.

[1] Further aspects of the term 'feeling' in connection with emotion are in Chapter IX where feeling appears as a quality, and Chapter XV where feeling appears as signification, as an indication of 'something else' in the sense of Sullivan. See also footnote p. 60, and Part III, p. 269.

[2] Sullivan, H. S., *The Interpersonal Theory of Psychiatry*, London, 1955.

of parts of the personality, but of the whole personality in its attitude at any given moment.

> . . . *emotion is the positive or negative after-effect of attitude.* By attitude we mean the whole complex of conscious processes as well as what is for the moment nonconscious, but which nevertheless enters into the organization of the complex, a *unity* sometimes segmented for descriptive purposes into the cognitive, the conative . . . and the affective aspects of experience.—R. S. Malmud, 'Poetry and the Emotions', *J. Abn. Soc. Psychol.*, 1927–8, p. 449.

Daly King[1] considers emotion the accompaniment of physiological events. He, and Masserman, hold for an epiphenomenal point of view which understands an 'accompaniment' as ontologically lesser or secondary.

> . . . emotions are 'subjective' epiphenomena that accompany stressful adaptations, and are expressed in the behaviour patterns that range in complexity from the relatively simple and constant bodily dysfunctions of anxiety to the highly elaborate and variable concomitants of complex affective states such as pity, enthusiasm, esthetic appreciation, etc. The expression of emotion, further is determined not only by the cultural and experiential history of the subject but by various contingent circumstances. . . .—J. H. Masserman, *Principles of Dynamic Psychiatry*, Philadelphia, 1946, p. 17. (See also p. 33 above for a more recent view of Masserman's which attempts to get rid of this bothersome 'epiphenomenon' altogether.)

Therapeutically, of course, these theories offer little. Emotion-therapy really means dealing with something other than emotion—attitude, physiology, instincts, etc.—because emotion is only an accompanying epiphenomenon like a whistle from the tea-kettle.

The difficulty in all these views is the relationship between emotion as an accompaniment and that which it accompanies. The explanation of emotion will have to depend on the explanation of this relationship, that is, whether it be a causal one, or an energetic one, or one in which there operates a third factor such as repression, conflict, etc. One way of solving the problem of relationship between two orders of events is to maintain that these two orders are isomorphic. For example, we might assume that the accompaniment called emotion is the same thing as a tendency, an instinct, or a physiological occurrence expressed in another language. The accompaniment and the thing accompanied would then have no causal relationship as suggested by some of the views here, but would be equal aspects of the same event. This brings us to the theories of the next chapter where isomorphism is used to explain the mental and physical aspects of emotion.

[1] King, C. D., *The Psychology of Consciousness*, London, 1932, p. 118.

IV

EMOTION AND ISOMORPHISM

THE CONCEPT of isomorphism originates in mathematics and the natural sciences. In the former discipline it means 'identity of form and of operations between two or more groups'; in the latter, it means 'the property of crystallizing in the same or closely related forms, especially as exhibited by substances of analogous composition'. In psychology, it is a concept invoked to heal the mind/body wound, that chronic split which appears both as subjective events/observable behaviour and as bio-psychological life/anorganic nature. Although the concept is particularly evident in Gestalt psychology, some sort of what we might call isomorphic thinking appears in those areas of psychology where the unity of the organism (organismal view) is stressed and where the problems of the mind/body relationship are understood as two aspects of the same thing or as two languages expressing the same thing. Thus we find it in the Gestalt theory of Koffka:

> Subjective feeling and objective observation of behaviour or of physiological symptoms are in the best possible agreement. This is fundamental for our theory of emotions. If there were no such agreement, if we could feel excited . . . when our psychophysical field were . . . calm . . . our theory of emotions, nay our whole psychology would have to be entirely different. Then it certainly would not be isomorphic, whereas the real facts support our isomorphic methodology.—K. Koffka, *Principles of Gestalt Psychology*, London, 1935, p. 402. (See also Chapter XI, below.)

In Bekhterev's reflexology:

> Reflexology regards emotional states as somato-mimetic reflexes, in which the subjective and objective aspects represent one and the same indivisible process.—V. M. Bekhterev, 'Emotions as Somato-Mimetic Reflexes', FE 28, p. 276. (See also Chapter XII, below.)

And also in Dunbar's psychosomatic medicine:

> The organismal theory provides the fundamental concept . . . in . . . psychosomatic medicine . . . the idea that the psychic and somatic are

48

not two different universes, but the same one viewed from different approaches. . . .—F. Dunbar, *Psychosomatic Diagnosis*, N.Y., 1943, p. 649. (See also Chapter VI, below.)

In short, isomorphism is a monistic refinement of parallelism which tries to avoid the dangers of classic parallelism, epiphenomenalism, occasionalism, interactionism, and the like.

In the last part of the last century, Ribot and James each present a theory of emotion which is based on this assumed analogous composition between an order of events called physical and an order called mental.

> In my view, there would be great advantage in eliminating . . . every notion of cause and effect . . . and in substituting for the dualistic position a unitary and monistic one. The Aristotelian formula of matter and form seems to me to meet the case better, if we understand by 'matter' the corporeal facts, and by 'form' the corresponding psychical state: the two terms . . . only existing in connection with each other and being inseparable except as abstract conceptions. . . . No state of consciousness can be dissociated from its physical conditions: they constitute a natural whole, which must be studied as such. Every kind of emotion ought to be considered in this way: all that is objectively expressed by movements of the face and body, by vaso-motor, respiratory, and secretory disturbances, is expressed subjectively by correlated states of consciousness. . . . It is a single occurrence expressed in two languages.
> —Th. Ribot, *The Psychology of the Emotions*, London, 1897, p. 112.

This is Ribot's fundamental hypothesis which he identifies in substance, though not in formulation, with the theory of James and Lange.

There are many ways of understanding James' theory of emotions,[1] depending upon which aspect is considered the essential one. We can sketch below some of the ways:

(1) Emotion is an *accompaniment* of instinct: '*Instinctive reactions and emotional expressions thus shade imperceptibly into each other.* Every object that excites an instinct excites an emotion as well' (*op. cit.*, p. 442).

(2) Emotion is composed of *sensations:* '. . . whatever moods, affections, and passions I have are in very truth constituted by, and made up of, those bodily changes which we ordinarily call their expression or consequence. . . . They are *sensational* processes, processes due to inward currents set up by physical happenings' (pp. 452–3).

(3) Emotion is composed of *elements*: '. . . each emotion is the resultant of a sum of elements, and each element is caused by a physiological process of a sort already well known' (p. 453).

[1] James, W., *The Principles of Psychology* (1890), Dover edn., N.Y., 1950.

49

(4) Emotion is based upon *reflex* (stimulus-response) acts which underlie the elements or sensations: 'The elements are all organic changes, and each of them is the reflex effect of the exciting object' (p. 453). '. . . the genesis of an emotion is accounted for, as the arousal by an object of a lot of reflex acts . . .' (p. 454).

(5) Emotion is based upon *visceral* reflexes, requiring no seat in the brain: 'Supposing the cortex to contain parts, liable to be excited by changes in each special sense-organ, in each portion of the skin . . . muscle . . . joint . . . viscus, and to contain absolutely nothing else, we still have a scheme capable of representing the process of the emotions. An object falls on a sense-organ, affects a cortical part, and is perceived. . . . Quick as a flash, the reflex currents pass down through their preordained channels, alter the condition of muscle, skin, and viscus; and these alterations, perceived, like the original object . . . combine with it in consciousness and transform it from an object-simply-apprehended into an object-emotionally-felt. No new principles have to be evoked . . .' (pp. 473–4).

The essential view of James to which these other views are accessory is that physiological events are simultaneously apprehended by consciousness so that the mental and physical events are the same thing:

> My theory . . . is that *the bodily changes follow directly the perception of the exciting fact, and that our feeling of the same changes as they occur* IS *the emotion* (p. 449).
>
> . . . *every one of the bodily changes, whatsoever it be, is* FELT, *acutely or obscurely, the moment it occurs* (pp. 450–1).

But when James says: 'Now the general causes of the emotions are indubitably physiological' (p. 449), and then proceeds to identify his view with that of Lange, he overlooks one difference between their views which makes his view 'isomorphic' and which makes Lange's 'visceral'. For James, emotion is the feeling and the changes in the body together at the same moment; for Lange, emotion is bodily changes the feeling of which is secondary and consequent (Chapter X B).

Claparède expresses the principle of isomorphism even more clearly:

> The emotion is nothing other than the consciousness of a form, of a 'Gestalt', of these multiple organic impressions. In other words, the emotion is the consciousness of a global attitude of the organism. . . .
>
> What the consciousness seizes in emotion is . . . the form of the organism itself—that is to say—its attitude.
>
> This peripheral conception which regards the emotion as the consciousness of an attitude of the organism is, besides, the only one which

can take account of the fact that the emotion is immediately 'understood' by him who experiences it. The emotion contains in itself its significance. —E. Claparède, 'Feelings and Emotions', FE 28, pp. 128–9.

His negative evaluation of emotion ('Feelings are useful . . . emotions serve no purpose', p. 126) is only incidental to his theory based on the isomorphic principle of identity of operations between body and mind.

The logical consequence of this theory is that for every emotional state of mind there is a corresponding physiological emotional pattern and vice versa. This idea is presented by James: 'The various permutations and combinations of which these organic activities are susceptible make it abstractly possible that no shade of emotion, however slight, should be without a bodily reverberation as unique, when taken in its totality, as in the mental mood itself' (p. 450). Recent experiments claim this to be demonstrable:

> The results of this study suggest that each attitude is associated with its own unique set of bodily changes. . . . Nothing is implied in this connection about a cause-and-effect relation between 'mental' and 'physical' events, and, indeed it seems unprofitable to look at the matter in this light.
> These considerations suggest the advisability of defining the word emotion, so that it means an attitude and the associated bodily changes. —W. J. Grace and D. T. Graham, 'Relationship of Specific Attitudes and Emotions to Certain Bodily Diseases', *Psychosom. Med.* 1952, p. 248.
> These results provide further evidence for the psychophysiological unity of the organism in the sense that even the finest nuances of psychological acts may be found to have a corresponding differentiation at the physiological level.—A. Ax, 'The Physiological Differentiation between Fear and Anger in Humans', *Psychosom. Med.* 1953, p. 441.

This of course implies, as Grace and Graham point out, that emotion is going on all the time. If this be so—and we find this statement made again and again (Chapters I, VI, IX, X B, etc.)—then we ask: when is an emotion an emotion? How does isomorphism explain emotion? Explanation as such is not given on this view, instead it is a philosophical position upon which specific and divergent explanations are based. James and Ribot ultimately refer emotion to bodily events, Grace and Graham to the criterion of intensity, Claparède to a notion of disorder, while others suggest conflict or the stimulus situation as the criteria.

The philosophical position itself divides into two kinds: simple and sophisticated isomorphism. Simple isomorphism as a direct parallelism between two orders of events or as aspects (languages) of a third thing, the whole, leaves one with the problem of specifying this relationship. This must be done by examining such philosophical questions as the nature of relations, part-and-whole, dualism, as well as the 'reason' for these poles, orders, languages. (The metaphor of 'languages' brings in as many new complications as it resolves old ones.) Furthermore, the assumption must be specifically tested in regard to the facts of emotion. For example, can isomorphism account for the pathological splitting of physiological pattern from conscious event; or the experimentally produced states of 'sham' or 'cold' emotion; or the results of Asian meditation techniques in which there appears to be such a radical independence between the two orders of events. It would seem we run up against something contrary to Ribot: 'no state of consciousness can be dissociated from its physical conditions', and James: 'every one of the bodily changes . . . is FELT . . . the moment it occurs', and Koffka: 'subjective feeling and objective observation . . . are in best possible agreement'. There lurks an idealistic hope of wholeness and order in this assumption that we are always aware of the world about us and of what is occurring within us. The psychotherapist knows full well that emotion can be objectively present in tone of voice, facial expression, gesture and gait, and yet be subjectively absent in the consciousness of the patient and also in his habitat. Man is split; bodily pattern, outer situation and consciousness can all be exhibiting different worlds. Simple isomorphism, as a philosophical position, would deny that *psyche* and *physis* are relatively independent and that they can at times even be opposed to each other.

Sophisticated isomorphism goes beyond the appearances of divergent facts, such as the splitting of consciousness, body and world, by positing a single order behind these facts. Things do not have to appear alike to be isomorphic. For Kohler[1] there are mathematical principles operative both in anorganic bodies and in the nervous system. Metzger[2] suggests isomorphic laws for vision, the fluids of the body and anorganic liquids. Thus sophisticated isomorphism harks back to an older model of meeting these problems. In Hobbes we find the hypothesis that the world ultimately consists of motions which are 'pressed' upon our organs of sense and, via the system of animal spirits (nervous system), they set up corresponding motions which are perceived by consciousness as sensible qualities. A single order of motions (dynamics) stands behind the qualities in objects and the qualities in consciousness:

> All which qualities, called *sensible*, are in the object that causeth them, but so many several motions of the matter, by which it presseth our organs diversely. Neither in us that are pressed, are they any thing else,

---

[1] Köhler, W., *Die physischen Gestalten in Ruhe und im stationären Zustand*, Erlangen. 1924.
[2] Metzger, W., *Gesetze des Sehens*, Frankfurt a/M, 1953 (last chapter).

but divers motions; for motion produceth nothing but motion.—
Leviathan, I, 1.

And these motions follow definite laws of geometry. This is not a
mechanical explanation either in Gestalt theory or in Hobbes, but
a *rational idealism* that posits the union of consciousness and world
in supra-psychic and supra-physical laws deducible by reason.

Some hold isomorphism is proved; others deny it. We leave the
matter open, accepting it as a fundamental model for thinking about
the problem of emotion. For us the question is not whether or not
there is a single occurrence expressed in two languages (Ribot) or that
'the body is the manifestation of the mind, the mind the meaning of
the bodily manifestation' as two poles of the same event (Klages).
Rather it is a matter of interpreting the meaning of this model used
to explain emotion to see what it has to tell us about emotion. Since
this point of view must be invoked by some as a ground for a theory,
evidently adequate explanation of emotion requires taking into
account events in several fields of operations which, during emotion,
are intimately connected, if not identical. Thus at best isomorphism
proposes the possibility that in emotion man can be one with himself,
his body and his world. This in turn implies that therapy of emotion
is a total therapy, a constellation of factors yielding *mens sana in
corpore sano in mundo sano*. It further indicates that it is not a
rational philosophy of isomorphism which heals the split between
psyche and physis, but the experience of emotion itself.

EMOTION AND THE UNCONSCIOUS

RETURNING to the conclusions of Chapter II, i.e. that emotions are invisible forces which form character according to laws of relationship, then we need only postulate for them a region or manifold (to use the term of Wundt and Allport) somewhere 'outside' or 'below' the region of awareness and we have the basis of explanation of the theories of this group. This is how Grossart proceeds. For him emotions are 'ultimate, real existents, psychic forces or tendencies, independent of consciousness', so that 'the search for the essence of emotion leads necessarily to the question of the unconscious, or better said, of unconscious psychic forces'.[1] Thus emotion here will be explained by means of the concept of the unconscious. Other explanatory ideas are brought in, such as: conflict, accompaniment, representations, energy, etc., but what differentiates the theories here from those which depend upon these other ideas is the explanation through the unconscious. This concept is essential to these views.

Freud takes up the question of unconscious emotions and discusses how it is possible for us to speak of them in such a way:

> It is surely of the essence of an emotion that we should feel it, i.e. that it should enter consciousness. So for emotions, feelings and affects to be unconscious would be quite out of the question. But in psycho-analytic practice we are accustomed to speak of unconscious love, hate, anger, etc., and find it impossible to avoid even the strange conjunction, 'unconscious consciousness of guilt', or a paradoxical 'unconscious anxiety' . . . .
>
> To begin with it may happen that an affect or an emotion is perceived but misconstrued. By the repression of its proper presentation it is forced to become connected with another idea, and is now interpreted by consciousness as the expression of this other idea. If we restore the true con-

---

[1] Grossart, Fr., 'Gefühl und Strebung', *Arch. f.d. Ges. Psychol.* 79, 1931, p. 392. '*Sie müssen vielmehr allgemein als letzte, vom Bewusstsein unabhängige, real existierende, von ihm aber erfassbare seelische Kräfte oder Strebungen begriffen werden. Die Frage nach dem Wesen des Gefühls führt so notwendig zu der Frage des Unbewussten, besser gesagt der unbewussten seelischen Kräfte.*'

nection, we call the original affect 'unconscious' although the affect was never unconscious but its ideational presentation had undergone repression. In any event, the use of such terms as 'unconscious affect and emotion' has reference to the fate undergone, in consequence of repression, by the quantitative factor in the instinctual impulse. . . . In every instance where repression has succeeded in inhibiting the development of an affect we apply the term 'unconscious' to those affects that are restored when we undo the work of repression. So it cannot be denied that the use of the terms in question is logical; but a comparison of the unconscious affect with the unconscious idea reveals the significant difference that the unconscious idea continues, after repression, as an actual formation in the system Ucs, whilst to the unconscious affect there corresponds in the same system only a potential disposition which is prevented from developing further. So that, strictly speaking, although no fault can be found with the mode of expression in question, there are no unconscious affects in the sense in which there are unconscious ideas. But there may very well be in the system Ucs affect-formations which, like others, come into consciousness. The whole difference arises from the fact that ideas are cathexes—ultimately of memory-traces—whilst affects and emotions correspond with processes of discharge, the final expression of which is perceived as feeling. In the present state of our knowledge of affects and emotions we cannot express this difference more clearly.—S. Freud, 'The Unconscious' (1915), (*Coll. Papers*, Vol. IV, London, 1949, pp. 109–11).

In understanding this passage about the nature of emotion, it might be helpful to use an analogy. Let us conceive of these 'cathexes—ultimately of memory-traces' as bombs and the affect as the quantitative explosive potential of the bombs. The bombs 'exist' 'in' the unconscious, but the affect is only a potential which is not discharged until the bomb is released, i.e. repression is lifted by one means or another. The bomb and the explosion, the idea and the emotion, are intimately connected; but the emotion is ultimately rooted in the body's physiology as 'the quantitative factor in the instinctual impulse'.

This explosion if taken by itself is essentially an internal event and different from motility:

> Affectivity manifests itself essentially in motor (i.e. secretory circulatory) discharge resulting in an (internal) alteration of the subject's own body without reference to the outer world; motility, in the actions designed to effect changes in the outer world.—*Op. cit. supra*, p. 111 fn.

Elsewhere he phrases emotion as:

> . . . a motor or secretory function, the key to whose innervation lies in the ideas in the *Ucs.—The Interpretation of Dreams*, London, 1954, p. 582.

And in another statement, he again brings ideas into connection with emotion, emphasizing its value and significance.

> We remain on the surface so long as we treat only of memories and ideas. The only valuable things in psychic life are, rather, the emotions. All psychic powers are significant only through their fitness to awaken emotions. Ideas are repressed only because they are connected with liberations of emotions, which are not to come to light; it would be more correct to say that repression deals with the emotions, but these are comprehensible to us only in connection with ideas.—*Delusion and Dream*, London, 1921, p. 159.

Freud's writings on emotion are reported on fully in the psycho-analytic literature and further statements from and about him are not essential here. Before proceeding to the theory of affect which later psycho-analytic writers have drawn from his statements, we can point to several ideas of Freud's which shall occupy us in later sections: (1) Freud notes the significance of the idea (representation) in relation to emotion; (2) he looks at emotion as a kind of physiological quantum; (3) he notes a double function of emotion—that it be felt in consciousness and that it internally alter the body; (4) he holds that it is opposite to object reference and to motivated behaviour in regard to the outer world; and (5) Freud stresses the value of emotion. From this we can see that it is no simple matter to state Freud's theory of emotion, and the controversies among the theories of the psycho-analytic writers which follow take their rise in his richness of view. The one frame of reference which contains his insights, however, is the division of the psyche into dynamic structures and the operation of the function of repression.

The development of the orthodoxy called the psychoanalytic movement gave rise to many formulations[1] for a theory of affects, a term which has been equated with both feelings and emotions by these people.

Glover's theory depends upon that idea of Freud's that zones and organs of the body could become 'erogenized':

> Study of the affective reactions following frustration of different component impulses provides a valuable line of inquiry. Variations in the distribution of libido or of aggressive charges throughout the different body organs or zones are responsible for characteristic affective experiences. And no doubt these could be traced back to differences in the

---

[1] See: F. Alexander, 'The Logic of Emotions', *Int. J. Psycho-Anal.*, 1935; M. Brierley, 'Affect in Theory and Practice', *ibid.*, 1937; K. Landauer, 'Affects, Passions and Temperament', *ibid.*, 1938 (see, p. 158, below); S. Novey, 'A Clinical View of Affect Theory in Psycho-Analysis', *ibid.*, 1959; H. Nunberg, *Allgemeine Neuroslehre*, 1932; O. Fenichel, 'The Ego and the Affects', *Psychoanal. Rev.*, 1941.

nature of sensory excitation and of stimulation of the sympathetic system.—E. Glover, 'The Psycho-Analysis of Affects', *Internat. J. Psycho-Anal.*, 1939, p. 301.

Glover's theory has the classic stamp. It is reminiscent of all those views which used to explain the characteristic differences of the passions in terms of movements and distribution of spirits and humours (here called libido and aggressive charges) throughout different body organs and zones.

Jacobson's theory depends upon another set of Freud's ideas: the structural division of the psyche into ego, super-ego, and id:

> We may consider replacing . . . [Glover's] with a classification that employs our current structural concepts. Even though all affects are ego experiences and develop in the ego, one of their qualitative determinants must be the site of the underlying energetic tension by which they have been induced and which may arise anywhere within the psychic organization. Practically, certain affects have always been characterized in this way; guilt feelings, for instance, are commonly defined as arising from a tension between ego and super-ego. There is no reason why we should not introduce this kind of classification for affect types in general. Thus we might distinguish:
>
> (1) simple and compound affects arising from intrasystemic tension:
>   (*a*) affects that represent instinctual drives proper, i.e. that arise directly from tensions in the id (e.g. sexual excitement, rage);
>   (*b*) affects that develop directly from tensions in the ego . . .
> (2) simple and compound affects induced by intersystemic tensions:
>   (*a*) affects induced by tension between ego and id (e.g. fear of the id, components of disgust, shame, and pity);
>   (*b*) affects induced by tension between the ego and the super-ego. . .
>
> As will be noticed, I have not included tensions between ego and reality. These represent conflict, that is affective responses to reality. The underlying energetic psychic tension can only arise within the psychic organization and not between it and the outside world.—E. Jacobson (MS., 1951, quoted by D. Rapaport, *Int. J. Psycho-Anal.*, 1953, p. 193).

This theory does not discuss 'pleasant' or 'positive' emotions, and could be labelled a 'conflict' theory with specific reference to a structural conflict, rather than a conflict between two opposing dynamisms.

Federn also depends upon Freud's ideas on the structure of the psyche, but combines in his theory topographical views from Gestalt psychology. He differs from Jacobson in so far as the structural tensions which give rise to affect are not between the three sections of the psyche, but are all within the ego.

Affects always develop between two ego boundaries acting on each other, and differ according to the kind of drive cathexis of the ego at these boundaries: . . . Therefore, affects are the mutually developing sensations which the drive cathexis of the ego arouses in the drive cathected ego. In this way we understand the manifold nuances of affects of the same kind, their manifold mixture and shading, their displaceability, and their simultaneously centripetal and centrifugal nature of the discharge in their excitation. We must presume that they arise precisely at the ego boundaries because frequently, the affects are subject to specific and very peculiar sensations of estrangement.—P. Federn, *Ego Psychology and the Psychoses*, London, 1953, pp. 334–5.

Every affect is a characteristic sensation apart from topography, dynamics and economics. It is the specific mode of sensation of the manner in which the adjustment at the ego boundaries occurs, whether it fails or succeeds, is rapid or delayed, expands or shrinks, and depending precisely upon the specific, highly differentiated types of drive cathexes involved.—*Op. cit.*, p. 340 fn.

As Rapaport[1] points out, Federn's concept of the ego is not the usual psychoanalytic one, and his theory does not explicitly depend upon a concept of the unconscious. It is nevertheless implied since all the various ego boundaries are not conscious at the same time. What is obscure in his theory is the nature of the 'specific, highly differentiated types of drive cathexes' which qualify emotion. Emotion is due to conflict at the ego boundaries, but the *kind* of emotion, i.e. its characteristic sensation, is not really explained.

Of all these writers none seems to have got more involved in the problems of theory of emotion than Rapaport. In a detailed, drawn-out and difficult paper he reviews the whole field of psycho-analytic theory of affect. He divides the history of psycho-analytic thinking into three phases, each phase laying hold of one theory of affect.

The dominant concept of affect of the beginning phase of psycho-analysis, in which no sharp differentiation between the theory of cathartic-hypnosis and that of psycho-analysis had as yet occurred, equates affect with the quantity of psychic energy, which was later conceptualized as drive-cathexis.—D. Rapaport, 'On the Psycho-Analytic Theory of Affects'; *Int. J. Psycho-Anal.*, 1953, p. 179.

The major implication of the affect-theory of the second phase of psycho-analysis is that affect-expression is the outcome of the discharge of part of the accumulated drive-cathexes when direct discharge in drive-action *cannot* take place.—*Op. cit.*, p. 183.

The Ego and the Id, which officially ushers in the third phase of psycho-analytic theory contains a simile which . . . forecasts the view that, owing to structure-development, processes which are originally related to the conflicts of the id recur and involve higher levels of psychic structure.—*Op. cit.*, p. 186.

[1] EM, p. 31.

He then rephrases these three views into a summary and attempts to integrate the three into the outlines of a theory:

> In the first theory, affects were equated with drive-cathexes; in the second theory, they appeared as drive representations, serving as safety-valves for drive-cathexes the discharge of which was prevented; in the third theory they appear as ego-functions, and as such are no longer safety-valves but are used as signals by the ego . . .—*Op. cit.*, p. 187.
>
> The theory of affects, the bare outlines of which seem to emerge, integrates three components: *inborn affect discharge-channels* and dis-charge-thresholds of drive-cathexes; the use of these inborn channels as safety-valves and indications of drive-tension, the modification of their thresholds by drives and derivative motivations prevented from drive-action, and the formation hereby of the *drive-representation* termed *affect-charge;* and the progressive 'taming' and advancing ego-control, in the course of psychic structure-formation, of the affects which are thereby turned into *affect-signals* released by the ego.—*Op. cit.*, p. 196.

Rapaport does not seem blessed with the happy gift of clarity, and his statements hardly fulfil the meaning of the word 'explain'—to unfold or make plain. But it seems that the three components of his theory of affects refer to (*a*) inherited patterns of behaviour having a quantitative 'threshold' for release; (*b*) these ways of releasing energy are modified into affective-expression when the inborn pattern of emotional behaviour cannot be directly released; (*c*) in the growth of the individual a hierarchy becomes established and the ego controls these ways of releasing this energy in a significative way. It is actually a theory which explains in terms of *development*; bringing together the three ideas of emotion as phylogenetically inherited patterns, as expression of conflict, and as signification.

Jung, like Freud, has been writing about emotional phenomena for many years and, like Freud, has no single explicit theory of emotion. Both consider it of first importance and both understand it through that system of operations called the unconscious. But where Freud was influenced in his explanation by a neurological and biological background, Jung's first views on emotion take rise in psychiatry and his association with Bleuler.

> The essential basis of our personality is affectivity. Thought and action are only, as it were, symptoms of affectivity.—C. G. Jung, *Ueber die Psychologie der Dementia praecox*, Halle, 1907, p. 42 (translation mine).

But where Bleuler continued to treat emotion or affectivity as a kind of molar, quantitative and generalized event—we shall come to his theory in Chapter VIII—Jung, in this same early work, showed an interest in the differentiation of this general affectivity.

The elements of psychic life, sensations, ideas, images and feelings, are given to consciousness in the form of certain entities, which if one may risk an analogy to chemistry, can be compared to a molecule.—*Idem*, p. 43.

This mention of elements, this interest in structure, shows another influence on Jung, that of Wundt.

His early work on the association experiment and the theory of complexes treated emotion—and feeling—as an energetic, quantitative charge, the formal aspect of which was the idea or molecular group of ideas. To put it simply: the 'molecule' or complex was a form of energy, or formed energy. The energy appeared as the feeling tone, or emotional tone, of a pattern of ideas. The energy of the complex was the emotional tone which could be experienced as felt value, yet this emotional tone was not separable from the way in which the ideas or memory-images were associated. In this way, the energy and the pattern were dependent upon each other, as if two aspects of the same thing. This was demonstrated by the fact that resolution of complexes freed energy.

The energetic view of emotion, in spite of this emphasis upon the formal aspect, remained the dominant theme. The emotional tone of the complex was also called 'association readiness', that is, the energetic drawing power of a complex to increase its size and strength. The energetic point of view was also furthered by correlations with physical energy by means of the psychogalvanometer. Nevertheless, just as Jung did not identify emotion and energy, he also kept distinct physical and psychic energy. He also distinguished later between feeling and emotion (affect); unlike Bleuler and Freud who did not make this distinction.[1] In this way, the concept of emotion became separated out from a host of related concepts—feeling, psychic energy, physical energy, affectivity—and came to be a concept closely related to the concept of the complex, as in his later

---

[1] As H. Rohracher (*Einführung in die Psychologie*, 1951, p. 441) and R. Heiss (*Allgemeine Tiefenpsychologie*, 1956, p. 243) complain, neither psychology nor psychiatry—nor philosophy—have been able to achieve a simply formulated demarcation between feelings and affects. Jung agrees (at least in his earlier work, *Psychological Types*, definition 'Affect') 'that no definite demarcation exists'; nevertheless he points the way for clarifying the two concepts. Feeling is a function of consciousness; as Harms says ('A Differential Concept of Feelings and Emotions', FE 50, p. 153) '. . . Ego control effects a phenomenological differentiation between them, relegating "feelings" to the actual Ego-controlled activity and "emotions" to the Ego-uncontrolled feelings; we possess our feelings but we are possessed by our emotions.' (Affects, for him, are Ego-uncontrolled willings, while Jung uses 'affect' and 'emotion' interchangeably.) Other criteria for the differentiation of these concepts shall become clearer as we go along, e.g. emotion is total, feeling not (Chapter VIII); emotion involves gross, perceptible physiological changes, feeling not (Chapter X B); emotion involves drive activities, feeling not (Chapter X C); emotion is symbolic, feeling rational; emotion transforms, feeling evaluates; etc. See further, Part III, p. 269.

writings where the autonomy of emotion as a distinct entity is emphasized.

As a matter of fact, an emotion *is* the intrusion of an unconscious personality. The unconscious contents it brings to light have a personal character, and it is merely because we never sum them up that we have not discovered this other character long ago. To. the primitive mind, a man who is seized by strong emotion is possessed by a devil or a spirit; and our language still expresses the same idea, at least metaphorically. There is much to be said in favour of this point of view.—*The Integration of the Personality*, London, 1940, pp. 19–20.

And these distinct entities appear spontaneously (compare Jorgensen, Chapter II) out of the unconscious.

Emotions are not 'made', or wilfully produced, in and by consciousness. Instead, they appear suddenly, leaping up from an unconscious region.—*Op. cit.*, p. 10.

Jung takes up the autonomy of emotion in another passage in relation to the formation of complexes, where emotion is conceived under *two aspects*: *energetic force and image*:

Psychologically we should say, every affect tends to become an autonomous complex, to break away from the hierarchy of consciousness, and, if possible, to drag the ego after it. No wonder, therefore, that the primitive mind sees in it the work of a strange invisible being, a spirit. Spirit in this case is the image of an independent affect, and therefore the ancients appropriately called spirits also *imagines*—images.—'Spirit and Life', in *Contributions to Analytical Psychology*, London, 1928, pp. 89–90.

A late statement makes explicit the double view of emotion held all along:

Affectivity, however, rests to a large extent on the instincts, whose formal aspect is the archetype.—'Synchronicity: An Acausal Connecting Principle' in *The Interpretation of Nature and the Psyche*, C. G. Jung and W. Pauli, London, 1955, p. 34.

Here, instinct is both energy and formal pattern and provides the ground—both as energy and form—for emotion. Hence, it becomes apparent why certain forms, those which are archetypal, i.e. archaic, collective, universal, are so emotionally charged and give rise to emotional reactions. These forms or images are but the formal side of instinct. (For further discussion of this, see Chapter XIV.)

Finally, Jung adds another aspect to his views in discussing the relation of emotion to extra-sensory phenomena and synchronistic events.

. . . an emotional state . . . alters space and time by 'contraction'. Every

61

emotional state produces an alteration of consciousness which Janet called *abaissement du niveau mental:* that is to say there is a certain narrowing of consciousness and a corresponding strengthening of the unconscious which, particularly in the case of strong affects, is noticeable even to the layman. The tone of the unconscious is heightened, thereby creating a gradient for the unconscious to flow towards the conscious. The conscious then comes under the influence of unconscious instinctual impulses and contents. These are as a rule complexes whose ultimate basis is the archetype, the 'instinctual pattern'.—*Op. cit.*, pp. 42–3.

Jung quotes Albertus Magnus to the same effect:

> When therefore the soul of a man falls into a great excess of any passion, it can be proved by experiment that it (the excess) binds things (magically) and alters them in the way it wants, and for a long time I did not believe it, but after I had read the nigromantic books and others of the kind on signs and magic, I found that the emotionality (affectio) of the human soul is the chief cause of all these things. . . .—Alb. Magn., *De Mirabilibus Mundi* (no date), quoted by Jung, *op. cit. sup.*, p. 45.

With this passage Jung points to the fascinating question of the relation between emotion and parapsychological events. He observes that emotion as a state of relative unconsciousness is a magical kind of behaviour altering the subject-object relation, a view given also in the theories of both Sartre (Chapter XV) and Jonas (Chapter XII). Collingwood (Chapter XVIII) also connects magic and emotion.[1] Among the 'nigromantic books' which Albert read most probably were works of Avicenna, since he was indebted to the Arabic philosopher for much else. Gruner puts Avicenna's view as follows:

> *Emotional states as a basis of occult phenomena.* Strong emotional states may impress places and things sufficiently to affect other persons in the absence of the original impressor. Obsessions and haunted houses are accounted for in this way. 'A place or thing . . . which has played a part in the events that aroused very intense emotional activity . . . becomes itself saturated as it were with the emotions involved. . . .'—O. C. Gruner, *The Canon of Medicine of Avicenna*, London, 1930, p. 150.

Schopenhauer, too, found the basis for occult phenomena to be in emotion, although he expressed his theory of magic in terms of manipulations of the Universal Will through our access to it in our unconscious ('the secret depths inside man himself').[2] He quotes Roger Bacon, Paracelsus, Jacob Böhme and many others in support of his hypothesis of the Will, but the operative concept in these quotations qualifies this Will in terms of emotion as it is generally understood

---

[1] Collingwood, R. G., *The Principles of Art*, Oxford, 1938, p. 66.
[2] Schopenhauer, A., 'Animalischer Magnetismus und Magie', *Ueber den Willen in der Natur* (Coll. Works, Frauenstädt/Huebscher edition), Leipzig, 1938, p. 115—'. . . geheimnisvollen Tiefen seines eigenen Innern. . . .'

(e.g. *Gemüth, Begierde, ardenter desideret, appetitum animae, affectio animae,* etc.). Further, he explains magic events as ending the isolation of the subject, through *actio in distans* (overcoming the principle of individuality due to space and time) much in the same way as noted by Jung, Sartre, Jonas and Rhine. For Rhine maintains that psi effects, although voluntary, are unconscious and not localized organically. He stresses the overriding importance of 'interest', 'drive' or 'motivation' in achieving Psi effects. 'Instances are on record in which subjects produced extremely high scores during intervals of intense interest and enthusiasm'. 'It is, in fact, necessary for almost everyone to be keenly inspired to exercise his psi-ability to a marked degree.' [1] It is evident in all these statements that the emotional state of the individual is of first importance in the exercising of 'magical' effects.

We are left then with the problem of explanation. Let us conceive of emotion, following the views set forth here, as an autonomous complex or unconscious partial personality having both energy and formal quality, an organized dynamism rather like a 'trait' of Chapter II. The emotion would be located 'in' the unconscious. But the unconscious must be taken in Jung's sense of a collective unconscious, or objective psyche of archetypal constellations which transcends the categories of inner and outer. Then the unconscious would no longer be conceptually confined within the individual and emotion would belong to the unconscious aspect of an entire situation rather than only to the individual's subjectivity. The 'idea-pattern' of Tyrrell and the 'persistent and dynamic entities' of Price attributed to the mid-levels of the personality which have been offered as hypothetical explanations[2] for parapsychological events might be taken in this light.

Two conclusions emerge from this digression into the occult: one for parapsychologists, the other for therapists. Research in parapsychology might do well to take more into account what Murphy calls 'human needs', that is the emotional component often exorcised from the test situation. This emotional factor in turn might better be conceived not as 'unscientific' or as something personalistic and idiosyncratic, but perhaps as the very ground of the still inexplicable union of subject and object as exhibited by psi-events. Therapy of emotion must take into account the extraordinary power of emotion, its magical effect in binding the world, so that the reordering of the

---

[1] Rhine, J. B., and Pratt, J. G., *Parapsychology*, Springfield, Ill., 1957, pp. 86–96.
[2] Tyrrell, G., *Apparitions*, London, 1953, pp. 83–115; Price, H. H., 'Haunting and the "Psychic Ether" ', (*Proc. Soc. Psychical Research*, XLV) reprinted in *Tomorrow*, 5, 1957, pp. 107–26.

patient's emotional life goes well beyond his immediate intra-psychic structure and its past history, but is in fact a reordering of the world at large even beyond the space-time limits imposed by consciousness.

With this, then, we can pass on to Neumann, one of Jung's pupils, who tries to 'root' the instinct or lowest reaches of the psyche in the phylogenetically older regions of the brain.

> Emotions and affects are bound up with the lowest reaches of the psyche, those closest to the instincts. The feeling tone basic to what we shall hereafter describe as the 'emotional-dynamic' components has its organic roots in most primitive parts of the brain, namely the medullary region and the thalamus. Since these centres are linked up with the sympathetic nervous system, the emotional components are always intimately associated with unconscious contents.—E. Neumann, *The Origins and History of Consciousness*, London, 1954, p. 330.

It is important to observe here that Neumann in support of his theory of consciousness assumes a kind of equation between energy-source, thalamus, primitivity, unconscious and instinct. He fails to keep separate these concepts each of which has a meaning within a different field of operations. In his attempt to ground the emotional part of the psyche in a special part of the brain, he shifts from psychological to physiological language, assuming a one-to-one equation between cortex and consciousness over against medulla and unconscious (emotion).

> The trend of evolution makes it clear that the medullary man is superseded by the cortical man. This can be seen from the continuous deflation of the unconscious and the exhaustion of emotional components. It is only now, in the present crisis of modern man, whose over-accentuation of the conscious cortical side of himself has led to excessive repression and dissociation of the unconscious, that it has become necessary for him to 'link back' with the medullary region.—*Op. cit.*, p. 331.

This kind of approach comes under fire from Jung since it biologizes the psyche. His criticism is directed against Bleuler's term *psychoide*, the ambiguities of which are due to this kind of organological thinking represented equally well by Neumann. Jung writes thus:

> The confusion obviously springs from the organological standpoint, still observable in Bleuler, which operates with concepts like 'cortical soul' and 'medullary soul' and has a distinct tendency to derive the corresponding psychic functions from these parts of the brain, although it is always the function that creates its own organ, and maintains or modifies it. . . . It is extremely difficult, if not impossible, to think of a psychic function as independent of its organ, although in actual fact we experience the psychic process apart from its relation to the organic

substrate. For the psychologist, however, it is the totality of these experiences that constitutes the object of investigation, and for this reason he must abjure a terminology borrowed from the anatomist.—C. G. Jung, 'The Spirit of Psychology', in *Spirit and Nature, Papers from the Eranos Yearbooks*, N.Y. and London, 1957, p. 388.

We find in conclusion that this group of theories holds on to many threads: emotion has to do with drives and instinct; with energy and quantities; with conflicts and repression, due mainly to a psyche structurally divided—ego, id, super-ego, ego-boundaries, complexes; with signs; with organs and zones and sensations; with time, magic and extra-sensory perception; with ideas and images; with primitivity; with spirit. This huge conglomeration of hypotheses is contained within one overall frame—the unconscious. This attests to the strength and weakness of such an explanation. All depends upon how this unconscious is conceived, which in turn brings in that host of explanatory concepts just reviewed. We need not try to clear up the concept of the unconscious here. Critical attacks have been spent against it regularly for half a century, ever since Freud first brought it before the world. Its variety of meanings makes it a difficult and shifting ground for explanation. Each way in which it is conceived will give a different kind of theory of emotion which can be more carefully discussed in appropriate chapters.

The positive results of these views can be stated simply: whatever else emotion might be, take rise from, point to, or bring about, it is always a phenomenon which bears witness to another, an unconscious, moment of life. Therapy of ill or inadequate emotion must therefore involve practices which investigate the unconscious and which allow it to have its say. To put it another way round, allowing emotion its say is the way to investigate the unconscious. How exactly one lets emotion have its say cannot be taken up here since it will be amplified—as will the concept unconscious itself—through later chapters, particularly Chapters X, XI, XIV, XV and XVIII, as well as in Part III. This more definite denotation gives the unconscious the meaning of a field of significations and representations, and even energy, potentially present to, but not under the control of, ego consciousness.

VI

EMOTION AS ENERGY

WE HAVE already seen the concept of energy brought into relation with the concept of emotion in many of the views in previous chapters. But in these views following, emotion is explained in terms of energy and this concept is used to solve many of the mind-body, organic-inorganic, subject-object problems attendant upon explanations of emotion.

Jacobson (Chapter V) found one of the determinants of emotion to be underlying energetic tension within the subject. The view was psychological and based on Freud's ideas. Bousfield, here, broadens the concept of energetic tension to a metaphysical idea. He hints that the tension present as an element in subjective feeling might be connected with tension states which underlie all objective organic and inorganic phenomena.[1] His theory can be summed up in these three of his 'essential axioms'.

(1) In the conscious animal pain is the conscious affect accompanying tension, and it is proportional to the tension but modified by the sensitivity of the cell or individual on the one hand and by the kind of stimulus on the other hand.

(2) All tension tends to cause those affects which can be classified as painful, and all stimuli therefore tend to cause pain.

(3) Pleasure is that affect which results in the conscious animal as a result of the discharge, or neutralization of tension. It is not, however, proportional to the amount of tension as in the case of pain, but has a relation to the rate of discharge of tension modified by the sensitivity of the cell or individual on the one hand, and the type of stimulus on the other hand, together with possible determinants.—P. Bousfield, *Pleasure and Pain*, London, 1926, p. 93.

This theory is also an attitude toward life which Kant endorsed[2] and

---

[1] Bousfield, P., *Pleasure and Pain*, London, 1926, pp. ix–x.
[2] Kant, I. *Anthropologie*, 60: 'Also muss vor jedem Vergnügen der Schmerz vorhergehen; der Schmerz ist immer das erste.'

which can be traced back as far as Anaxagoras,[1] and which can be detected in the homeostatic views of the human being.[2] In brief, the point of view is: all stimuli disturb stability; an increase of stimuli increases tension and increases pain; pleasure accompanies a reduction of tension and a return to a well-balanced, homeostatic paradise. Reality is painful. Life with its slings and arrows of fortune is a shower of painful stimuli. Subject and object irritate each other as opposites. The world is not meant for man. Bousfield makes this clear by holding pain accompanies tension and that tension underlies all the phenomena in the world. That such a view inadequately values pleasure, tension, and stimuli is evident; more trenchant analysis has recently been excellently made by Flugel.[3] Here it is the aim to point out the attitude of mind involved in such a theory which unites energetic tension with the problems of hedonism.

Where Bousfield leaves open the nature of this underlying tension, Prince and McKinney call it energy. Their theories connect emotion to energy directly, not in the manner of Bousfield via concepts of sensation and affective tone.

The postulate of physical science of an entity called anthropomorphically energy is, by all criteria of matter, *immaterial*. Its nature is unknowable by the objective methods of science. It is inferred from and postulated to explain the happenings of the so-called 'physical world'; it is only known, therefore, by its manifestations or behavior—by what it does. It is known from without, not from within.

As kinetic energy it manifests itself in many forms—as mechanical, electrical, thermal, chemical, etc., and perhaps neural energy, and each may be transformed into another form. Many of its forms, it is agreed, are the resultants of the complexities, collocation, combination, number, and organization of its units. The present thesis is that psychical energy is another form. . . .

Now according to our thesis emotions may be conceived as emerging as consciousness out of energy in either one of two ways. (1) They may be discharging complexes of units of energy associated with the electrons of the highly complex atomic structure of the nervous system. That is to say, the discharges emerge (by the principle of 'emergent evolution') as emotion because they are energy itself—energy from *within* not as observed from without, of the *extremely complex organization of enormous*

---

[1] EGP, pp. 273–4. Burnet says: 'It was a happy thought of Anaxagoras to make sensation depend upon irritation by opposites, and to connect it with pain. Many modern theories are based upon a similar idea.'

[2] See in particular F. Alexander, 'Three Fundamental Dynamic Principles of the Mental Apparatus and of the Behavior of Living Organisms', *Dialectica* 5, 1951, pp. 239–45. In Alexander's trinity, the creative principle, though opposed to the principles of inertia and stability, still remains a servant of them in the name of 'homeostatic balance'. Balance is the preferred pleasant state, not creative tension. (See Chapters XVII and XVIII for further elaboration of these problems.)

[3] Flugel, J. C., 'The Death Instinct, Homeostasis and Allied Concepts', in *Studies in Feeling and Desire*, London, 1955, pp. 96–154.

numbers of units of neural energy. Observed from without they would be known only by what they do. Or (2) we can conceive that kinetic *afferent* neural energy, being *immaterial,* becomes transformed into its like, immaterial psychical energy, which in turn, as a link in the chain of events, becomes transformed into *immaterial* efferent energy, thus conforming to the physical law of the transformation of energy.

That which is the unknown and unknowable by the objective methods of science emerges as the known of psychology, as states of consciousness.—M. Prince, 'Can Emotion Be Regarded As Energy?' FE 28, p. 166.

McKinney discusses along just the same lines. If man is conceived as an energy system, as a physical field of force, then the 'dynamic changes within the organism which may or may not be aroused by external stimuli, we feel and appreciate as emotion'.[1] Science can only measure energy from without, but the mind can experience energy from within in its 'true nature'. This would account for the 'strange ability which enables the poet, the writer, the musician and the artist to gain insight into the true nature of things'.[2] If energy were the underlying substrate of the universe, i.e. its 'truth', and if emotion were the way in which it manifested itself to the mind, then the creative artist through his emotion would be apprehending this truth from within. This at once raises the essential question of inner images and how they relate to energy and to emotion, a question which McKinney neglects but which we shall have to deal with in detail in Chapter XIV and again in Part III.

Marston's[3] theory of emotion is also based upon an identity of energy and consciousness. He limits however his concept of energy to a specific local definition. Byrne, a student of his, sums up his position briefly:

> He supposes that the type of energy developed upon the junctional tissue, or synaptic membrane at the synapses, is a different type of energy from disturbances of propagation within the nerves themselves (following, in this, the authorities Sherrington and Herrick). He calls the junctional tissue at each synapse a 'psychon', and the energy developed thereon 'psychonic energy'. This psychonic energy, he says, *is* consciousness. He then shows structural differences between sensory and motor nerves, and concludes that two types of synaptic membranes, or psychons, also exist, sensory and motor. Therefore, he suggests that we have two basic types of consciousness, sensory and motor.—O. Byrne, *The Evolution of the Theory and Research on Emotions* (unpubl. M.A. Thesis), Columbia Univ., N.Y., 1927, p. 100.

[1] McKinney, J., 'What Shall We Choose to Call Emotion?', *J. Nerv. Ment. Dis.* 1930, p. 56.
[2] *Ibid.,* p. 57.
Marston, W. M., *Emotions of Normal People,* London, 1928, pp. 23–4, 68, 106–7.

This psychonic energy, or motor consciousness, is affective consciousness, a scientific description of which is the psychology of emotion. Such a description, he says, involves an account of the interaction of two kinds of causes—mechanistic and vitalistic—both of which operate in the field of emotion and are central to the problem of theory-forming. The mechanistic set of causes, i.e. the energy aspect of the psychon, is also called the 'motor stimulus'. It is phasic and of reflex origin. The vitalistic set of causes, i.e. the consciousness aspect of the psychon, is also called the 'motor self'. This is a continuous activity of tonic motor origin. Emotion depends upon the interaction of these two energetic phenomena, which are also two kinds of causes. This interaction produces four primary emotions: 'compliance', 'dominance', 'inducement' and 'submission'.

In this theory we find again a concept of energy upon which everything turns. Even though Marston precisely limits his concept to 'psychonic' energy, and interprets the two aspects of this energy in psychological terms (motor self and motor stimulus), this energy is of two distinct kinds. Locating the energy in microscopic points in the nervous system does not explain the two aspects, or two kinds of energy, the inter-relation of which is the basis of his theory. Just what enables the vitalistic motor self to dominate and act purposefully at one moment, while at another it is inferior to the motor impulse with its mechanistic set of causes? We are up against a basic problem in the theory of emotion as energy: if consciousness is energy, how can this consciousness free itself from the laws of energy and obey other laws which energy does not obey?

We might come to a solution of this by pausing over the concept of energy, which need not be conceived only along the lines of the mechanical physics of Newton and Descartes. Energy is an unknown, immaterial abstract; it is a *meta*physical hypothesis. And recent thinking on the part of physicists about energy is less and less inclined toward causal-mechanical metaphysics. Thus we are led to the position of Whitehead whose finely worked out philosophy could be used to substantiate the more limited theories of Prince and McKinney. Whitehead refuses the notion of two different sets of laws, a causal one operative in nature and a vital one in life. In a lecture called 'Nature Alive' [1] he proposes a hierarchical monism, a sketch for the construction of a 'systematic metaphysical cosmology'. 'The key notion from which such a construction should start is that the energetic activity considered in physics is the emotional intensity entertained in life.' [2]

Ultimately emotion in this view is the very ground, reality or first

[1] Whitehead, A. N., *Modes of Thought* (Lecture VIII), Cambridge, 1938.
[2] *Ibid.*, pp. 231-2.

principle for a monistic ontology. Rather than explaining emotion in terms of other more basic categories, emotion becomes the central concept for explaining everything else. It is the first, undoubtable reality. Descartes' 'Cogito, ergo sum' becomes 'Patior, ergo sum' [1]— and here is the point of departure for a new metaphysical cosmology. The 'Cogito' sets the subject apart from the object; it cuts nature and body off from consciousness and life. The 'Patior', however, is nothing else than the subjective experience of the flow of universal energy. Events are not mere energetic facts without aim; they are emotional intensities with intention. If energy is the one universal reality present everywhere, then emotion is too. Thus waves of energy are, perhaps, as well waves of emotion.—With this we shall stop, for the view of energy here set forth fast dissolves into the grander notion of spirit.

Returning then to the main phenomenological problems involved with the conception of emotion as energy: If the same universal energy can be now physical, now chemical, neural or psychical (as for Prince and McKinney), or if the same psychonic energy can be obedient both to mechanistic laws as well as vitalistic laws, then the central issue becomes one of *conversion* or *transformation.*

Such are the problems of psychosomatic medicine. Originally, with Freud, a conversion symptom was a symbolic phenomenon, not an energetic one. Dunbar, however, who considers emotion as energy, makes such symptoms outright energetic:

> Emotion is rather the psychological name for a flow of energy which permeates (though not in equal measure) all parts of the organism.— F. Dunbar, *Psychosomatic Diagnosis,* N.Y., 1943, p. 657.

> The basic law of Freud's work, which now is a basic law of general psychiatry as well, may thus be called the 'first law of emotional thermodynamics', or conservation of vital energy.

> But this law . . . has implications which have not until recently been fully apprehended. . . . It is often assumed that his dynamic conception of emotion referred only to the transformations of vital energy into various patterns of emotional or mental behavior. Yet many of his cases and observations reveal the transformation of vital energy into physical symptoms, and vice versa. . . . In this respect also the law of the conservation of vital energy is analogous to the physical conservation law, which postulates the transformation of energy not only into crude motion and work but also into heat, electricity and chemical changes. One can regard the bodily symptoms which sometimes retain and bind discharges of vital energy as the counterpart of heat, or of the electric

[1] Whitehead, A. N., *Modes of Thought* (Lecture VIII), see p. 228. ' "Cogito ergo sum" is wrongly translated, "I *think*, therefore I am". It is never bare thought or bare existence that we are aware of. I find myself as essentially a unity of emotions, enjoyments, hopes, fears, regrets, valuations of alternatives, decisions—all of them subjective reactions to the environment active in my nature.'

and chemical changes which embody some of the transformations of physical energy. Indeed, the analogy is extraordinarily close, since recent physiological research has shown us that changes in the body which are associated with emotional stimuli are, in sober fact, basically changes in temperature, electric potential, and chemical composition.—*Ibid.*, pp. 650–1.

This transformation of vital energy into bodily symptoms where it is so closely analogous to thermal, chemical and electrical energy, she conceives in terms of a short circuit.

> When a somatic short circuit occurs, it means simply that the cerebral cortex, which normally would have utilized a certain quantum of energy in a certain organization of external behavior, instead has to discharge this energy through the only other channels open to it, that is, through the involuntary and vegetative parts of the organism. It therefore should occasion no surprise to discover that when a person subjected to an unresolved emotional conflict, attempts to discharge energy in action or to develop defenses against it in the form of a certain pattern of behavior, and then this pattern is found to be an insufficient channel of discharge, or is denied by the circumstances of the environment, the resulting short circuit in somatic processes should also occur in a certain pattern, specific in each case to the pattern of impulse and reaction which has become insufficient or is blocked.—*Ibid.*, p. 657.

The job then in psychosomatic diagnosis is to correlate the symptom pattern with the emotional pattern. The job in psychosomatic therapy is to 'reverse' this flow of vital energy into appropriate channels of outlet before it causes permanent structural damage in the organs affected by the improper flow.

This theory of Dunbar has already been taken to task by Alexander who challenges the application of the laws of thermodynamics in this way to the theory of emotion.[1] In addition, we might point out that the theory of Dunbar rests upon the dubious concept 'vital' energy, in which lies the hidden hypothesis of isomorphism. It simply covers over the differences between the two orders of events, physical and psychic, by assuming a single life force called vital energy. A single life force begs the question. As soon as it is manifest it has two aspects which are different and which the very term 'psychosomatic'—awkward as it may be—expresses most justly. Her theory rests further on an analogy between physical events occurring in the body of man endowed with consciousness and physical events occurring in other bodies. These events are identical in some respects (measurements), but are different in others. It is in this difference that the problems lie. And even if, as she suggests, it might someday become possible to

[1] Alexander, F., Book Review of *Psychosomatic Diagnosis* by F. Dunbar, in *Psychosom. Med.*, 1945, p. 64.

'impart a measurable impulse to a human organism, and then to trace and measure all its effects in terms of speech, action, or bodily changes' (p. 653) we would learn nothing whatsoever about the psychic aspect of that speech, action or bodily change.

A corollary to the theory of emotion as energy, which does not involve transformation or conversion, is the idea that energy must be *discharged* or *released*. Energy must find a channel of discharge so that a proper energy balance of the organism is maintained. Ways of ordering the energy are, for example: catharsis, abreaction, exorcism, physical or chemical shock therapy. In all, emotion is viewed as energy which must be let out. It is conceived on the model of electricity in a circuit, or water in a set of pipes. We encounter problems of 'pressure', of 'heat', of 'tension'.[1] Therapeutic techniques for emotional disorders are aimed at regulating this 'flow'.

Two recent descriptions of abreaction conceive of emotion in this way.

A fundamentally different management of the abreactive technique has led to interesting and invaluable results. This consists in adding to and stimulating the patient's excitement rather than damping it down, when it will often reach a climatic phase and pass into a state of temporary general inhibition. Relief from tension and hysterical symptoms, when it occurs after this, is often very dramatic.

More important than the nature of the real life experience, or even than the emotional response it occasioned at the time, is the nature and degree of the patient's emotional excitation during the course of the therapeutic interview.—W. Sargant and E. Slater, *An Introduction to the Physical Methods of Treatment in Psychiatry*, 2nd. edn., Edinburgh, 1948, p. 139.

[Induction of Tension.] In simple terms, the aim of all anxiety-provoking therapy is to mobilize this emotion, to liberate it and to direct it into socially useful channels. . . .

As mentioned in the introduction, the object of excitatory group psychotherapy is the deliberate excitation of tension. . . .—J. Merry: 'Excitatory Group Psychotherapy', *J. Ment. Sci.*, 1953, p. 518.

The group situations described bear a resemblance to those obtaining at the meetings of various religious or political sects. There, a crowded group in an emotionally charged setting results in changes of attitudes in some members of the group due to an acceptance of new beliefs in the

---

[1] This 'hydrostatic' model is also used by Klein and Alexander (RDPM, pp. 12, 14, 19); and by Klopfer (*Developments in the Rorschach Technique*, Vol. I, by B. Klopfer, M. Ainsworth *et al.*, p. 585)—'The conceptual model for emotional intensity is the concept of 'pressure' in hydrodynamics. . . . Intensity of emotion is subjectively felt primarily as 'heat' of feeling. . . .' This in turn is associated with 'depth', but no explicit theory of emotion is provided by this important text in which the term 'emotion' appears again and again.

period of increased suggestibility that immediately follows a rise of emotional excitement.—*Idem*, p. 520.

Mesmer used such techniques based on theories of universal energy. He, too, excited his patients to emotional crises which came to a climacteric in an attempt to mobilize not only the patient's emotion, but the balance of energy between the patient and universe. He described energy like Prince—as universal and immaterial:

> A universally distributed and continuous fluid, which is quite without vacuum and of an incomparably rarefied nature, and which by its nature is capable of receiving, propagating and communicating all impressions of movement . . .—F. A. Mesmer, *Mémoire sur la découverte du magnétisme animal*, Genève, 1779; Eng. transl. by G. Frankau, *Mesmerism*, London, 1948, p. 54.[1]

A newer formulation of this point of view is presented in the works of Reich and the Orgone school. There is a 'universal primordial energy' called 'orgone energy' which in the realm of the organism is called 'bio-energy'. The emotions, which Reich considers the central problem of all psychiatry, are 'manifestations of a tangible bio-energy', which is the 'background and origin of every type of emotion'.

> Literally, 'emotion' means 'moving out', 'protruding'. It is not only permissible but necessary to take the word 'emotion' literally in speaking of sensations and movements. Microscopic observation of amebae subjected to slight electric stimuli renders the meaning of the term 'emotion' in an unmistakable manner. *Basically, emotion is an expressive plasmatic motion.* Pleasureable stimuli cause an 'emotion' of the protoplasm from the center towards the periphery. Conversely, unpleasureable stimuli cause an 'emotion'—or rather, 'remotion'—from the periphery to the center of the organism. These two basic directions of the biophysical plasma current correspond to the two basic affects of the psychic apparatus, pleasure and anxiety. As the experiments at the oscillograph have shown, the physical plasma motion and the corresponding sensation are functionally identical. They are indivisible. . . .—W. Reich, *Character Analysis*, 3rd edn., N.Y., 1949, pp. 358-9; also pp. ix-x.

Reich makes a functional identity (isomorphism) between the motions of expansion and contraction and the affect-sensations of pleasure and pain in a way reminiscent of Bousfield's identification of the two primary affect sensations with tension states. Their interpretations are different in so far as Bousfield considers all stimuli to

---

[1] Un fluide universellement répandu, et continué de manière à ne souffrir aucun vide, dont la subtilité ne permet aucune comparaison, et qui, de sa nature, est susceptible de recevoir, propager et communiquer toutes les impressions du mouvement. . . .— Mesmer, *Mémoire sur la découverte du magnétisme animal*, Prop. 2, Genève, 1779, p. 74.

be painful, while Reich considers some stimuli to be pleasurable. The goal for Bousfield is the reduction of tension and the reduction of pain (Stoicism), and the goal for Reich is the creative pleasurable expansion as represented by the orgasm (Hedonism). Both base their arguments upon the same implied functional identity between cells of protoplasm and conscious human beings, arguing from the simple to the complex. This leads to problems of genetic explanation which we must put off until the appropriate place (Chapter XIII).

Reich's description of therapy is in terms of energy, where the notions of 'release' and 'mobilization' are important.

> No matter whether we release the emotions from the character armor by way of 'character-analysis', or from the muscular armor by ways of 'vegetotherapy', in either case we cause plasmatic excitations and motions. What moves is essentially the orgone energy with which the body fluids are charged. *The mobilization of the plasmatic currents and emotions, then, is identical with the mobilization of orgone energy in the organism.—Ibid.,* p. 359.

Where Mesmer spoke of a therapeutic crisis, Merry of the 'induction or tension', Sargant and Slater of 'stimulating the patient's excitement', Reich speaks of the sexual orgasm which, when it occurs without obstruction, has the therapeutic effect of bringing the individual's energy in harmony with the primordial energy of the universe.

The critical role of emotion in respect to energy balance is blatant in the views presented so far in this group. More subtle is the role which notions of emotion as energy perform in providing a background for the many radical methods of treatment for 'emotional disorders'. If emotional disorder is conceived as energy disorder and the concept of energy is not carefully differentiated and qualified, the patient can be subject to any sort of 'energetic' treatment—chemical, electrical, physical, etc. And, as energy is essentially a concept of the quantitative sort, i.e. meaningless without measurement, *good* tends to be seen as *more*. Hence, a certain preference for the most violent methods which have yet to be adequately explained and which are always unqualified and unspecific,[1] that is, only quantitative. They resemble a blind and hostile attack which the early military meaning of the word 'shock' brings out—a sort of violent disordering impact such

---

[1] Kalinowsky, L. B. and Hoch, P. H. (*Shock Treatments and Other Somatic Procedures in Psychiatry*, N.Y., 1946, Chapter VII) review all current theories and concepts of shock and conclude: 'The therapeutic action of shock treatment is still obscure. . . . At present we can only say that we are treating empirically disorders whose etiology is unknown with shock treatments whose action is also shrouded in mystery' (pp. 242–3). The earliest exponent of 'shock' was perhaps the Roman physician, Celsus, who recommended for the insane a treatment based on torment, terror and startle.

as the sudden collision of two enemy armies. Treatment based on a quantitative concept alone tends to neglect, to say the least, whatever qualitative and specific factors might also be present. Whether emotion is or is not energy is less the debate, than whether emotion includes something over and above energy, in the sense of form, quality, content, or meaning, which energetic treatment cannot comprehend and might even destroy.

Let us return now to that image of emotion as a *flow of energy* which we have found in the views of Dunbar, Reich, Mesmer, Merry, and in the hydrostatic model of the libido concept used by Glover, Klein, Alexander, and Klopfer. Such was the model from Galen until Galvani for the spirits of the soul which were considered to be the basis of emotion, as the flow of energy is so considered by these views today. During the centuries this fluent model of the soul evolved into a highly differentiated set of hypotheses, the main concerns of which were the relations of this soul to the world spirit (universal energy) on the one hand and to the body (symptom formation) on the other. The solution of the latter problem was made in the eighteenth century by identifying the fluid model of the soul with the fluid model of the nervous system (Malpighi, Sömmering, Haller).[1] The title of Flemyng's book (*The Nature of the Nervous Fluid, or Animal Spirits, Demonstrated*:) shows the extent of the unification of these two models. This passage, from that book, is a translation from Haller and is a succinct description of this model:

... there is a fluid, which comes from the brain, and flows down through the nerves to the extreme parts, the motion of which fluid being accelerated by irritation, acts solely in the direction of its current, and cannot produce convulsions upward, as new fluids issued from the brain, prevent that effect.—A. Haller, *Primae lineae physiologiae*, 1747, quoted in

[1] By the eighteenth century this identification had become possible because the image of the animal spirits as a *flow* had become concretized into the image of a *fluid*. For Descartes, the flow was akin to fire; for Thomas Aquinas, it was a vapour akin to air and water; for Albertus Magnus (*Parva Naturalia*, Trac. I and II) it consisted of all elements, but having the form of air. For Augustine it was a kind of air, or nerve-ether, or light (A. Schneider, 'Die Psychologie Alberts des Grossen', Münster, 1903, p. 384), which echoes the notion of the circulation of the 'light' in Chinese yoga (R. Wilhelm and C. G. Jung, *The Secret of the Golden Flower*, London, 1931, as the immaterial principle of consciousness. See further on the doctrine of animal spirits, B. Hollander, *In Search of the Soul*, London, n.d., Vol. I, p. 67 (Erasistratos' distinction between *pneuma psychikon and pneuma zootikon*); p. 99 (Avicenna's division into three kinds of spirits); pp. 192–3 (seventeenth- and eighteenth-century controversies as the doctrine came to a close). The term, *psychikon pneuma*, originates with Philistion of Syracusa, Plato's friend (EGP, p. 249, fn. 4). FE 37, p. 118, gives further references to medieval variations of the doctrine. A Symposium sponsored by the Wellcome Foundation (*The History and Philosophy of Knowledge of the Brain and its Functions*, ed. F. N. L. Poynter, Oxford, 1958) brings together excellent and recent short papers with bibliographies on early views of nervous energy, hydrostatic models, animal spirits, etc.

Eng. transl. by M. Flemyng, *The Nature of the Nervous Fluid, or Animal Spirits, Demonstrated:* 1751, London, p. 7.[1]

In this little passage lies much that is still with us in the contemporary models of energy as the source of emotion: (*a*) the familiar notion of the downward discharge, (*b*) the notion of irreversibility, implying that there must be a discharge, and (*c*) the notion that stimuli act as irritants.

Flemyng then opens out the other side of the question: the connection between the spirits of the soul now become materialized as nervous fluid which we might call today neural energy, and the immaterial world spirit which we might call today 'immaterial energy' (Prince), 'orgone energy' (Reich), 'underlying tension states' (Bousfield).

> There may be in animal fluids in general, and that of the nerves in particular, some subtle aether, fire, or spirit, or whatever other name it may be called by, diffused through the atmosphere and perhaps over our whole system, acting by laws unknown to us, and in a particular manner in organised bodies; I say, there may be such a spirit necessary to cause muscular motion in co-operation with the proper fluid of the nerves. . . .
> —Flemyng, *op. cit. sup.*, p. 27.

According to Sherrington,[2] this ancient and complex model of the spirits of the soul finally broke up over the modern split between mind and matter. The material aspect, the nervous fluid, became electricity. The immaterial aspect, the spirits of the soul, became mind which was denied location in space by Kant. But it is our suggestion here that this doctrine has not disappeared, but has rather taken on new substitute models: Galvani's flow of electricity, Bergson's flow of élan vital, Freud's flow of libido.[3] The various

---

[1] 'Sic demonstratur liquidum esse, quod a cerebro adveniat, in nervos descendat, ad extremas partes effluat, cujus motus ab irritatione acceleratus, secundum directionem fluenti sui unice operatur, neque sursum convulsiones remittere potest, quibus novum a cerebro adfluens fluidum resistit.'—A. Haller, *Primae Lineae Physiologiae* (Chapter XII, Section 389), Gottingae, 1747.

[2] Sherrington, Sir Charles, *Man on His Nature*, 2nd edn., N.Y., 1953 p. 205.

[3] The term 'libido' is a complex image which Freud's genius struck upon to bring together a group of ideas which were already contained, so to speak, in the word itself. In the Roman god, *Liber*, we have the notion of a procreative, phallic principle. In *libet, lubet* (*libens, lubens*) we have the notion of pleasure. Libido as a flow of energy is found in the Latin root, *libare* = to pour liquid (OET, p. 473). The notion that a repression, restraint (damming) of libido is a loss of liberty, normal health and life (neurosis) is expressed in the Roman idea that '. . . freedom was the affair of the procreative spirit in man . . . and slavery in some sense denied or put out of action the latter, one may guess that *liber*, the term applied to a man or to his head when the procreative spirit in him was naturally active thus, and *Liber* . . . fertility god, were one, and that it originally expressed a natural state, a distinctive activity or attribute of the procreative spirit or deity.'—OET, pp. 472–3). As Onians points out, 'the attainment of membership of the community as a free citizen was identified with the attainment of procreative power' signified by the *toga virilis* or *libera* put on at the festival

energy concepts we have been looking at here are also models of what Sherrington calls the spirits of the soul: a confounding of 'two incommensurable things'. This doctrine has not disappeared because it cannot disappear; without it there is no meeting of the two incommensurables. So that where the soul is often denied a place in modern psychology, the soul is still represented in all its classic ambiguity by such concepts as psychonic energy, vital energy, bioenergy, nervous energy and the like, all combinations of mind and matter. Although these concepts are dubious to logic and inductive science, they are psychologically accurate in the sense that they represent meaningfully the double nature of the events which they describe. In short, it is our contention that the flow of energy model as an explanation of emotion has replaced the soul model and that the energy model, untenable logically and empirically, is only intelligible on the basis of the earlier model, the soul.

Another example of the way in which emotion is conceived as energy and the intricacies it leads to is in the discussions of emotion and *heat*. Ordinary speech retains innumerable expressions for this way of thinking of emotion, particularly when emotion is conceived as a sthenic expansion. Dunbar described her theory in terms of

---

of *Liber* (*idem*, p. 473, fn. 1). In other words, major ideas of Freud's psychology, i.e. pleasure, freedom, membership in society, creativity (sublimation), love, and sexual fertility are all immanent in this term 'libido'. But these considerations of Latin roots and cognates do not decide the main argument as to whether a sexual or an energetic interpretation of 'libido' is to be preferred. The latter view can be found in Jung's *Symbols of Transformation* (Coll. Works, V, pp. 129–31) based largely on classical (Latin) contexts.

If we turn to the *Greek* root we find that the sexual and energetic interpretations are united in the word *lips*, which means both 'desire' (sexual) and 'a pouring of liquid, a stream' (OET, p. 473). The same ideas are united in the word *ero, eros* = being moved sexually and 'I pour out (liquid)' (OET, p. 202, fn. 5); also in *deliciae*, delicious, used for sexual pleasure and for 'a water course', originally 'down-flowings' (p. 473); and also in the north-European word-complex of *freó, freón, Frig, free, frodig*, etc., uniting ideas of freedom, love, liquid, pleasure, and a Fertility Goddess (pp. 475–8). This does not mean, however, that the flow of liquid can be reduced to sexual liquids, which the close association of the two ideas in the same word might imply. Rather just the contrary is true: the sexual liquids are only a specification of a general, liquid lifestuff manifested for the ancients in the cerebro-spinal fluid or marrow, the joints (especially the knees), as well as in tears, sweat and semen. The general life liquid was not only sexual. Onians identifies it with Homer's *aiōn*. (As this idea is a main theme of his book, we can only bring it as a conclusion, foregoing the wealth of evidence upon which it rests.) This liquid soul (pp. 208–9) was conceived as akin to transpersonal fluids, such as the sap of plants (p. 177), wine (p. 216) and the flow of rivers (pp. 220 ff.). It was raised to a metaphysical, universal fluid by Thales at the foundation of Western thought. In other words, the sexual liquids are only one manifestation of the general liquid principle of life, just as sexuality is but one aspect of life, and as the sexual libido is one specification of an energetic, non-specific libido 'akin' to the universal flow of life. The root metaphor remains the same—from Homer and Thales (and Kant, too, uses the model of a river in discussing emotion) to the writers in this chapter who use the libido concept—a liquid model of the flowing stuff of life.

77

'emotional thermodynamics'. Cason[1] distinguishes between feeling, emotions and moods on the one hand which are 'warm', and thinking, perceiving and speaking on the other hand which are 'cold'. Krapf[2] links the experiences of 'coldness' and 'warmth' in the transference with such concrete physiological events as colds, skin sensations of temperature, etc. White[3] makes an analogy between resistance in an electrical circuit giving rise to heat, and conflict in a mental circuit giving rise to consciousness. But especially when emotion is explained in the spatial language (Chapter IX) of the 'depths', the 'center', and the 'inner'—in short, with the heat which distinguishes the living from the dead—do we find the concepts of emotion and heat invariably joined. The heat of emotion is the heat of life.

The great Harvey, who overthrew so much of the old physiology, 'attributed life to an animating principle, a *calidum innatum* in the blood, totally different in its operations from ordinary heat, and analogous to the element of the stars'.[4] In Hindu psychology, emotion and heat are also linked. The concentrated meditation for the building up of *tapas* is an attempt to contain and develop emotional heat, but this heat is different from ordinary or physical heat. The aim of such an exercise is the light of consciousness associated with heat of emotional energy. Heat and light, emotion and awareness, have long been associated. Hippocrates, for example, wrote: 'It appears to me, that what is called heat, the elemental fire, is immortal and omniscient; that it sees, and hears, and knows all things, present and to come.' [5]

Again we are involved in the ambiguity of a concept which tends to bring together in connection with emotion three different systems of operations: the metaphysical, the psychological, and the physiological. The *calidum innatum* or *calor inclusus* is different from warmth of feeling and hotness of passion, both of which are different in turn from the measurable changes in temperature representing changes in combustion during emotional emergency reactions. Just how these three modes of operating, here represented by the three ways of using heat in connection with emotion, relate with each other is the

[1] Cason, H., 'An Interacting-Pattern Theory of the Affectivities', *Psychol. Rev.*, 1933, p. 282.
[2] Krapf, E. E., 'Ueber Kälte- und Warmeerlebnisse in der Uebertragung', in *Entfaltung der Psychoanalyse* (ed. A. Mitscherlich), Stuttgart, 1956, pp. 216–21. Also B. Mittelman and H. G. Wolff, 'Affective States and Skin Temperature', *Psychosom. Med.*, 1943, p. 243.
[3] White, W. A., 'The Frustration Theory of Consciousness', *Psychoanal. Rev.*, 1929.
[4] See T. Laycock, *A Treatise on the Nervous Diseases of Women*, London, 1840, pp. 88 ff. (Others who have used analogies with heat, or explanations through heat are: Lucilius Balbus (*calor inclusus*), John Gerson, Descartes, Fernel, Thomas Aquinas—Aristotle perhaps being the common source.)   [5] Laycock, *op. cit. sup.*

fundamental problem of all the energy views. Always the question arises: just what kind of heat (energy) are we talking about? It is again our contention that the confusions arise legitimately because they are based on an earlier model of heat—the soul as animating and vital heat. Even if the soul has disappeared as an explanatory principle and as the meeting place of these various systems of operations, or realms of being, it is represented by one of its classic attributes: heat.

Appropriate here to the views of emotion as energy is the imaging, quite concretely, of emotion as an *animal* spirit. We need not go into dream symbolism, the symbolism of religious sacrifice, or the theriomorphic allegories of the passions, because we can find within the realm of theory of emotion the energy view presented as horse-power. The image of the charioteer with two horses—one white and good and amenable to reason, the other dark, ungovernable and ugly—is well known from Plato's *Phaedrus*. MacLean, whose theory we shall come to later (Chapter X A), uses the image of the horse and rider in a similar way:

> One might imagine that the neopallium and the limbic system function together and proceed through the world like a man on a horse. Both horse and man are very much alive to each other and to their environment, yet communication between them is limited. Both derive information and act upon it in a different way. At times the horse may shy or bolt for reasons at first inexplicable to his rider. But the patient and sympathetic horseman will try to find out and understand what it is that causes the panic, so he can avoid disturbing situations in the future or reassure and train the beast to overcome them.[1]

This beast, or brute brain as MacLean also calls it, represents emotion as energy. But the energy is not mechanical; the horse is alive to the environment. It is aware. Again we have an image similar to the concepts of 'heat' and 'nervous fluid' in which energy and consciousness are combined. Again we suggest that this image of the horse as a vital and animating principle can be taken as a substitute for the concept of the soul.[2]

In this long chapter, we have chosen to draw conclusions where

[1] MacLean, P. D., 'Studies on Limbic System . . .', Chapter VI in RDPM, p. 121.
[2] See also E. Rothacker, *Die Schichten der Persönlichkeit*, Bonn, 1948, p. 14, for another such horse metaphor. H. Benoit (*The Supreme Doctrine*, London, 1955, pp. 153–60) analyses in the light of Zen Buddhism the image of the horse and rider as a representation of the dynamic and rational sides of the personality. He suggests the image of the centaur as being more true; but the point of view in all is the same: emotional horse-power has a kind of consciousness. (It is also curious to note that the area of the brain said to be instrumental for emotion is called the hippocampus, named afte a morphological similarity to the sea-horse.)

they are pertinent rather than to bring them at the end. The problem, all along, has been the nature of the concept of energy which was being used as the explanatory principle. Wherever the concept was not specifically qualified, e.g. neural, psychic, electrical, etc., but used ambiguously as vital, psychonic, bio-, confusions arose as to just what kind of energy was meant. A statement from Adrian well sums up this issue:

> ... if we use the word 'energy' in its purely physical sense, the conception of nervous energy is unnecessary, and that of mental energy is impossible. If we use it in another sense, we must be careful to define its meaning exactly or we run the risk of assuming that it must necessarily follow the rules which have been found to govern the transformations of physical energy in material systems. But it would be foolish of me to suggest that psychologists as a whole are not alive to these risks, and I am quite ready to believe that the conception of mental energy, properly defined, may be as necessary to psychology as that of physical energy is to physiology.—E. D. Adrian, 'The Conception of Nervous and Mental Energy', *Brit. J. Psychol.*, 1923-4, p. 125.

Psychologists, however, have often not been alive to these risks and have often used the concept of energy without proper qualification, or in a pointedly ambiguous manner—as a mechanical causal energy endowed with vitalistic conscious intentions. (Whitehead's hierarchical monism is an exception.) We suggest the reason for this lies in the substitution of an ambiguous energy concept for the ambiguous soul concept. As Adrian points out, the energy concept must be precisely qualified if it is used correctly. The soul concept is legitimately ambiguous, since by definition it is involved with the body, the mind and that universal immaterial principle which we can call spirit. Therefore we suggest that the older concept of the soul is no less adequate than the newer conceptual model of energy for the explanation of the interaction of these several aspects of emotion.

If we ask what these theories have to tell us about emotion, we can further conclude that their main contribution to our amplification is, first, either implicitly or explicitly emotion is here taken to be central to the interaction of body, mind and spirit, and, second, emotion is as fundamental and as unknown as energy. Our own interpretation of the relation of emotion and energy must wait until Part III.

VII

EMOTION AS QUANTITY

THE THEORY of Pieron makes the transition from the views of the last chapter to those of this chapter:

> Now the idea of emotion seems to be associated with a quantitative aspect, a certain level, of the affect. The difference between a moderate interest taken in a theatrical performance and the keen emotion which it arouses, whatever may be the precise nature of the feelings involved . . . is essentially a quantitative one.—H. Pieron, 'Emotion in Animals and Man', FE 28, pp. 285–6.

> Thus it seems to us that emotion may be described as an extreme level of affect, tending toward the pathological as a limit. It consists essentially in an abnormal discharge of nervous energy, a discharge which exceeds the amount which can be used for the normal reactions of the individual, and which occurs even when there is no occasion for reaction. It consequently involves a diffusion of excitatory impulses into the viscera, which on the whole, seems to be not only useless, but harmful, and even pathogenic. . . .—*Idem*, p. 294.

The diffusion of excitatory impulses of which Pieron speaks is similar to the downward discharge of energy in a somatic short circuit which causes symptoms such as we reported in the last section. There, the emphasis was on the energy concept; here, the emphasis is on the idea of abnormality, extremity, in short, upon *quantity*. Emotion is distinguished by quantity which, in Pieron's theory, is a quantity of neural energy. In other views, it may be a quantity of feeling conceived as intensity; or simply 'strength' may be the criterion of affect.[1] The theories of this group have in common this approach to the understanding and explaining of emotion by means of quantitative concepts.

Thus Thalbitzer writes:

> Whatever feeling-process we investigate, it will be seen that it differs from all other such processes only in increased or decreased feeling, increased or decreased motor activity, and increased or decreased intellectual activity; or (as I have expressed it elsewhere) human emotion is

[1] Messer, A., *Psychologie*, Leipzig, 1934.

81

the expression of the quantitative side of mental life. Its differences rest exclusively on quantitative differences in the activity of the cerebral cortex, or rather, of its centers.—S. Thalbitzer, *Emotion and Insanity*, London, 1926, pp. 75–6.

He locates the function of feeling in specific feeling cells in the 'hinder part of the brain', thereby making consistent the quantitative notion of emotion with quantitative ideas of nerve cell discharge.

Another quantitative view is that of Troland, but expressed mathematically:

> The data of modern introspective psychology permit us to define a variable, which we may call *affective intensity*, as an algebraic quantity positive magnitudes of which are to be identified with the degrees of pleasantness of conscious states, while negative magnitudes represent the degrees of unpleasantness of such states. A zero value stands for indifference. This quantitative conception is supposed to be capable of formulating any possible affective value in consciousness regardless of the nature of the consciousness in respects other than the affective.—L. T. Troland, 'A System for Explaining Affective Phenomena', *J. Abn. Psychol.*, 1920, p. 376.
>
> *The affective intensity of any individual consciousness is proportional to the average rate of change of conductance in the synapses the activities of which are responsible for that consciousness.* This postulate may be expressed mathematically. If c is the average conductance of the synapses and a is the affective intensity, then: $a = k\dfrac{dc}{dt}$, k being a constant, and $\dfrac{dc}{dt}$ being the usual expression for the rate of change of c with respect to the time t (p. 377).
>
> Whether a given experience is called an emotion or not seems to depend upon its intensity, and in particular upon its affective intensity (p. 386).

Brown and Farber[1] and Beebe-Center[2] bring this mathematical kind of approach up to date so that emotion becomes a variable or function expressed in graphs or equations.

Affective intensity is also the criterion of Klages, understood not in terms of nervous energy, but in terms of 'drive activity'. However, the principle is the same: emotion means 'more'.[3]

---

[1] Brown, J. S. and Farber, I. E., 'Emotions conceptualized as intervening variables', *Psychol. Bull.*, 1951, pp. 465–95.

[2] Beebe-Center, J. G., 'Feeling and Emotion', Chapter VI in *Theoretical Foundations of Psychology*, ed. by H. Helsen, N.Y./London/Toronto, 1951.

[3] Klages, L., *Grundlegung der Wissenschaft vom Ausdruck* (7th edn.), Bonn, 1950, p. 154:
'Nachdem man im wissenschaftlichen Sprachgebrauch den Namen Gemütsbewegung oder Wallung oder Erregung durch Fremdwörter wie Affekt und Emotion zu ersetzen für gut befunden hatte, ist der Streit nicht mehr zur Ruhe gekommen, was eigentlich Affekte *seien*, ob etwa eine besondere Klasse von Gefühlen oder Zustände ganz anderer Art oder vorwaltend körperliche Erscheinungen, wenn auch im Verhältnis

Duffy (Chapter I) also held a quantitative view in respect to one of the basic concepts (intensity or 'energy mobilization') to which she said the term emotion could be reduced. Schlosberg follows her by equating this quantitative concept with Lindsley's (Chapter X A) 'levels of activation'. He considers emotion as having three dimensions, two of which are qualitative and are not yet carefully worked out theoretically, but the third is quantitative. It can be called variously 'level of activation', 'degree of energy mobilization', or the 'intensive dimension'. The important point in his view is that emotion does not differ qualitatively from other states. As an index of the level of activation, Schlosberg[1] recommends measurements of electrical skin conductance. Here again, we find the quantitative view coupled with concepts of physical, neural, or physiological processes as part of the explanatory procedure. This is particularly so in the cases of those authors who, in viewing emotion as quantity, measure what they call emotion by means of psychogalvanic experiments. For example, Whately Smith says:

> There seems, then, no *a priori* reason for doubting that the psychogalvanic reflex will give a correct measure of the intensity of the emotion (or affective tone) elicited by a stimulus-word, or that the emotion is genuinely correlated with the latter in kind and in degree.—W. Whately Smith, *The Measurement of Emotion*, London, 1922, p. 27.

Farmer and Chambers[2] and Wechsler[3] write to the same effect, correlating emotion or affective tone with a psychogalvanic reflex. Waller even goes beyond the notion of correlation and simply identifies emotion with the measurements:

> . . . 'Emotivity', or, to put it more specifically, the electrical resistance

zu Seelenvorgängen aufgefasst usw. Mit Hilfe nur *eines* Blickes auf die deutschen Bezeichnungen, denen die fremdwörtliche nachgebildet sind, haben wir inzwischen die Frage bereits entschieden: die Gefühle heissen Wallungen, Gemütsbewegungen, Emotionen, je mehr die Antriebsbeschaffenheit gegenüber der Artung hervortritt; im entgegengesetzten Falle heissen sie Stimmungen. Niemand wird das Gefühl tiefer Versunkenheit eine Wallung, niemand das Gefühl heftigen Erschreckens eine Stimmung nennen.'

[1] Schlosberg, H., 'Three Dimensions of Emotion', *Psychol. Rev.*, 1954, p. 87: 'The activation theory of emotion brings together many of the theories and facts of emotion, at least as far as the intensive dimension is concerned. Instead of treating emotion as a special state, differing qualitatively from other states, the theory locates emotional behavior on a continuum that includes *all* behavior. This continuum, general level of activation, has its low end in sleep, its middle ranges in alert attention, and its high end in the strong emotions.'

[2] Farmer, E., and Chambers, E. G., 'Concerning the Use of the Psychogalvanic Reflex in Psychological Experiments', *Brit. J. Psychol.*, 1924–5, p. 251. '. . . we are safe in assuming that an affective tone above a certain level has a psycho-galvanic reflex corresponding to it. . . .'

[3] Wechsler, D., 'Further Comment on the Psychological Significance of the Galvanic Reaction', *Brit. J. Psychol.*, 1925–6, p. 137.

of the palm of the hand.—A. D. Waller, 'Concerning Emotive Phenomena, Part III', *Proc. Royal Soc.*, Series B, 1920, p. 32.

There is another area where the concept of emotion plays a role and where correlations are made between energetic frequencies and emotion. This is in the field of electro-encephalography. Strictly, of course, these writers are not presenting a theory of emotion, or even an attempt to 'explain' the pregnant correlations which they make. Hill writes:

> Theta rhythm has been associated with emotional activity by a number of workers. Walter (1950) found it was possible to induce bursts of this activity by depriving young children of pleasureable stimuli—(sweets suddenly removed from the mouth). The writer has provoked bursts of theta rhythm by the presentation of psychological material carrying a high emotional charge to psychiatric patients. . . . Mundy-Castle (1951) found an increased incidence of theta rhythm when subjects were embarrassed, frustrated or discomfited during the carrying out of mental tasks.—D. Hill, 'Electroencephalography', Chapter XII in *Recent Advances in Neurology and Neuropsychiatry* by Brain and Strauss, (6th edn.), London, 1955, pp. 194–5.

Gastaut does attempt a 'psychological classification of cerebral rhythms'[1] correlating in a table characteristics of EEG records and characteristics of personality in the form of emotional syndromes. Correlations are not causal relations. This obvious truth must be continually kept in mind else we begin to explain emotion as specifically patterned brain frequencies or as changes in the electrical resistance of the skin. 'Bursts', 'waves' and 'excited states' refer equally to physical and psychological data—but that is all that can be said.

With this we are at the end of another chapter of inadequate explanations. We can agree with Thorndike when he says, 'Whatever exists, exists in some quantity, and can therefore ultimately be measured'.[2] Emotion, if we agree it exists in some way or another, exists in some quantity and can therefore be measured. That the quantitative aspect of emotion is essential is evident in the naïve, everyday use of the term. Warnock,[3] following Hume, points this out; emotions often have no qualitative names but refer to unspecified excessive agitations. Emotion is a term which refers to 'more' of

---

[1] Gastaut, H.: 'The Brain Stem and Cerebral Electrogenesis in Relation to Consciousness', in *Brain Mechanisms and Consciousness, A Symposium* (ed. by J. F. Delafresnaye), Oxford, 1954, p. 272. For other such correlations see also L. Saul, H. Davis and P. Davis, 'Psychologic Correlations with the Encephalogram', *Psychosom. Med.*, 1949, pp. 361–76; and M. Kennard, 'The Electroencephalogram in Psychological Disorders—A Review', *Psychosom. Med.*, 1953, pp. 95–115.

[2] Thorndike, E. L., *Mental and Social Measurements*, N.Y., 1913.

[3] Warnock, M., 'The Justification of Emotions' (Symposium), *The Aristotelian Society*, Suppl. Vol. XXXI, 1957, pp. 43–58.

something, not 'less'. We can agree therefore that quantity may be an essential characteristic of emotion and a quantitative explanatory hypothesis may be *necessary* for theory, yet such an hypothesis is not *sufficient*. Something else also enters in which gives an emotional event its specific character. For example, Knapp[1] raises the question of the difference between irritation and fury. Is it one of quantity —fury being 'more' irritation? Or, as the ancients might have put it: fury involves more yellow bile than does irritation. Knapp says: 'I think that the answer is not going to be in the discovery of more or less quantity of any substance but in terms of the maturation of mechanisms which are grouped together under the heading of "ego-psychology".' This means that the so-called quantitative basic determinant (Chapter I) as a differentiating criterion between emotions is in itself really qualitatively determined by the quality of the personality (maturation of the ego). Irritation and fury are not to be conceived as points on a scale reading from apathy to manic seizures, like degrees of temperature; they are rather individual conditions of the personality as a whole.

Without a criterion of quality, emotion conceived in terms of intensity alone does not differ from other states or behaviour as Schlosberg holds. In the same way, Klages' theory fails to differentiate emotion from other states of intense drive activity, since it is not the drive activity as such which is the criterion, but the quantity. Such a theory requires a system of measurements; at a certain reading on a scale behaviour is defined as emotional. But what would be measured? According to Klages, drive activity; according to Schlosberg, electrical resistance of the skin; according to Pieron and Thalbitzer, neural energy. What is said to be measured, this quantity, is not emotion, but only a partial aspect, a factor of emotion, or maybe even less—only a correlate, which may or may not be present and is not the infallible criterion.

For all this, common sense persists in labelling emotion by the mark of excess and it does not care whether this excess is of neural energy, feeling, drive activity or yellow bile: emotion means simply *too much*. This complaint, as a fact of the consulting room, can lead the therapist unaware that emotion is not just a quantitative phenomenon into a therapy of emotion based on quantitative views. His therapy becomes a method of dealing with excess. The aim is to reduce emotion, to lower the emotional temperature. And thus begins a programme of repression, sublimation and substitution—and tranquillizers—all of which fails to acknowledge the quality of the emotion

---

[1] Knapp, P. H., 'Conscious and Unconscious Affects: A preliminary approach to concepts and methods of study', in *Research in Affects* (Psychiatric Research Reports, 8, 1957), p. 86.

and *the significance of the excess*. This last is of over-riding importance. It is the fundamental issue arising from this chapter on emotion as quantity. The meaning of excess and intensity is bound up with the problem of disorder which we must come to in due time, but which does not belong here.

VIII

EMOTION AS TOTALITY

SOME LIGHT is shed on the 'excess' aspect of emotion by the theories of this group. They bring out another interpretation of quantity—that of massiveness. But here massiveness, the molar nature of emotion, is not to be understood as a quantity in the sense only of a *big* event, but rather as a totality in the sense of a *kind* of event. The massiveness of an emotional event takes its meaning not just in the volume, but because this volume expresses a totality. Since the concept of totality carries with it connotations of size, total events are sometimes muddled with big events. But this distinction must be kept in mind in order to perceive the difference between the theories of this group and those in the chapter preceding.

Beck's definition of emotion does not make this distinction between quantity and totality:

> This is a complex of organic sensations, the stimulus to which is some larger life situation, of great—usually critical—importance to the organism. An affective quality is always present in emotion so defined. . . . Emotion is a massive experience setting the entire individual into action or into preparation for it; i.e. it is *emotive*.—S. J. Beck, 'Emotional Experience as a Necessary Constituent in Knowing', FE 50, p. 95.

Presumably he makes this statement upon the basis of the Latin origin of the word emotion, *emovere* = 'to move away or to move much'. This 'much moving' is a massive moving, from which he seems to conclude that it necessarily is a total or 'entire moving'.

Sherrington points up nicely the distinction between size and totality, bringing emotion into line with the latter idea:

> The process by which a reaction of merely 'quantum' order is biologically raised to molar dimensions is called by some biologists 'amplification'. A means to 'amplification' is emotion. As physical stimulus a ghost may be barely of threshold power; but given emotion, and it can convulse the whole individual.—Sir C. Sherrington, *The Integrative Action of the Nervous System*, 1947 edn., Cambridge, 1952, p. xxii.

The view of Bleuler is comparable:

> An intellectual process, a perception, an action in response to a stimulus, and a thought, are all in a certain respect partial functions. . . . In contradistinction to this, the affective processes signify an *assumed attitude of the whole person*. . . . Intellectual and affective processes are related parallel manifestations; they represent the local and the general side of the same psychism.—E. Bleuler, *Textbook of Psychiatry* (transl. by A. A. Brill; Dover reissue of 1924 edn.), N.Y., 1951, p. 36.

> An affect generalizes a reaction or we may express it quite as correctly by saying: *An affect is a generalized reaction.*—E. Bleuler, *Affectivity, Suggestibility, Paranoia* (Eng. transl. by C. Ricksher), Utica, N.Y., 1912, p. 11.

Bleuler sees this general reaction as positive; apart from exceptional conditions it 'contributes to the general advance of the individual'.[1] Stern interprets the general or total nature of emotion otherwise. He presents emotion as a total event:

> The manifestations of feeling life fall easily into two groups. On the one side are the 'emotions', i.e. those states which for a time completely fill out experience and *subjugate* all the rest of psychic life; on the other side, 'the feelings', those movements which join with and *serve* other kinds of psychic events and contents, and which therefore have a more special and limited character.—W. Stern, *Allgemeine Psychologie*, Haag, 1935, p. 706.[2]

Affects, too, he describes as similar to emotions: both are complete or total events. But in this 'total convulsion' direction is lost, and meaning too.[3] The result of his view is this: although emotion is a total event completely overwhelming all aspects of experience, it is a disorder. Totality, in short, is excessive; it is something negative.

Yet, if we turn to that condition called in electro-encephalography 'compulsory normalization' (*forcierte Normalisierung*) we might risk another interpretation of these apparently chaotic, meaningless reactions of excess. Landolt reports on cases of abnormal EEG pictures in epileptics and schizophrenics when the patients themselves appear psychically calm and normal, whereas there is a normalization of the EEG in the same patients during states of high emotional tension and rage (epileptics)[4] and during a psychotic episode (schizo-

---

[1] Bleuler, E., *Textbook of Psychiatry*, p. 37.

[2] Stern: 'Die Erscheinungen des Gefühlslebens gliedern sich zwanglos in zwei Gruppen. Auf der einen Seite stehen die Gemütsbewegungen oder 'Emotionen', d.h. solche seelische Verfassungen, die zeitweilig das Erleben ganz ausfüllen und alles übrige Seelenleben sich *unterwerfen*; auf der anderen Seite solche Regungen, die sich an Seelenvorgänge und Inhalte anderer Art *dienend* anschliessen, daher, einen spezielleren, begrenzteren Charakter haben, die "Gefühle".'

[3] *Ibid.*, p. 761.

[4] Landolt, H., 'Ueber Verstimmungen, Dämmerzustände und schizophrene Zustandsbilder bei Epilepsie', *Schweiz. Arch. f. Neurol. u. Psychiat.*, 1955, pp. 313–21.

phrenics).[1] He states: 'It seems in other words as if, to put it bluntly, there are epileptics who must have a pathological EEG in order to appear psychically normal.'[2] The essential element in the normalization of the EEG seems to Landolt to be emotional tension which can also be of a positive or happy nature.[3] *Perhaps, then, the total convulsion of an emotional reaction is profoundly therapeutic.* The very excess and massiveness is to generalize, amplify, mobilize the person as a whole, thus contributing to the 'general advance of the individual' (Bleuler). This hypothesis that emotion has to do with wholeness can only be introduced here. It will reappear again in other formulations in later chapters and will be discussed more fully in Part III.

The definition of emotion as a total event helps understand the excess aspect of emotion, but further theory is required for explaining why and how the person can perform like this and whether or not this general reaction has a central system of organization. Those who follow along these lines approach emotion by means of some sort of centralization concept—either psychological or physiological. This leads us over to the theories of the next groups which can be taken as consequences of a molar or total view of emotion.

[1] Landolt, H., 'Elektroenzephalographische Untersuchungen bei nicht katatonen Schizophrenien', *Schweiz. Zeitschrift f. Psychol. u. ihre Anwendungen*, XVI ,1, 1957, pp. 26–30.

[2] Landolt, H., 'Ueber Verstimmungen . . .', p. 318.

[3] *Ibid.*, p. 314.

IX

EMOTION AND PSYCHOLOGICAL LOCATION

THE PROBLEMS of location will be occupying us in this and the next few chapters. We have already met spatial figures of speech in explaining emotion, e.g. as energy *in* a system, as entities *in* the unconscious, as zones, as borders between psychic structures. Here, the general concern is with the place of the emotion in the organization of psychic life. Placing, here, means qualitative position within an order of values, or a scale of being, where certain positions are primary and essential and others are secondary and accidental. Spatial concepts are used to express these ideas because spatial concepts lend themselves to statements which combine value and structure. 'Peripheral' and 'central', 'deep' and 'shallow', 'inner' and 'outer' have meanings other than only the description of physical space. Because of this interest in value, distinction, position, a view of emotion as *quality* also appears in this section.

Let us turn to some views which make use of spatial expressions in describing and explaining emotion. For example, Kühn[1] states in spatial metaphor the hypothesis that emotion performs the function of 'bridging the gap' between intellect and instinctual life. Heiss[2] speaks of emotion as the mediator between 'inner' and 'outer'. Haisch and Lewin use the concept of the 'centre':

> It is of great central importance whether a psychological process belongs to more central or to more peripheral strata. Dembo's experimental investigations on anger have shown the significance of this factor for emotions. If only peripheral strata of the person are touched, manifestations of anger occur more easily. The outbreaks of anger are then more superficial. If more central strata are involved an open outbreak of affect is more rare. . . . Therefore expression usually occurs more

---

[1] Kühn, H., 'Die Bedeutung des Fühlens für den Erlebnisbau', *Der Nervenarzt*, 1947, p. 7.

[2] Heiss, R., *Allgemeine Tiefenpsychologie*, Bern/Stuttgart, 1956, p. 261 f. (See further Chapter XVIII for quotation of Heiss's theory.)

readily when events of more peripheral strata are concerned.—K. Lewin; *Principles of Topological Psychology*, N.Y., 1936, p. 180.

Emotional life represents, so to speak, the interior and the actual centre of man, the basic source which serves the higher levels for the experience of the world. Even thought is produced in a qualified milieu, already emotionally selected, which prescribes for it its direction and its form.—E. Haisch, 'Sur l'importance de la psychologie de la sphère affective', *L'Union Med. Canada*, 1954, p. 545.[1]

The 'central' position of emotion is often conceived as *deepest* or as *innermost*. This is particularly so where architectural or geological language is used to image the personality as concentric spheres or in terms of strata. (Knapp combines the geological model with the fluid model. Emotion becomes a kind of pool of petroleum which can be 'drained off' or 'tapped' at different layers.[2]) That emotion has to do with the central depths of the person would account, on these views, for the view that emotion is a molar event: when the deepest, central, innermost 'place' is aroused, the whole structure is moved.

Lersch calls this deepest layer of experience the 'endothymic ground'—endo = inner, thymic = feeling. He locates all emotional life there.

Here belong above all those events and states of the soul which we habitually designate as affects, emotions, feelings, moods and passions as well as drives, desires and tendencies. They all have the characteristic of the subterranean and of intimate inwardliness. . . .

Self-reflection gives witness that the endothymic contents of our experience present a special layer which we describe as the endothymic ground. . . . The German words 'Gefühl' and 'Gemüt' as well as the scientific concepts 'emotional' and 'affective'.are not enough to comprehend the complex variety of that—as we shall see—which is meant by the words endothymic ground.

The endothymic ground is thus the deepest and inner sphere of experience, in so far as we look at it phenomenologically. Ontologically the organic ground of life comes first upon which all experience rests.— P. Lersch, *Aufbau der Person*, München, 1952, p. 81.[3]

---

[1] Haisch: 'La vie émotive représente pour ainsi dire l'intérieur et le centre concret de l'homme, la source fondamentale qui sert à l'élévation de l'expérience du monde. Même le penser se produit dans un milieu qualitatif déjà émotivement élu qui lui prescrit sa direction et sa formation.' (Compare Bleuler, Chapter VIII).

[2] Knapp, P. H., 'Conscious and Unconscious Affects: A Preliminary Approach to Concepts and Methods of Study', *Research in Affects* (Psychiatric Research Reports 8, 1957), p. 72.

[3] Lersch: 'Hierher gehören vor allem diejenigen seelischen Vorgänge und Zustände die wir als Affekte, Gemütsbewegungen, Gefühle, Stimmungen und Leidenschaften zu bezeichnen gewöhnt sind, desgleichen aber auch die Triebe, Begierden und Strebungen. Sie alle haben das Merkmal der Untergründigkeit und der intimen Innerlichkeit; . . .

'Die endothymen Gehalte unseres Erlebens stellen somit nach dem Zeugnis der Selbstbesinnung eine besondere Schicht dar, die wir als den endothymen Grund

And, according to Lersch, the various kinds of experiences—whether they be passions, moods, affects, feeling-states, feeling-processes, or emotions—are each aspects of this inner area of the person. He carefully qualifies each, making his distinctions with particular reference to strength of impulse and intention, or object-reference. In respect to the latter concept, he holds that what we might call in general 'feeling life', signifies not only objective values, but also signifies the values of our own inner selves. He notices, too, in connection with affect, the vegetative and 'symptomatic' side. His explanation of emotional phenomena, however, depends upon concepts of psychological location expressed in this notion of the endothymic ground.

Bresser follows Lersch in placing emotion in the innermost endothymic ground which he calls the 'Gemüt'.[1] He claims this concept is untranslatable and is peculiar to the German language and people. As for Lersch, this region is the phenomenological ground of experience and so for Bresser it is the equivalent of the soul. Soul and spirit are a polar unity, but soul and body are opposites. In this way, this region is the way to 'Verinnerlichung', 'Verwesentlichung', 'Vergeistigung', and to God. In his positive enthusiasm for this region which he describes in spatial language ('. . . das Gemüt ein ganz eigenartiges Inneres, nämlich gleichsam das innerste Innere des Menschen ist'—p. 19), he tends to neglect both the bodily aspects of emotion and the so-called 'negative' emotions which too take their rise in the same inner place and which too must be related—if his theory is to be consistent—to the higher life, to inwardness and to God. For example, Nietzsche, who also, it might be said, knew something about the German Gemüt, writes of the 'Verinnerlichung' of man in terms of violent and 'negative' emotions.[2]

Bollnow's theory of mood is similar to Lersch's idea of the endothymic ground. Again, we find emotional life described in terms of spatial location: 'Als die unterste Stufe liegen dem gesamten seel-

---

bezeichnen . . . die deutschen Wörter "Gefühl" und "Gemüt" als auch die wissenschaftlichen Begriffe "emotional" und "affektiv" reichen nicht aus, die ganze Mannigfaltigkeit dessen zu erfassen, was – wie wir sehen werden – mit der Rede von endothymen Grund gemeint ist.

'Der endothyme Grund ist also eine tiefste und innere Sphäre des Erlebens, sofern wir es phänomenologisch betrachten. Ontologisch ist ihm der Lebensgrund vorgeordnet, auf dem ja alles Erleben aufruht.'

[1] Bresser, P., *Das Gemüt*, unpubl. Ph.D. Diss., Univ. of Munich, 1950, p. 59. (The 'inner theory of emotion' for which Bresser is a contemporary advocate runs right through German psychology and can be said perhaps to begin with J. G. F. Maass' emphasis on the subjectivity, the movement of the 'innere Sinn', of affect (*Versuch über die Gefühle, bes. über die Affekten*, Halle/Leipzig, 1811-12; *Versuch über die Leidenschaften*, Halle/Leipzig, 1805-7).)

[2] Nietzsche, F., *Der Wille zur Macht*, ¶ 376.

ischen Leben die "Lebensgefühle" oder "Stimmungen" zugrunde.'[1] This lowest, most fundamental level determines (bestimmen), or has a voice in (Stimme) or gives a tone or mood (Stimmung) to all experience. This 'layer' of emotional moods is the 'underground support' of all psychic life.[2] Bollnow differentiates feelings from emotional moods (Stimmungen). The former are always object-directed, while the latter have no object-referents. They point to nothing outside of themselves.[3]

Krueger, too, refers the emotional to the inner. Emotion is to be understood not only as a total reaction in the molar sense of Bleuler and Stern, but also as the quality of that total reaction. The accent is on the *quality* of the whole experience: ('. . . feelings are the complex qualities of the experienced total-whole . . .', p. 70, *op. cit. inf.*) Thus, the emotional becomes the way in which the 'inner' qualifies each experience.

> Whatever pleases one, whatever interests him, whatever depresses him, whatever excites him, whatever he perceives as the comic; even more, how easily and how continuously he is moved internally in these ways— this is the particular characteristic of his 'being', his character, and his individuality. Such has pre-scientific thought unanimously been since ancient times. Feelings embrace or penetrate all other mental events in some way. The 'emotional' testifies in a unique way to the structure of the 'inner', the mental life. Apparently it is generally typical of life itself. —F. Krueger, 'The Essence of Feeling', FE 28, p. 58.

This statement is perhaps as close as we can get to an articulated theory of emotion, because Krueger foregoes explanation in so far as every explanatory analysis is destructive to the experienced event as such, and therefore can hardly be said to explain anything. But in this view against explanation, he attests further to the description of the emotional in terms of location. Whatever is located most inwardly and most deeply is consequently hardest to bring to light —and is altered upon exposure.

Because feeling and emotion are conceived in terms of qualities of the subject which remain inaccessible to explanation (Aufklärung), one must also forego examination in terms of cause and effect:

> No constellation of stimuli can ever predict that it will positively initiate feelings at all, to say nothing of releasing this or that definite feeling. On the contrary, every intentional change of psychophysical

---

[1] Bollnow, O. F., *Das Wesen der Stimmungen*, Frankfurt a/M, 1941, p. 17.
[2] *Ibid.*, p. 25.
[3] 'Die Stimmungen . . . haben keinen bestimmten Gegenstand. Sie sind Zuständlichkeiten, Färbungen des gesamtmenschlichen Daseins, in denen das Ich seiner selbst in einer bestimmten Weise unmittelbar inne wird, die aber nicht auf etwas ausser ihnen Liegendes hinausverweisen' (pp. 18–19).

experience can be an initiating (komplementär) condition of every kind and intensity of emotions ... (p. 72).[1]

Krueger's notion of the unpredictability of emotion is different from the notion of spontaneity of Jorgensen (Chapter II). There, emotions were conceived as distinct energy forces capable of behaving autonomously; here, the emotion is not autonomous or a distinct substance. It is a quality and as such depends on the whole experience which in its manifold complexity cannot be reduced to a single set of causal stimuli. Krueger's view here is more like that of Wenger and Dunlap (Chapter X B), who contend that emotion is always going on as part of all experience. They however conceive this as an *activity*, while for Krueger it is a *quality*.

Gerard, like Krueger, conceives emotion as a quality ('flavor or tone or color') of the totality of an experience;[2] while Schultz-Hencke takes the finer emotions as qualities which accompany perceptions, but this quality is not an epiphenomenon easily reduced to something else (as in Chapter III). The quality is essential to experience; without it there would not be experience. An experience lives 'by the grace of our accompanying emotion'.[3] Above all in his view, as with Krueger, Lersch, Bollnow and Bresser, emotion attests to the inner.

Thus Hoisington, in reporting on the investigations of affective experience done by Nafe, Horiguchi, and others, treats emotions as a quality located inwardly. This quality is described as the experience of different kinds of pressure which are localized in different regions of the body introspectively experienced. For example, the essential affective quality is a bright or dull pressure; the dull pressure localizes in the region of the abdomen, the bright pressure in the region of the neck and shoulders. Again, the dominant idea is that affective experience is entirely inward and subjective, so much so that Hoisington writes:

... with specific object reference the affective quality drops out. ... This means that we are not pleased or displeased with this or that object as such, but with this or that kind of experience.—L. B. Hoisington, 'Pleasantness and Unpleasantness as Modes of Bodily Experience', FE 28, p. 237.

We are led by this to the extreme position of these 'inner' theories. Emotion is locked within. As soon as any object reference occurs, there is no longer any emotion. Lipps'[4] view of empathy also flounders upon this problem. Locating the affective life within the subject, he

---

[1] The translation of 'komplementär' as 'initiating' is questionable.
[2] Gerard, R. W., in discussion following 'The Central Mechanism of the Emotions', Spiegel, Wycis, *et al.*, *Am. J. Psychiat.*, 1951, p. 431.
[3] Schultz-Hencke, H., *Der Gehemmte Mensch*, Leipzig, 1940, p. 86.
[4] Lipps, T., *Leitfaden der Psychologie*, Leipzig (1903), 3rd edn. 1909.

tries to get over to the outer object by the theory of feeling *into* the other. But basically, for him, all feelings are self-feelings, or as Hoisington puts it: 'We are not pleased . . . with this or that object, but with this or that kind of experience.' Empathy is only a projection of my inner self into the other. I am always left feeling myself. Emotion remains inside the subject. An emotional mood tells me something only about myself (Bollnow).

We get into such straits because of muddling the inner with the subjective. When the inner is identified with the subject and emotion is located there, then the outer-other-object has no inherent connection with the inner. The world out there and my private world of subjective emotional experience have no necessary relation, and elaborate theories have to be developed, such as Lipps' theory of empathy, in order to correlate these two distinct worlds. These views all flow naturally from the method of introspection for, naturally, if we turn our backs to the outer in order to introspect, the outer remains shut out. And naturally, too, by looking only inward for emotion we find it only inside. Therefore, Krueger can say: 'The emotional testifies in a unique way to the structure of the inner.' But does this mean 'to the structure of the inner', *exclusively*? Does emotion have anything to do with the object? Hoisington would say, No: 'With specific object reference the affective quality drops out.' And Lipps can only take aesthetic 'pleasure in the object, but not the object as such, but only so far as I have felt myself into it.' This is solipsism.

The other extreme we have already seen in Chapter I, where emotion as an inner event was denied outright. The two different methods of procedure—introspection and behaviourism (empirical observation of outer events)—lead to this dilemma: emotion is only inner *vs.* emotion is never inner. We suggest, here, that this dilemma is due to using outdated models for the subject-object, inner-outer relation.

In the last century, the inner and the subjective were identified and were distinct from the object which was identified with the outer. This was before the discovery of the unconscious 'within' and the realm of micro-physics 'without'. In this century, due to these discoveries, the subject has moved to a middle position between the inner, no longer wholly subjective world, and the outer, no longer wholly objective world. Today, depth psychology asserts that the inner world is by no means the possession of the subject, and that the contents and events encountered upon introspection do not belong wholly to the subject. (In fact, identification with these contents and events is a 'de-personalization' of the subject and is a form of emotional confusion and possession as demonstrated by psychopathological states!) On the other hand, contemporary physics asserts that the outer object is not wholly distinct from the subject but is relative to it.[1] In this way, to put the matter in a paradox, the new model of the subject-object relation puts the inner world as much 'outside' the subject as the hitherto outer world which has now taken on a high degree of 'subjectivity'. On this new model, behaviourism and introspection are *strategically*, or theoretically, alike and are not two different ways of approaching two different realms. Both are concerned with the strategy of engaging the object—whether 'within' or 'without'—always and only relative to the subject. Both retain, of course, different *tactical* techniques which have evolved from experience based on earlier models. With this, this part of the behaviourist-introspectionist dilemma might perhaps be laid to rest.

All this means for the theories we are discussing here that the 'inner' must be understood in this new way, where it is relatively distinct from the subject which is, in turn, not cut off from and opposed to the object. Emotion on this model can still be located in the 'inner' and remain relatively independent of the subject. In this way, it is no longer legitimate to claim as do these theories here that the emotional qualities, emotional tones, the 'intimate inwardliness' (Lersch) are the possessions of the subject. They may take rise in and attest to the innermost regions of psychic functioning which Bresser calls the soul, but on the new model, this region—this soul—is relatively independent of the subject. The problem of emotional solipsism is also resolved since the inner world of emotion is objectively given, as sense data are objectively given by the 'outer world', available to all alike. Hence, emotional events are at once apprehended by others, which could not be so if the emotional inner world were subjective and private.

From this we shall hazard a conclusion: the emotional qualities bound up with all experience attesting to the innermost region of the personality are the gifts of the soul. To claim them for the subject goes against both the traditional view of the soul as a relatively independent psychic function and against the new model of the 'inner' as a relatively independent psychic function. And further, to claim them as a possession of the subject is a hubris indicating a subject identified with and possessed by the soul.

Let us now return to other descriptions of emotion in terms of

[1] Jeans, Sir James, *Physics and Philosophy*, Cambridge, 1942, p. 143; Pauli, W., 'The Influence of Archetypal Ideas on the Scientific Theories of Kepler', *The Interpretation of Nature and the Psyche*, London, 1955, pp. 208 ff. Concerning the non-subjectivity of the unconscious see, besides the works of Jung, M. Geiger, 'Fragment über den Begriff des Unbewussten und die psychischen Realität', *Jbch. f. Phil. u. phänomen. Forsch.*, 1921, pp. 1–137. Also, C. A. Meier, 'Moderne Physik—Moderne Psychologie', in *Die Kulturelle Bedeutung der Komplexen Psychologie*, Berlin, 1935.

psychological location concepts. Clinical description makes much of 'closeness' and 'nearness' and of 'distance' and 'detachment' when referring to emotional conditions. Lewin, above, writes of 'peripheral' and 'central' emotions. Tow speaks of 'emotional shallowness' following frontal leucotomy.[1] Stern brings together the concept of depth with the concept of *seriousness*, finding a 'gradation of affective seriousness' in emotional life.[2] B. Lewin discusses *false* emotion, similar to delusion (false idea) and hallucination (false perception).[3] Whitehorn writes of *conventionalized* emotions by means of which the patient can be deceptive and escape from real emotionality.[4] All of this implies gradations within this region of emotion from the shallow, conventional—even false, downwards and inwards to the deepest, most central and serious emotion, where the core of the personality is thought to lie. We might of course, in the light of what has gone before, interpret this inner region as the soul, but more useful to understanding this entire chapter is an approach to these depth views by means of an historical perspective, so that with the critical analysis behind us, we might come to an appreciation of what is being expressed in this group of theories.

As we have seen when the same spatial language is used to express the order of quality, the order of values, the order of being and the order of functional anatomy, we can be led into muddles and diffi-culties.[5] But if we try to go beyond these semantic obstacles in order to look at what is being said and what has always been said by theories of this kind—and by common speech which so often iden-tifies the emotional, the vital, the valuable, and the inner—we come to this conclusion: *emotion is the essence of life.* Where emotion is, life is. Thus, as we know from the work of Spitz and others in infant psychology, a baby becomes 'dehumanized' and actually dies without emotional contact, no matter how correct the technical care might be. Thus, the common man's popular literature correctly interchanges the terms 'life problems' and 'emotional problems', while novelists in the great tradition have been principally concerned with the exploration of human emotions in their attempts to hold the mirror

---

[1] Tow, P. MacD., *Personality Changes Following Frontal Leucotomy*, Oxford, 1955.

[2] Stern, W., ' "Ernstspiel" and the Affective Life', FE 28, p. 328.

[3] Lewin, B. D., *The Psychoanalysis of Elation*, London, 1951, p. 166.

[4] Whitehorn, J., 'Physiological Changes in Emotional States', *The Inter-relationship of Body and Mind*, Baltimore, 1939, p. 263.

[5] See J. Nogué, 'Le symbolisme spatial de la qualité', *Rev. Phil.*, 102, 1926, pp. 70–106; 269–98, where a philosophical examination of some of these difficulties is attempted. H. W. Gruhle, *Verstehende Psychologie* (2nd edn.), Stuttgart, 1956, p. 42, also notes the confusions arising from the use of spatial language in describing the psyche. Much of the trouble here comes from 'Schichtentheorie'. A review of this problem and pertinent literature can be found in S. Strasser, *Das Gemüt*, Utrecht/Antwerpen/Freiburg, 1956, pp. 10–17; 88–101. In English, see A. R. Gilbert, 'Recent German Theories of Stratification of Personality', *J. Psychol.*, 1951, pp. 3–19.

up to life. And thus, the eradication of all emotion is the central doctrine of certain ascetic practices aiming at Nirvana, since emotion means attachment to life. This attack on emotion, Hartmann notes,[1] accounts for the 'ethical poverty of ascetics' who, in their destruction of emotion, extirpate the very life of the soul.

This innermost depth called the soul or more precisely that aspect of the soul involved with emotional consciousness, has often been located in the midmost darkness of the body. For the Greek trage-dians it was the liver; for Aristotle, the blood around the heart. In the Kundalini yoga system, the Manipura chakra—the emotional centre—is 'located' just below the diaphragm. In Homer, Plato and Hippocratic medicine this centre was the *phrenes*.[2] These are represen-tations for the dark, inexplicable (as Krueger maintains in our times) inner essence of life, or core of the personality, expressed concretely as 'essential organ'. (The word 'core', coming perhaps via *cœur, cor,* from *kēr* retains this idea[3]. Reymert, editor of the Wittenberg and Mooseheart symposia on emotion, uses the same image: '. . . I feel now, that this field constitutes the very "heart core" of man's prob-lems in relation to himself and other men . . .'[4] But we have here not so much the old argument for a cardiac theory of emotion— although a fascinating presentation of such views has been made by Lhermitte, and by others in the same volume.[5] Rather, it is a matter of understanding the continuity of the same explanatory image which links emotion with the essence of life, whether in the modern theories where it is called 'Gemüt', 'endothymic ground', 'soul' and con-sidered inexplicable and located in an unphysiological sense in the body (Hoisington) or 'inside' the subject, or whether in classic Greece, India, Egypt, or China.[6]

For if we look at this essence of life, not through the spatial lens where it becomes localized and static, but through a temporal lens where it becomes an activity, we find the same relation of emotion and vital essence. Emotion, in the German language, is generally called *Gemütsbewegung* = movement of the *Gemüt*,[7] that untrans-

---

[1] Hartmann, N., *Ethik*, 3rd edn., Berlin, 1949, p. 437.

[2] See OET, Part I, in particular Chapter II on *phrene* and *kēr*; Chapter V on the liver and Chapter III on *thymos*.

[3] Funk and Wagnalls' dictionary.

[4] FE 50, p. 579.

[5] *Le Cœur*, Les Études Carmélitaines, Paris, 1950.

[6] In Chinese, 'the ideographs used to denote the prefix "psycho" as in psychoanalysis, psychology, etc., are still today *hsin li* which can be translated approximately as "the reasons or principles of the heart" . . . the heart and its ideograph continues to "minister" the mind, even in today's technical literature of psychoanalysis and psychol-ogy'.—I. Veith, 'Non-Western Concepts of Psychic Function' in *The Brain and its Functions*, ed. by F. N. L. Poynter, Oxford, 1958, p. 33.

[7] Gruhle, H. W., *Verstehende Psychologie* (2nd edn.), Stuttgart, 1956, p. 39, writes: 'Gemüt ist der Sammelname für alle Gefühlsregungen.'

98

latable, intimate ground of all experience which can be identified with the soul. (*Mut*, itself means in short, 'courage', again referring to *cor*.) In Hindu thought, the activity of life is imaged as a dancing movement, a kind of rhythmical play of conflict, exemplified in the midriff by the expansion and contraction of the heart and the rising and falling of the diaphragm. These movements of the *kēr* and *phrenes* have always been associated with emotional phenomena. In ancient Egypt, the word *ib*, in its narrower sense of 'heart', signified certain emotions, wisdom and courage.[1] The word *ib* meant actually 'dancer'.[2] In other words the locus of emotion was seen through the temporal lens as an activity.[3] We continue to revolve around this inexplicable essence which links soul, heart, life, liver, diaphragm and central darkness, with emotion.

And so it is incidental whether we use abstract spatial concepts (inner, deep, central), or concrete spatial concepts (liver, heart, lungs) or mixed concepts (*phrenes*, soul, *Gemüt*) in order to conceive this essential core of the personality, as long as we keep in mind this vital image which seems to require such complexity of expression. This complexity of expression must also involve the order of quality as we have seen, since the essence of life—although described spatially —belongs to that order as well in these descriptions. Emotion is both that 'place' and that qualitative essence which makes experience possible.

Today, our times' most urgent and dramatic emotional demonstrations are covered by the diagnostic category of schizophrenia, primarily an affective disorder.[4] Coined in this century, the term means generally 'splitting of the personality' and etymologically 'splitting of the *phrēn*'. It is a poignant coincidence of the same expressive image: again we are told that the complex core of the personality, its living essence, is emotion.[5]

---

[1] ERE, entry 'Heart'.   [2] OET, p. 28, fn. 1.

[3] It is interesting to note that, although this activity can be conceived as a dance, or as a state of tension, or as a conflicting play of tendencies, all these terms have a single root. *ten = 'to draw, to pull, to stretch' is the common source of 'dance' from the Old High Germ. *dansôn* = 'to draw, to stretch out'; the Latin *tendo -ere*, from which come 'tension' and 'tendency'; the Latin *tempus* = 'time'; and also the Norwegian dialect *tinder*, Old Danish *tan* both meaning 'diaphragm'.—A. Wilde, *Vergleichendes Wörterbuch der Indogermanischen Sprachen*, Berlin/Leipzig, 1928.

[4] Henderson, D., and Gillespie, R. D., *A Textbook of Psychiatry* (7th edn.), Oxford, 1952, p. 295.

[5] Thus ends Sergi's historic paper ('Ueber den Sitz und die physische Grundlage der Affekte', *Ztschft. f. Psychol. u. Physiol. d. Sinnesorg.*, 1897, p. 100): '. . . so lässt sich feststellen, dass das Zentrum des Lebens oder der Lebensphänomene auch das Zentrum der Affekte ist, und diese entsprechen der wahren, ursprünglichen Funktion, dem Schutze des Lebenden.'

X

EMOTION AND PHYSIOLOGICAL LOCATION

A. THE BRAIN

THE THEORIES in this group use the language of spatial location in its physical sense. We are not dealing here with images of value or with orders of being or of quality, but with the perennial idea of the physical *seat* of psychic functions. Emotion is to be understood through understanding its location in the body. The first group of these theories takes its cue from Hippocrates: 'Men ought to know that from nothing else but the brain come joy, despondency, and lamentation . . . and by the same organ we become mad and delirious and fears and terrors assail us . . .' [1]

Let us begin with the important theory of Hess which depends upon the concept of the centre which he discusses in the following way:

> It is a burning problem to arrive at a clear concept of the structure of a so-called center. Center is a word in universal usage. However, it is very difficult to find out what notion a person has of the functioning of a center. It is clear that a system of synapses must be involved here. This provides the coordinated connections between definite reflexogenous areas, or patterns of cortical association, and definite effectors. The nervous apparatus mediating the coordination of the effectors is the central representation of a definite performance or, in brief, its center as a physiologic concept. As this paraphrase indicated, the physiologist does not connect a topographic focal but a topologic notion with the term center. . . .—W. R. Hess, *Diencephalon*, London and N.Y., 1954, p. 48.

Again:

> In actual fact, a center in its physiologic aspect unites the functions of individual effector organs for the performance of a definite task. Its

[1] SS, p. 63 ('The Sacred Disease', Section 17).

most important components are thus *connections* between elements, irrespective of whether these elements are located in close vicinity to each other or are widely separated from one another (pp. 60–1).[1]

He then explains how the diencephalon fulfills the requirements of this concept of the centre. Affectivity is dependent upon the diencephalon because of that organ's superordinate position to the autonomic nervous system. After summing up his evidence, Hess concludes:

> Therefore I conclude this treatise with a repetition of my conviction that true autonomic regulation finds its highest level of direct and automatic co-ordination in the diencephalon (p. 63).

Where Hess seems to use the concept of centre in terms of *function*, that is, in the topologic sense as 'the central representation of a definite performance', he seems to end up with the notion of the centre as a *seat* in the topographic sense of location *in the diencephalon*. He chides his colleagues who search for the centre 'as a collection of ganglia visible on histologic examination' (p. 60), yet although the diencephalon is not principally a collection of ganglia, it is a place, a physiological structure. And so in this first encounter with physiological location we come upon the central problem which will appear in one way or another again and again. These theories all conceive of functions in terms of structures where the function is located and on which the function depends for explanation.

Thus we have Cannon:

> It becomes a matter of interest, therefore, to inquire regarding the seat of the neural mechanism which operates the action complex of rage. —W. B. Cannon, 'Neural Organization for Emotional Expression', FE 28, p. 258.

His theory of emotion locates this 'seat' definitely in the thalamus:

> The localization of the reaction patterns for emotional expression in the thalamus—in a region which, like the spinal cord, works directly by simple automatisms unless held in check—not only accounts for the sensory side, the 'felt emotion', but also for the impulsive side, the tendency of the thalamic neurones to discharge. These powerful impulses originating in a region of the brain not associated with cognitive consciousness and arousing therefore in an *obscure* and *unrelated* manner the strong feelings of emotional excitement, explain the sense of being seized, possessed, of being controlled by an outside force and made to act without weighing of the consequences.—W. B. Cannon, 'The James-Lange Theory of Emotions: A Critical Examination and an Alternative Theory', *Am. J. Psychol.*, 1927, pp. 123–4.

[1] He makes the same point elsewhere: 'Symposion ü.d. Zwischenhirn', *Hel. Physiol. et Pharmacol. Acta* 8, Suppl. 6, 1950, pp. 10–13.

This passage presents the fundamentals of Cannon's theory. The well-known 'emergency' function of emotion in fulfilling a 'homeostatic' requirement as part of the 'wisdom of the body'[1] is widely presented and discussed in detail in the literature. But it is important to note here that his purposive interpretations of the function of emotion as well as his explanations of the nature of emotion depend on the location of the emotional seat in the thalamus, i.e. separate from the cortex in a phylogenetically ancient part of the brain[2] where such patterns are congenitally inwrought and are ready for simple automatic release[3] upon suspension of cortical inhibition.

This theory, also called the Cannon-Bard theory, is presented briefly by Bard as follows:

> ... this theory proposes that at the same time that the diencephalon discharges the motor impulses which produce the emotional behavior it discharges upward to the cortex afferent impulses which throw into action the cortical processes which underlie emotional consciousness. As stated by Cannon the essence of this theory is that '*the peculiar quality of the emotion is added to simple sensation when the thalamic processes are aroused.*[4]—P. Bard, 'The Neuro-Humoral Basis of Emotional Reactions', in *The Foundations of Experimental Psychology* (ed. C. Murchison), Clark Univ., U.S.A., 1929, p. 483.

The Cannon-Bard theory depends on two different kinds of arguments. The first is an argument which interweaves hypotheses from different areas of evidence—ontogenesis, phylogenesis, animal experimentation, clinical experience. The second argument is based on a mechanistic model of the relation of structure to function. An example of the first kind of argument is given in simple clarity by Schou:

> The result then arrived at is that the emotions are regulated from the mesencephalon where all the vegetative phenomena accompanying the emotions have their centre. This is in conformity with the phylogenetic view of the diencephalon as the oldest part of the brain, being the seat of the primitive emotional life. Likewise it is in conformity with the ontogenetic view according to which children, whose cerebrum is a comparatively uncultivated field, have a richer and more unrestrained emotional life. The perception is also confirmed by experiments on animals, in which the cerebrum can be removed simultaneous with a complete conservation of the expression of the emotions. And lastly, it coincides with the modern clinical experience from chronic epidemic encephalitis and the surgery of cerebral tumors respectively, confirming that the

---

[1] Cannon, W. B., *The Wisdom of the Body*, N.Y., 1932.
[2] Cannon, W. B., 'Neural Organization for Emotional Expression', FE 28, p. 263.
[3] Cannon, W. B., *Bodily Changes in Pain, Hunger, Fear and Rage* (2nd edn.), 1929, Boston (1953 printing), p. 369.
[4] Bard's quotation of Cannon is from *op. cit., loc. cit. sup.*

mesencephalon is the seat of emotions.—H. I. Schou, *Some Investigations into the Physiology of Emotions*, Copenhagen and London, 1937, p. 92.

The second argument in terms of structure and function uses three different conceptual systems of operations. These are: the structures (cortex, diencephalon or thalamus); the neurological impulses or processes which are considered to be functional discharges of the structures: which, in turn, 'underlie emotional consciousness' (Bard). So we see, the psychological function (emotional consciousness) depends on the physiological function (processes) which take place in anatomical structures (cortex and thalamus). The argument therefore depends entirely upon a mechanistic view of the relation of these three orders of events.

This kind of argument is given clearly by Papez, who is considered to be the first to present a newer and more complex theory of physiological location. In his view, only this mechanistic view of the relation of structure and function is 'scientific'.

> Is emotion a magic product, or is it a physiologic process which depends on an anatomic mechanism? An attempt has been made to point out various anatomic structures and correlated physiologic symptoms which, taken as a whole, deal with various phases of emotional dynamics, consciousness and related functions. It is proposed that the hypothalamus, the anterior thalamic nuclei, the gyrus cinguli, the hippocampus and their interconnections constitute a harmonious mechanism which may elaborate the functions of central emotion, as well as participate in emotional expression. This is an attempt to allocate specific organic units to a larger organization dealing with a complex regulating process. The evidence presented is mostly concordant and suggestive of such a mechanism as a unit within the larger architectural mosaic of the brain. . . .
>
> Emotion is such an important function that its mechanism, whatever it is, should be placed on a structural basis.—J. W. Papez, 'A Proposed Mechanism of Emotion', *Arch. Neurol. Psychiat.*, 1937, p. 743.
>
> Taken as a whole, this ensemble of structures is proposed as representing theoretically the anatomic basis of emotions (p. 725).

These mechanisms of emotion have become more and more differentiated as the methods of observation have become elaborated and refined. The 'activation theory' of Lindsley shows how complex Papez's 'harmonious mechanism' has become. He refers to a drawing which is a 'schematic representation of principal central nervous structures and probable pathways involved in emotional behavior'.[1] Fourteen different connections are elaborated which link up cortex, thalamus, hypothalamus, pituitary body, mid-brain, brain-stem, etc.

[1] Lindsley, D. B., 'Emotion', in *Handbook of Experimental Psychology*, ed. by S. S. Stevens, NY. and London, 1951, pp. 504–07.

E.—H   103

These make 'clear the extent of hierarchical arrangement of reflex pathways involved in emotion. Most of the interconnections . . . are supported by both anatomical and physiological evidence, although a few of them are merely inferred from suggestive data. The activation theory requires all the possible mechanisms schematized . . .' (p. 506). 'Thus it may be seen that, through the mechanisms illustrated . . . varying degrees and complexity of activation are possible as a hierarchy of reflex responses progressively involves higher levels of the neuraxis' (p. 508).

Theoretically, the problem here is similar to the problem in the hypotheses of Papez, Cannon and Bard: psychological function, physiological function and anatomical structure are conceived mechanistically. Emotion depends upon the 'interaction of the cerebral cortex and subcortical structures', described here in great detail. And yet, in spite of the intricacy of the hypotheses, they do not take us very far:

> Beyond the relatively simple startle response, involving mainly a brain-stem level in the hierarchy of response mechanisms, the nature of the more complex emotional responses is less clear (p. 508).

And he concludes:

> . . . it is not profitable on the basis of present experimental evidence to attempt to account for all the varieties of emotional expression. . . . Many of the nuances of behavior undoubtedly depend upon learning and habituation, which reinstated through memory and ideation and operating through the complex network of intracortical connections, make possible emotional responses that represent varying gradations between maximal excitement and its opposite—relaxation and sleep. In short, the activation theory appears to account for the extremes, but leaves intermediate and mixed states relatively unexplained as yet (p. 509).[1]

Lindsley's theory depends not only upon the fourteen hypothesized pathways but also upon circulatory and hormone influences which affect the electrical activities of the cortex.[2] It is these rhythmically patterned electrical discharges of nerve cells in the cortex which 'activate' and are 'activated' by sub-cortical structures by means of the enumerated pathways conceived as feedback circuits. With this we have come a long way from Papez' harmonious mechanism of a few structures. And we can question whether the intricacy of such physiological description is not self-defeating. The further the investigation proceeds, the more mechanisms seem to be required in the explanation and the less localized they become (e.g. hormones, neurosecretions, and blood circulation are also involved).

---

[1] Bloch, V. ('Sur les conceptions actuelles de l'émotion', *Journ. de Psychol. Norm. Pathol.*, 1954, pp. 79–90) mainly follows the theory of Lindsley.

[2] Lindsley. D. B., 'Emotions and the Electroencephalogram', FE 50, p. 245.

Let us pause here and ask why the locus of emotion has become so intricate and diffuse. On the one hand this is due to the refinement of brain-mapping techniques, but on the other hand—and this is fundamental—it is due to the nature of emotion as Lindsley conceives it:

> Emotion is one of the most complex phenomena known to psychology. It is complex because it involves so much of the organism at so many levels of neural and chemical integration. Both subjectively and objectively its ramifications are diffuse and intermingled with other processes. Perhaps therein lies the uniqueness, and possibly the major significance, of emotion (p. 473).

Any explanation of a complex whole spread through many levels of integration at any given moment requires an inordinate amount of description of that whole in order to be adequate, let alone satisfying. No partial system of functions or structures will be adequate. The concept of feedback circuits of which Lindsley makes use points this up very well. Emotion, as a complex phenomenon intermingled with other processes involving so much of the organism, cannot be localized in any specific partial functional system owing to the complex interaction of these circuits and levels of integration. This is an observation which Lindsley himself makes about the measurement of the bodily changes of emotion: 'The complexity of these interactions makes it clear that the measurement of bodily change in emotion can never be definite or exhaustive' (p. 474). If this is true for one level of integration (quantitative measurement of bodily changes), it is even 'more true' for the entire complex of emotion. Therefore, Lindsley's theory fails to account for emotion, not because of the empirical difficulties involved in locating all the mechanisms, but because emotion, as he defines it, cannot be equated with any localized mechanisms. 'Perhaps therein lies the uniqueness, and possibly the major significance, of emotion.'

Turning now to the theory of MacLean, we find he takes the theory of Papez as his point of departure:

> Broca, in 1878, demonstrated that a large convolution which is called the great limbic lobe is found as a common denominator in the brain of all mammals. . . . Broca chose the word limbic to indicate that this lobe *surrounds* the brain stem. In accord with the theory of Papez, recent experimentation has shown that the limbic lobe is also, physiologically speaking, a common denominator of a variety of viscerosomatic and emotional reactions in the mammal. Furthermore, it has been found that the limbic lobe and its subcortical cell stations constitute a functionally integrated system which may be appropriately designated as *the limbic*

system. . . . Thus it has evolved that the limbic system is not only an anatomical but also a physiological entity, . . .

On the other hand, there is evidence that the rapidly evolving neo-cortex . . . could be likened to an expanding numerator, representing in phylogeny the growth of intellectual function. It is because of the presumed primacy of the role of the limbic system in emotional behavior that in psychiatric parlance I have used the term 'visceral' in its original sixteenth-century meaning and applied it to the brain included in this system.—P. D. MacLean, 'The Limbic System ("Visceral Brain") in Relation to Central Gray and Reticulum of the Brain Stem: Evidence of Interdependence in Emotional Processes', *Psychosom. Med.*, 1955, p. 355.[1]

In spite of MacLean's differentiation between the limbic lobe as a structure and the limbic system as a physiological system of functions, he uses interchangeably the terms: 'visceral brain', 'animalistic brain', 'limbic system', and 'primitive structure', thereby losing the differentiation he was first careful to make. Not only does he merge anatomical (structural) concepts with physiological (functional) concepts,

---

[1] Although we shall be coming later to discuss phylogenetic theories (Chapter XIII), a note on one of the more apparent dangers of this kind of approach might be in place. It does not necessarily follow that because there is a part to part similarity between two different biological species there is also a function to function correlation. That the rat and rabbit have a limbic lobe basically similar to man's does not necessarily mean that the limbic lobe in man performs in the same way as in the rat or rabbit. The limbic lobe of the rat is in the rat, part of the total organism of the rat, and serves the rat's being and way of life. The limbic lobe in the man is always a man's limbic lobe. So too, the patterns of behavior which we might just here call emotions, even if they be phylogenetically similar to the emotions in the rat, are always, nevertheless, emotions of and in a man. Thomas Aquinas states it like this: 'To inquire into the meaning of animal is one business, to inquire into the meaning of human animal quite another.' (*Summa Theol.* Ia. xxix, 4.) Spinoza says: '. . . emotions of animals . . . differ only from the emotions of man inasmuch as their nature differs from the nature of man. Horse and man are filled with the desire of procreation; the desire of the former is equine . . . of the latter is human' (*Ethics*, III, note to Prop. 57). Tertullian remarks bitterly against those who try to prove the location of the soul by observing the functioning of animals after the experimental removal of hearts and brains: '. . . let all those, too, who have predetermined the character of the human soul from the condition of brute animals, be quite sure that it is themselves rather who are alive in a heartless and brainless state' (*De Anima*, XV). The same argument—that fundamental differences between animals and humans can invalidate deductions concerning functional analogies—comes also from modern researchers, e.g.: 'One must keep in mind in any case the principally different coordination of eye, head and body motor movements, which probably also utilize different anatomical bases.'—Translation mine from R. Jung, 'Symposion ü.d. Zwischenhirn', *Helvet. Physiol. et Pharmacol. Acta* 8, *Suppl.* 6, 1950, pp. 53–4. See also, *idem*, p. 33, P. Matussek to the same effect.

The original quotations read as follows: Thomas Aquinas—'Unde aliud est quaerere de significatione animalis, et aliud est quaerere de significatione animalis quod est homo'. Spinoza—'. . . affectus animalium . . . ab affectibus hominum tantum differre, quantum eorum natura a natura humana differt. Fertur quidem equus et homo libidine procreandi; at ille libidine equina, hic autem humana.' Tertullian—'. . . et omnes iam sciant se potius sine corde et cerebro vivere, qui dispositionem animae humanae de condicione bestiarum praeiudicarint.' Jung—'Festzuhalten ist jedenfalls die *prinzipiell verschiedene Koordination von Augen-, Kopf-, und Körpermotorik bei Mensch und Tier, die wahrscheinlich auch verschiedene anatomische Substrate benutzt.*'

106

but when he theorizes about the psychological functions of these neural mechanisms he 'psychologizes' them. By failing to keep to terms appropriate to the field of investigation, MacLean psychologizes the brain by calling it 'brute',[1] just as Neumann (Chapter V, p. 41) biologized the psyche when speaking of 'cortical' and 'medullary' man. This becomes more evident when MacLean presents his interesting speculations about the psychological functions of these neural mechanisms:

> In his monograph on encephalitis lethargica, von Economo emphasized his belief that there are distinctive neural mechanisms that account for what one might refer to respectively, as 'feeling drive' and 'conceptual will'. The presumed primacy of the role of the limbic system in emotional behavior and the demonstration of the potential schizophysiology of the limbic and neocortical systems gives further support for such an assumption. It presents a situation that holds promise of shedding light on the nature of mechanisms concerned in hypnosis, hysteria, schizophrenia, and psychosomatic diseases. It has also therapeutic implications. For if . . . the limbic system is poorly discriminated and interprets experience largely in terms of feeling, it raises the question of whether or not sufficient attention has been paid to non-verbal methods in dealing with this animalistic brain.—MacLean, *Psychosom. Med.* 1955, p. 364.

Elsewhere, he describes in more detail the way in which this animalistic brain works.

> On the basis of these observations one might infer that the hippocampal system could hardly deal with information in more than a crude way, and was possibly too primitive a brain to analyze language. Yet it might have the capacity to participate in a non-verbal type of symbolism. This would have significant implications as far as symbolism affects the emotional life of the individual. One might imagine, for example, that though the visceral brain could never aspire to conceive of the colour red in terms of a three-letter word or as a specific wave length of light, it could associate the colour symbolically with such diverse things as blood, fainting, fighting, flowers, etc. Therefore, if the visceral brain were the kind of brain that could tie up symbolically a number of unrelated phenomena, and at the same time lack the analyzing ability of the word brain to make a nice discrimination of their differences, it is possible to conceive how it might become foolishly involved in a variety of ridiculous correlations leading to phobias, obsessive-compulsive behaviour, etc. . . . Considered in the light of Freudian psychology, the visceral brain would have many of the attributes of the unconscious id. One might argue, however, *that the visceral brain is not at all unconscious (possibly not even in certain stages of sleep), but rather eludes the grasp*

---

[1] MacLean, P. D., 'Studies on Limbic System ("Visceral Brain" and their Bearing on Psychosomatic Problems', RDPM, p. 120.

of the intellect because its animalistic and primitive structure makes it impossible to communicate in verbal terms.—P. D. MacLean, 'Psychosomatic Disease and the "Visceral Brain" ', *Psychosom. Med.*, 1949, p. 348.

Kubie, too, sees in this region of the brain the physiological mechanism for a host of psychological functions:

> Here then, in the depths of the temporal lobe, with its intricate connections, is a cross-road where the multipolar functions of the symbolic process can be integrated. It is impossible to over-estimate the importance of the fact that the temporal complex constitutes a mechanism for integrating the past and the present, the phylogenetically and ontogenetically old and new, and at the same time for integrating the external and internal environments of the central nervous system. Thus it is through the temporal lobe and the visceral brain that the 'gut' components of memory can enter into our psychological processes; and it is precisely here that the multipolar areas of reference of the symbolic function can be served. Consequently, we are justified in saying that the temporal lobe, with its deeper primitive connections, is a mechanism for the coordination of all the data which links us to the world of experience, both external and internal. It is through these mechanisms that we are able to project and to introject; and it is through these central structures which serve the multipolarity of the symbolic function that the central nervous organ can mediate the translation into somatic disturbance of those tensions which are generated on the level of psychological experience. It is this area of the brain then which deserves to be viewed as the organ which is essential for psychosomatic relationships.—L. S. Kubie, 'The Central Representation of the Symbolic Process in Relation to Psychosomatic Disorders', RDPM, p. 132.

These fascinating hypotheses indeed open magic casements. New perspectives unfold and it seems as if we have found at last the organ essential to the symbolic function, the unconscious, and psychosomatic relationships. Here, 'in the depths of the temporal lobe', tensions resulting from psychological experience are 'translated' into somatic disturbances (Kubie).[1] This hippocampal formation, 'too primitive a brain to analyse language', makes foolish correlations leading to all sorts of neurotic symptoms (MacLean). This brain is given such a set of mental attributes that it is no longer clear whether we are describing a physiological or a psychological order of events. The concept 'visceral brain', like the concept 'vital energy' (Chapter VI, p. 71) covers over the difference between two orders of events which it sets out to explain. And we suggest that it, too, like 'vital energy', is a substitute concept for the soul. These attributes: an affinity and sensitivity to symbolism, a connection to the ancestral past, a kind of dream consciousness which perhaps does not sleep,

[1] See also Kubie, L. S., 'Influence of Symbolic Processes on the Role of Instincts in Human Behavior', *Psychosom. Med.*, 1956, pp. 189 ff.

and a functional utility in joining mind and body, have also been, in different times and places, postulated for the soul. That the 'visceral brain' is considered 'primitive', 'crude', 'brute', and 'animalistic' is only further evidence for our view. These adjectives have been applied in other contexts to the contemporary soul and are perhaps especially apt in expressing the undervalued position of the soul in contemporary scientistic psychology.

The same kind of suggestive interpretations of physiological regions is made by Rof Carballo. In an excellently concentrated paper he integrates hypotheses from Cannon, Hess, Papez, Watson, Ruck-mick, Janet, Jung, Lewin, Sartre, and others in order to produce a general theory of emotion. The conceptual model which he uses is that of levels. He considers:

> . . . the emotions placed, on the one hand, within the major instinctive impulses of the living being, and, on the other, they form part of its defense mechanisms. One of the basic instincts of man, the one which, in a way, is a continuation of the instinct of growth, of development and self-affirmation is the instinct of *defense of the image which man forms of 'himself'*. One of the most powerful motivations of human conduct . . . is that of maintaining as high as possible the idea and image of oneself. . . . many emotional states can only be explained as a functioning of defense mechanisms against all which tends to lower, diminish or annul the image which man makes of his own value. From the neurological point of view we tend to localize this image . . . in the immediate vicinity of, or mixed with, the image of the bodily form.—J. Rof Carballo, 'Fisio-patología de la Emoción', *Medicina Clínica*, Barcelona, 1950, pp. 331–2.[1]

As in the view of Kubie and MacLean, in this area of the brain the body image is said to merge with the self image (which might also be called *amour-propre*; see Chapter XIII). In addition to the emotion centred on this image and its associated instinctive impulses, there is another sphere of higher moral values which also give rise to emotion. This second emotional area he locates neurologically in the pre-frontal cortex (p. 332).

And in spite of the passionately intelligent plea for an appreciation of the significance of emotion with which he concludes, the theory rests upon the same assumption that psychological functions can be located in physiological functions or structures. Upon this the whole attempt at a general integration of so many views stands or falls. This blurring of distinctions is partly due to the Spanish prefix *sub*, which provides a facile link for the *sub*-conscious, the *sub*-cortex, and the magical, ancient, *sub*-terranean depths of the personality.

We find now on looking back that essential to these views—to put

[1] Translation mine.

the matter in a gross simplification—is the identification of 'intellect' with cortex and 'emotion' with sub-cortical structures, between which operates a 'potential schizophysiology' (MacLean).[1] From the point of view of biological morphology, these two structures are interpreted as phylogenetically and ontogenetically younger and older (Schou). They are also said to have different sets of 'values' (Rof Carballo), and two different ways of integrating experience (Kubie, MacLean). In psychology, the opposition between two systems of mental functioning has been put forward in terms of abstract and concrete behaviour (Goldstein), ego and id (Freud), directed and dereistic thinking (Bleuler). In all these various formulations of the same kind of idea, the explanation of emotion does *not* rest upon its identification or location in one member of the conceptual pairs. It rests upon the way in which these two systems, fields, regions, structures relate. On Lindsley's view, there was a hierarchical pattern of activation of different levels. On the view of Cannon, Kubie and MacLean, the sub-cortical brain functions in a radically different way from the cortex, forming an almost separate system in itself. On Darrow's view, the emphasis falls definitely upon the *relation* of these two regions, here conceived in terms of cortical inhibition:

> If conflict is . . . essential to the release of subcortically controlled emotional behavior, and if, as seems apparent, the cortex does, except in emotion, maintain a high degree of selective inhibitory control over subcortical primitive automatic mechanisms, the probable neural mechanism of release of emotion by ideas is at once suggested. True, we do not know the exact nature of cortical inhibitory control. Whether it is by means of a potential gradient, by the maintenance of volleys of inhibitory nerve impulses, by the inhibiting effect of interfering nerve frequencies . . . can only be experimentally determined. The present hypothesis is that whatever the form of inhibitory control it is interfered with when perceptual patterns demanding or implying action conflict with patterns already identified with the individual's thought and action. It seems obvious that in conditions of active intracortical conflict there may be lessened (energy for?) control of subcortical functions and that the result is to set free the lower level activities. In other words, excited emotion may arise from a partial or relative *functional decortication* occasioned by dynamic cortical conflict.—C. Darrow, 'Emotion as Relative Functional Decortication', *Psychol. Rev.*, 1935, pp. 572–3.

Theoretically, then, emotion is the result of intracortical conflict. Yet the theory is not a conflict theory of the same kind as those in Chapter XVI, because it conceives the conflict physiologically: the brain 'functions causally in precipitating emotion' (*ibid.*).

[1] This idea, important to all *Schichtentheorie* (see above, Chapter IX, p. 97, fn.), seems to begin in modern times with F. Kraus (*Allgemeine und spezielle Pathologie der Person*, 2 Bde., Leipzig, 1919–26), who uses the concepts 'Tiefenperson' and 'Rindenperson'.

Kurtz distinguishes 'three general modes of evolvement for passions',[1] and his theory, too depends on the *relationship* of cortex and thalamus. He admits: 'passions may be of cortical origin'. Lindsley's view also offered this possibility. For Darrow, this is only possible when cortical inhibition is interfered with. This brings us to the view of Arnold, who challenges the notion of cortical inhibition and presents a theory in which the function of the cortex in emotion is seen as 'excitatory'.

It is possible now to present a sequence of events in emotional experience which will take into account Cannon's observations but use the alternative hypothesis of cortical excitation instead of cortical inhibition. We start not with the stimulus but with the autogenous activity of the cortex to which electroencephalograph (EEG) studies have accustomed us. To quote Papez: 'In the past, many of us have thought of the nervous system as a silent network of neurons activated only in response to sensory stimulation. We must now enlarge our thinking by assuming a preexisting and probably autogenous activity.'
Psychologically speaking, the stimulus does not break in on us; rather, we focus on it, an activity which can be called 'attention', 'set' or 'expectancy'. Neurologically speaking, this focusing may consist in the activation of cortico-thalamic fibers which . . . are interspersed among sensory thalamo-cortical fibers. The incoming sensory excitation could then be modified either in the thalamus or at arrival in the cortex. Thus we see what we have learned to expect by previous *sensory* experience . . . A similar focusing process may go on transcortically, and we now see what we expect to see *emotionally* (a flapping sheet becomes a ghost in the dark). This fusion of expectancy and sensation represents a psychological evaluation of the situation: 'How does this affect *me*?' The resulting emotional attitude (anger, fear, disgust, etc.) then initiates nerve impulses from the cortex to centers in the thalamus-hypothalamus, which touch off the appropriate pattern of emotional expression as well as the corresponding peripheral changes. The autonomic effects thus produced . . . are then reported back to the cortex via the afferent sensory pathways. Finally, this cortical perception of organic changes may again be evaluated as to 'how it affects me'. A complete emotional experience would include the whole sequence—evaluation, emotional attitude (or feeling), resulting in emotional expression, autonomic changes, and their cortical perception and reevaluation.—M. B. Arnold, 'An Excitatory Theory of Emotion', FE 50, pp. 18–19.

The same is said by Solomon: 'Emotion in its beginning is cortical and the reaction takes place from the cortex downward';[2] and by

---

[1] Kurtz, P., 'An Approach to Psychodynamic Appraisal', *J. Nerv. Ment. Dis.*, 1953, pp. 534–5.
[2] Solomon, M., 'The Mechanism of the Emotions', *Brit. J. Med. Psychol.*, 1927, p. 313.

Gellhorn: 'Emotional response in man, particularly in its highest forms, appears to be due to cortical excitation'.[1]

We are confronted here with psychological interpretations of sets of clinical and experimental observations. On the one hand we have a cortical theory of emotion, on the other a sub-cortical theory. We might say that the cortical theory is a formulation in physiological terms of the Scholastic position where emphasis lay on apprehension and evaluation,[2] which Arnold here calls attention, focusing or expectancy. It is also in general agreement with that aspect of the Stoic position which held that imagination alone calls emotion into being and that all emotion takes rise in man's reason.[3] In other words, the cortical theory presents again the view that there are relatively independent, self-activating (autogenic), higher levels which act as efficient causes upon (excite) lower levels. The sub-cortical theories have interpreted the evidence in accordance with another main stream of thinking about emotion. Here, through the diencephalon and autonomic nervous system, emotion is intimately interconnected with the body, man's corporeal nature. Like an unruly, unreasonable animal, it is held in check by the inhibiting activities of reason from which world it is all but cut off (schizophysiology).

One can surmount these alternatives by means of a hierarchical system of relations (Lindsley), or by allowing for two modes of emotion (Rof Carballo), or three (Kurtz). One can also surmount the problem by the use of a concept of multi-causality—such as we discussed in the Introduction. Careful distinctions between kinds of causes can avoid the pitfalls and waste of make-believe problems. Within the framework of physiological location of the cause of emotion, the cortex might be a necessary cause of one kind, and the sub-cortical systems a necessary cause of another kind. There is no need to choose between them, a need which gives rise to the surgical ablation of cerebral areas in order to prove the priority of one or another region. It is perhaps more useful to examine the concept of centre—as Hess does—than to search for the centre itself. A centre defined in one way is bound to turn up differently, if not in a different place, from a centre defined in another way.

The ultimate question in these theories is: Can the 'complex underlying process' (Lindsley) or the 'central representation of a definite performance' (Hess) be physiologically located for emotion? Here it depends entirely upon what concept of emotion we are

[1] Gellhorn, E., *Physiological Foundations of Neurology and Psychiatry*, Univ. of Minn., 1953, p. 360.
[2] FE 37, p. 103
[3] Zeller, E., *The Stoics, Epicureans and Sceptics*, London, 1892, p. 245.

trying to locate or represent. If we conceive of emotion as a *physiological* function (as vascular, glandular and autonomic activity) then structural location is inevitable. This is legitimate procedure in physiological explanation which says: 'In order to understand the function of an organ it is usually essential to have a knowledge of its structure.' [1] In this realm, mechanistic thinking seems still to reign, which would account for the mechanistic way of relating function and structure in the theories of these physiologists who, even when aware of these problems, seem driven by the logic of their methods to mechanistic conclusions.

But if we conceive emotion as psychological, at least in part, then the location of emotion turns on the problem of representation of psychic functions in somatic structures or systems. Here, it might be well to bring in those views which would deny, for one reason or another, that emotion can be so located. For example, Nielsen and Sedgwick claim to have found what they call instincts and emotions in an anencephalic infant without thalami.[2] Spiegel, Wycis, *et al.* conclude that it is 'not possible to refer emotional reactions to a single circumscribed nucleus within the diencephalon or to connections with the frontal lobes, but there exists a multiple representation of this function'.[3] Grinker reviews and concludes a recent symposium on emotion, by coming out strongly against 'line-to-point mechanisms' which are said to explain emotion in a direct cause-and-effect way.[4] And Gooddy examines the concept of cerebral representation in general. He says:

> With rejection of the principle of representation, we reject the idea of the brain as a diagram of an organ full of departments, each with some kind of technical equipment such as scientists have designed for . . . laboratories. . . . All those functions, hitherto believed to originate from particular parts of the brain, must depend upon the changing state of activity of the whole nervous system. A function does not originate in a specific region of brain tissue, where its 'representation' has been traditionally located.—W. Gooddy, 'Cerebral Representation', *Brain*, 1956, p. 186.

If we follow Gooddy and refuse representation of psychic functions in cerebral structures we can be driven back to the days before modern experimental anatomy where indeed, as Papez says, emotion is something 'magical', having to do perhaps with von Reichenbach's

[1] Best, C. H., and Taylor, N. B., *The Physiological Basis of Medical Practice*, Baltimore, 1943, p. vi.

[2] Nielsen, J., and Sedgwick, R., 'Instincts and Emotions in an Anencephalic Monster', *J. Nerv. Ment. Dis.*, 1949, p. 394.

[3] Spiegel, E., Wycis, H., *et al.*, 'The Central Mechanism of the Emotions', *Am. J. Psychiat.*, 1951, p. 430.

[4] Grinker, R. R., 'Discussion on Symposium on Neurohumoral Factors in Emotion', *Arch. Neurol. Psychiat.*, 1955, p. 140.

Od or Stahl's phlogiston. On the other hand, if we stress representation we can fall into the phrenological explanations of Gall and Spurzheim seeking to locate 'innate ideas' in little areas of the head. Cerebral localization of psychic functions is an old controversy, which turns fundamentally on the question of the 'divisibility of the soul'. Certain Church Fathers (Lactantius, Tertullian, Gregory of Nyssa) held that the soul was indivisible and permeated the whole body. Another line of tradition (Poseidonius, Nemesius, Arabic philosophy, Albertus Magnus, Mundinus) definitely localized distinct activities of the psyche.[1] Again, the resolution has to do with precision of the concept which is being located. Line-to-point mechanisms may give a satisfactory account of some phenomena; but locating emotion, when conceived as a molar event involving many levels of integration, becomes muddled with locating the psyche. As Malmo points out, ' "emotion" and "psychic" are terms which are frequently used interchangeably in the literature'.[2] And so we are up against the age-old attempt to locate the seat of the soul. This conclusion has already been drawn by Féré:

> The history of the encephalic localisations of the emotions confound themselves with that of the seat of the soul, which writers have for the most part placed in the median and unique organs of the encephalon like the pineal gland (Descartes), the corpus callosum (Bounet, Lapeyronie), the septum lucidum (Digby), the bridge of Varolius (Haller), the spinal cord (moelle allongée) (Boerhaave).—C. Féré, *The Pathology of Emotions* (transl. by R. Park), London, 1899, p. 418.

Tuke presents other choices in reviewing his contemporaries.[3] While Tertullian, for whom the soul was the source of emotion, reviews a host of options for the location of this soul:

> . . . so that you must not suppose, with Heraclitus, that this sovereign faculty . . . is moved by some external force; nor with Moschion, that it floats about through the whole body; nor with Plato, that it is enclosed in the head; nor with Zenophanes, that it culminates in the crown of the head; nor . . . in the brain, according to . . . Hippocrates; nor around the basis of the brain, as Herophilus thought; nor in the membranes thereof, as Strato and Erasistratus said; nor in the space between the eyebrows, as Strato the physician held; nor within the enclosure of the breast, according to Epicurus . . .—Tertullian, 'De Anima', Chapter XV, ANCL XV, pp. 441–2. ('Zenophanes' should read 'Xenocrates'.)

With this we can conclude, stating that the locus or loci of emotion has not been found because it cannot be found, either in spatial

[1] SS, pp. 77, 87–8, 96, 103, 129, etc.
[2] Malmo, R. B., 'Research: Experimental and Theoretical Aspects', RDPM, p. 87.
[3] Tuke, D. H., *Illustrations of the Influence of the Mind upon the Body*, London, 1872, pp. 112–21.

structures or in localized physiological functions, because the
'complex underlying process' or 'central representation of a definite
performance', i.e. that for which we are looking, is best understood
as the soul. Thus the cerebral structures and pathways involved in
emotion do not pin-point emotion to these targets, nor can such
areas even be said to operate centrally, release autogenically or
initiate emotion. They are but circuits of interacting servo-mechan-
isms (another way of putting the traditional concept of the circulation
of the psyche throughout the whole person). Surgical incisions
(leucotomy) or stimulation through electrodes only alters these
circuits and does not *post hoc, ergo propter hoc* establish the origin
of emotion in a special place. But of course the eminent investigators
in this field know this very well.

B. THE BLOOD, GUT AND GLANDS

The passage from Tertullian with which the last section ended continues on. After denying cerebral location, he affirms following
Aristotle that the soul, or sensing faculty, is located lower in the body
—*sanguis circumcordialis*.[1] Bichat, at the beginning of the last century,
puts the same kind of view so clearly that it is often quoted: 'le cer-
veau n'est jamais affecté par les passions qui ont pour siège *exclusif*
les organes de la vie interne . . .'[2] These organs of the internal life
can be understood, following Bichat, as the liver, the heart, the lungs,
etc. Or they can be understood, following Lange, as the cardio-
vascular system (*sanguis circumcordialis* and its extensions) by means
of which these inner organs are altered. Or the emphasis can fall on
the 'internal life' understood as *milieu interieur*, i.e. chemical-hor-
monal composition of the blood carried in the vascular system that
alters the inner organs. Even where they differ in degree of subtlety
and level, all these views attempt the same sort of explanation.
Emotion is to be explained by events in the body, not by events in
the head.

As Titchener[3] has shown, the bodily as opposed to mental explanation of emotion has a long history and can count among its supporters
Descartes, Malebranche, La Mettrie, Bichat, Cabanis, Domrich
and Lotze. (Ubeda Purkiss[4] gives evidence for the extension of

[1] Tertullian, *De Anima*, XV, ANCL XV.

[2] Bichat, F. X., 'Recherches physiologiques sur la vie et la mort' in *Anatomie
Générale*, Paris, 1818. D. Sennert (1572–1637) placed the seat of mental derangement
also outside the brain: *Cordis enim temperies corrupta corrumpit temperiem cerebri*. SS,
p. 126.

[3] Titchener, E. B., 'An Historical Note on the James-Lange Theory of Emotion',
Am. J.Psychol. 1914, pp. 427–47.

[4] Ubeda Purkiss, Fr.M., 'Desarrollo histórico de las doctrinas sobre las emociones',
II, *La Ciencia Tomista*, Salamanca, 1954, pp. 35–9.

Titchener's list to include Lamarck, Tracy, Blaud, Beraud, Dufour, Buffon, and in particular the Scottish-associationist, James McCosh (1880).) Looking back over this history of controversy between head and body, ranging from Tertullian to Bichat, appearing again in the central view (Sherrington, Cannon, Goltz) versus the peripheral view (James, Lange, Sergi), and appearing now most recently in the cortex versus thalamus discussions (Chapter X A), we can find the same dominant theme: *higher versus lower*. When emotion is explained by means of higher centres, no matter whether they be conceived as cerebral events or as mental events, the role of the body becomes only instrumental, only a means of expression at the service of higher processes which are in control and sit in the seat. Such were the views we have just seen. Here the theories champion the body. Visceral, vascular, and glandular changes constitute emotion. Without these bodily events, there is no emotion. Lange puts it like this:

> If from one terrified the accompanying bodily symptoms are removed, the pulse permitted to beat quietly, the glance to become firm, the color natural, the movements rapid and secure, the speech strong, the thoughts clear,—what is there left of his terror?—C. Lange, *Om Sindsbevaegelser*, Köbenhavn, 1885 (transl. from German translation of H. Kurella, by B. Rand, in *The Classical Psychologists*, London, 1912, p. 675).

With this he maintains that the bodily events are the emotion. The theory itself is put in the form of a suggestive question:

> Is it possible that the vasomotor disturbances, the changes in dimension of the blood vessels and thereby the amount of blood in the individual organs, are the real primary action of emotion, whereas the other events—abnormalities of movement, perception weaknesses, subjective sensations, changes in secretion, disturbances of intelligence—are only secondary disorders which have their cause in anomalies of vascular innervation?—(My rendering of Kurella edition, p. 41.)

Whereas Lange points to the vascular changes, Hunter uses 'the term emotion to refer to the visceral components of an instinct',[1] and Cameron also considers the term emotion directs our 'attention to visceral activities' in particular.[2]

For Stieler, a process is emotional due not only to the visceral or vascular components; but when consciousness reflects the body as a whole in a state of excitement, when an agitation of the whole psychophysical person is paramount. The more an experience is characterized by the *body as a whole*, the more can it be said to be emotional.[3] He then draws a curious, but classical, analogy to

[1] Hunter, W. S., 'The Nature of Instinct and Its Modifications', *Psychosom. Med.*, 1942, p. 167.

[2] Cameron, N., *The Psychology of Behavior Disorders*, Boston, 1947, p. 72.

[3] Stieler, G., 'Die Emotionen', *Arch. f. d. Ges. Psychol.*, 1925, p. 381.

strengthen his argument: God has no emotions like human emotions, because God has no body. ('One can indeed attribute to God knowledge and will and also inclinations, but no emotion analogous to human emotions, no excitement, feelings, affects, etc.'[1] Spinoza wrote to the same effect;[2] but Augustine maintained that Christ felt affects[3] and Lactantius wrote an important treatise on God's wrath.[4]

So far the position is: Emotion consists of bodily events. These events can be described as 'anomalies of vascular innervation' (Lange)—a forerunner of this view can be found in Crichton (1798);[5] or as visceral components (Hunter and Cameron)—compare Pinel (1801)[6] who located the seat of mania in the stomach; or simply the body as a whole (Stieler). Further specification of these bodily events gives more specific theories of emotion. For example, Allen (1877)[7] and Lagerborg (1905)[8] refer to *nutritional processes*. Lotze (1852)[9] lays emphasis on the *spinal cord*: the more intense the emotion the farther down the spinal cord is the activity. Spencer (1855)[10] holds that the amount of bodily movement is proportional to the intensity of the emotion. This view that the more 'body' is in the event, the more is the event emotional is similar to the view of Stieler, except that Spencer lays emphasis on the *muscles*. Both he and Lotze find weak emotions expressed by the small muscles of the face. Meynert (1892)[11] stresses the role of *breathing*, and he correlates vaso-dilation with sthenic emotions and vaso-construction with asthenic ones. Modern counterparts of the relation of emotion to specific body regions and processes is given in Dunbar's great volume (EBC).

Such specifications can lead to extremes of peripheral localization, such as Dunlap's well-known catch-phrase: 'the pain is in my toe'. From this it might seem that the peripheral view of emotion, i.e. emotion is referable to specific regions of the body, when driven to its logical conclusion dwindles into nonsense. But this is only nonsense when these peripheral events are taken as mechanistic causes of emotion, as is often the case in the nineteenth-century views just mentioned. It is far better to see, however, that the intention here is to stress the manifest phenomena of emotion, the gross bodily events,

[1] *Ibid.*,
[2] Spinoza, *Ethica*, V, Prop. 17.
[3] Augustine, *City of God*, XIV, 9.
[4] Lactantius, *De Ira Dei*, ANCL, XXII.
[5] Crichton, A., *An Inquiry into the Nature and Origin of Mental Derangement*, 2 vols., London, 1798.
[6] Pinel, P., *Traité médico-philosophique sur l'aliénation mentale*, Paris, 1801.
[7] Allen, G., *Physiological Aesthetics*, London, 1877.
[8] Lagerborg, R., *Das Gefühlsproblem*, Leipzig, 1905.
[9] Lotze, R. H., *Medizinische Psychologie*, Leipzig, 1852.
[10] Spencer, H., *The Principles of Psychology*, London, 1855.
[11] Meynert, T., *Sammlung von populär-wissenschaftlichen Vorträgen*, Vienna/Leipzig, 1892.

117

rather than subtle mental events or hidden cerebral mechanisms. As Dunlap says: '. . . visceral occurrences are demonstrable. Hence, when I use the term emotion I mean these things. This is the final *demonstration*'.[1] These demonstrable events—sweating, pallor, tachycardia—are not to be taken as causes of emotion, unless we revert to a very simplified kind of materialistic causation, but rather as emotion itself. This emotion, these demonstrations are then best grasped on the level of phenomenological understanding, rather than in terms of some central system of operations which hypothetically lies behind and is their explanation. The explanation lies in understanding the meaning of the manifestations. In this way, the older arguments between peripheral (body) and central (head) theories can be seen in the light of two contrary approaches: a phenomenological approach to the *manifestations* of emotion as opposed to a reductive-explanatory approach to the *hidden causes* of emotion.

Wenger's theory would seem to overlook this fundamental problem. He follows Lange and Dunlap in understanding emotion as visceral activity, that is as bodily manifestations, but he refers this activity to an hypothesis of the central type, the autonomic nervous system.

> For me, then, emotion became inner motion, i.e. visceral action, as elicited by these reverberating circuits—the autonomic nervous system. Since rereading Lange's early work I am inclined to believe that this point of view should be considered an extension of his original theory.—M. Wenger, 'Emotion as Visceral Action: An Extension of Lange's Theory', FE 50, p. 4.
>
> It is obvious that under this theory the term 'emotion' would undergo a semantic metamorphosis. It would be absolved of many of its current connotations and would acquire a meaning much more closely related to its Latin root *emovere* and to its early usage, which sought to describe an 'inner turbulence'. Emotion would be continuous, because autonomic activity is continuous, while the state of homeostasis would be regarded as a state of emotion, and we would speak of increased or decreased emotion from this basic pattern. We would distinguish between emotions per se only insofar as we can differentiate patterns of visceral change, and we no longer would speak of visceral changes induced by emotion.—*Ibid.*, p. 5.

We have seen already the hypothesis that emotion is always going on and can only be distinguished quantitatively (Chapters I and VII) or by patterns of visceral change (Chapter IV). If we accept this description of emotion as a continuous autonomic activity, emotion tends to become muddled with the life of the organism in general or what used to be called the psyche, so that this model is a definite iteration of a very old doctrine of the soul. The British scholar at the

---

[1] Dunlap, K., 'Emotion as a Dynamic Background', FE 28, p. 153.

court of Charlemagne, Alcuin, defined the soul as 'always in motion' (*semper in motu*),[1] and this notion was taken up again by Alexander of Hales and Albertus Magnus and it provides another amplification of the doctrine of the motions of the animal spirits.

The juxtaposition of a concept of the soul with the autonomic nervous system is also to be found in the theory of López Esnaurrízar. He examines several emotions (joy, love, desire, anger) to show that 'we feel emotion through the sympathetic system, and the internal changes which produce the emotion are functions of the sympathetic system'.[2] The sympathetic is said to be in 'intimate relation with or to be the finest instrument of the soul (comprising feelings and emotions, desires, impulses and appetites)'.[3] The soul and the sympathetic are both distributed throughout the body and are both of 'exquisite sensibility'. But the paper ends leaving us only with this 'correspondence', not specifying further the relation of the sympathetic, emotion and the soul.

A specification of this relation is made by De Crinis. Unlike López Esnaurrízar who suggests that the physiological system is an instrument of the soul, De Crinis reduces the soul to the physiological system:

> Vegetative processes are not open to 'psychic' influences, but are the very foundation of them. Psychic lability does not express itself in vegetative lability, but vegetative lability is the basis of 'psychic' lability. . . .—M. De Crinis, *Der Affekt und seine körperlichen Grundlagen*, Leipzig, 1944, p. 62. (Italics in original.) (My translation.)

Emotion is defined as 'Ergriffenheit' (p. 71), or state of being seized, touched or affected by the environment. But emotion does not depend on the environment:

> Events in the environment are not the psychic (mental) cause of an affect, but rather the bodily reactions which are going on in us. These are ordered by the vegetative system. The vegetative system is thus decisive in determining the way in which psychically apprehended events of the outer and inner world will be experienced.—*Ibid.*, p. 78.

The way in which events are received by the vegetative system depends particularly upon the way in which this system has been conditioned through memory traces of former experiences (p. 79), its rhythm (pp. 63–6) and also through constitutional factors such as organ inferiority (pp. 72–3). Individual inner organs (heart, liver,

---

[1] Schneider, A., 'Die Psychologie Alberts des Grossen', *Beitr. z. Gesch. d. Phil. d. Mittelalters*, IV, 6, 1903, pp. 370–80. Seydl, E., 'Alkuins Psychologie', *Jhbch. f. Phil. u. spek. Theol.*, 1911, pp. 34–55.

[2] López Esnaurrízar, M., 'Las Emociones y el Simpático', *Medicina México*, 1953, p. 457. (Orbeli's theory—according to London, 'Theory of Emotions in Soviet Dialectic Psychology', FE 50, p. 86—is also based upon the sympathetic system.)

[3] *Ibid.*, p. 459.

guts, etc.) are also embraced by the concept of the vegetative system and have specific relations to specific emotions (p. 77).

This theory brings together both peripheral and central kinds of arguments, but the central one is dominant since the vegetative system governs the peripheral organs to which are related the specific emotions (liver and depression, urinary system and ambition, etc.).

Another set of 'body' hypotheses of this central sort are those that explain emotion in terms of *glands*.

If we follow Dunbar in saying that the 'endocrine-hormonal system appears to supersede most other organ systems in its rheostatic control of biochemical equilibrium',[1] then it is easy to see how attractive it is to explain emotion in terms of hormones. Since emotion generally defined as movement appears so often as upset and disbalance, and since this disbalance is demonstrable biochemically, and further, if the highest regulatory control depends on the hormonal system, then why not link emotion to that system?

Berman does just that in an extraordinary fashion:

> The chemical mechanisms of the emotions described: sex libido, passion and jealousy in relation to the ovaries and testes, fear and anger in relation to the adrenals, sympathy and curiosity in relation to the pituitaries, suggests that a similar explanation will hold for the dynamics of the other instincts. In the closest relation to the thyroid appear . . . self-display and self-effacement, accompanied by emotions of pride and shame . . .—L. Berman, *The Glands Regulating Personality*, N.Y., 1930, p. 212.

Geikie-Cobb[2] does the same, giving emotional attributes to the endocrine organs, while Dorfman[3] attempts to make a 'correlation' between hormones and emotions. Wiener[4] suggests that the hormones in the blood might be the 'carriers' of emotion. Gray explains the relation of emotion and endocrine functioning as follows:

> Thus, emotion can be explained objectively as the intense but temporary bodily behavior initiated by some sort of stimulation sufficient to bring about immediate action of the endocrines (and a resultant change in blood chemistry), profound visceral activity, heightened muscle tonus, increased sensitivity, etc. These physiological changes (especially the changes in blood chemistry) then stimulate the internal receptors and the organism *feels* emotional. He feels himself behaving in that way called emotional. Different emotional feelings are distinguished because blood chemistry and other physiological changes are so

[1] EBC, p. 261.
[2] Geikie-Cobb, I., *The Glands of Destiny*, 3rd edn., London, 1947.
[3] Dorfman, W., 'Endocrines and Emotions', *N.Y. State J. Med.*, 1954, pp. 1331–7.
[4] Wiener, N., *The Human Use of Human Beings: Cybernetics and Society*, N.Y., 1954.

characteristically different for the various emotions that the proprioceptors are stimulated differently. This is no psychic state but physical
behavior in response to internal stimulation.—J. S. Gray, 'An Objective
Theory of Emotion', *Psychol. Rev.*, 1935, p. 116.

On this view emotion is physical behaviour caused by blood chemistry. The psychic aspect is secondary and reducible to physical
events. This is the main hypothesis presented by Berman, Geikie-
Cobb, Naccarati[1] and Gray in slightly different ways.

Braceland[2] takes a more cautious and differentiated view. He
warns against this kind of one-to-one, cause-and-effect relation. He
interprets the gross emotional reactions exhibited after hormone
therapy in Addison's and in Cushing's diseases as being due to 'violent
shifts in the internal environment' which constitute as much a situation of stress as do radical external changes. For him then emotion
is conceived as a reaction to environmental change, whether inner
or outer. The result is a view of emotion in terms of *situation*
(Chapter XI).

For M. Bleuler, the emotional and the hormonal are two aspects
of one substance:

> It is not that there are emotional and endocrine phenomena which
> influence each other; but rather these data are often better understood
> when one takes both the emotional and endocrine functions as different
> aspects of the same undivided living process.—M. Bleuler, *Endokrino-
> logische Psychiatrie*, Stuttgart, 1954, pp. 72–3. (My translation.)

Jores calls emotions effectors or realizers (*Realisatoren*).[3] And like
Bleuler he sees no causal relation between hormone and psyche, but
rather that they are two aspects of the same living process. The result
is a view of emotion in terms of isomorphism such as we interpreted
it in Chapter IV.

And so we find the relation of hormones and emotion can be conceived in different ways, depending upon the way in which emotion
is conceived and also upon the way in which the mind-body problem
is formulated. If human behaviour is chemical behaviour we have
one kind of theory; if human behaviour involves other kinds of
factors, then theories bring in other kinds of hypotheses such as
isomorphism or situation or energy-balance.

There are two conclusions which we can draw here: The first is
technical. Following Dunbar we have said that the endocrine system
has much to do with high-level control of physiological balance. But

[1] Naccarati, S., 'Hormones and Emotions', *Med. Rec.*, 1921, pp. 910–15.
[2] Braceland, F. J., 'Hormones and their Influence on the Emotions', *Bull. N.Y. Acad.
Med.*, 1953, p. 769.
[3] Jores, A., 'Hormone und Psyche', *Wien. Klin. Wchnschr.* 66, 1954, p. 4 f.

also following Dunbar, we do not know how this works, nor how it works in connection with even the most physiologically investigated emotions of rage and fear.

> Too little is known about the synchronization which is required to bring about healthy functioning of the endocrine-hormonal system. Even less is known about the type of disequilibrium that may be brought about by such emotions as fear and rage or by one or another type of disequilibrium in a personality.—F. Dunbar, EBC, p. 271.

The second conclusion is not a problem of empirical knowledge but of theory-forming. The relation between hormones and emotion ultimately depends upon the way in which the mind-body problem is conceived, as is shown by the different kinds of conclusions drawn by the different investigators in the field. And so, should we speculatively offer our own hypothesis (which would relate hormones to emotions not only in terms of balance-disbalance but also in terms of the concept of realization, that is in terms of a transforming function which makes happenings concretely real in so far as they become lived by the body, here and now) we cannot argue such a view without specifying the relation of hormones and emotion in terms of the mind-body problem. We can state that emotions are catalysts and that hormones are catalysts and that both are necessary to motion, process and change, but the nature of the relation between these kinds of catalysts remains in the dark.

The same body-mind problem occurs in the discussion of therapy of emotional disorders through bodily agents. As we have already seen, energetic views of emotion propose energetic methods of treatment. Theories in which a concept of the unconscious is the dominant hypothesis offer depth analysis while theories of cerebral location suggest lobotomy, etc. Here the proposals look to the body. Lange says:

> If emotional states can be released through the enjoyment of certain products or by means of other purely bodily methods, it follows that one can reduce and overcome annoying affects in the same way; as brandy and opium bring forth joy, so, too, are they effective against worry, etc. —C. Lange, *op. cit. sup.*, p. 56.

López Esnaurrízar suggests treatment via the sympathetic in keeping with his location of emotion in that system. Here we enter the field of psycho-pharmacology in which a body theory of emotion plays a major part. For, whether it be the spirits and opium mentioned by Lange, or the enigmatic beans of Pythagoras, whether it be tobacco,[1]

[1] See Sargant, W., 'On Chemical Tranquillizers', *Brit. Med. J.*, 1956, 4973, where tobacco and alcohol are compared with recent drugs.

tonics, herbs, diets, stimulants or tranquillizers,[1] the principle is the same.[2] A change in an emotional state can be brought about directly by a change in the bodily state. Even the old Stoic concept of *ataraxia* (freedom from the disturbance of passion) has been brought out again and been suggested as a fitting description for the new tranquillizing agents,[3] which points to how the problem of emotion is now being approached through the body.[4] The literature here is legion, but one fact stands out among the great lot of technical reports: there is some sort of third factor or intervening variable between the pharmacological and the emotional aspects. There is not a one-to-one relation between the drug and the reaction, since—as even such an enthusiastic drug protagonist as Himwich[5] admits—not all patients are affected equally by these chemical substances, something which might be expected if human behaviour were fundamentally chemical behaviour. Human behaviour involves something else, something personal or individual, demonstrable even chemically, since no two humans can be shown to have the same chemical composition.

Those who have looked into this third factor come up with different suggestions. Gold[6] speaks of the unconscious bias of the physician and of the patient's mood. Lasagna, *et al.*,[7] show how the prior personality pattern is an important variable. Sabshin and Ramot[8] emphasize the social field or total situation. Sarwer-Foner writes:

> A complex is formed by the interaction of pharmacologic effect on the one hand, and the psychological meaning of this pharmacologic effect, in terms of the patient's total situation, on the other. This is never a function of the drug alone. The resultant change in affect depends on this interaction and *not* primarily on the . . . drug concerned.—G. J. Sarwer-Foner, 'The Transference and Nonspecific Drug Effects in the Use of the

---

[1] Perhaps the earliest use of the term tranquillizer which one finds in psychiatric literature is in Benjamin Rush's *Medical Inquiries and Observations upon the Diseases of the Mind*, Philadelphia, 1812, p. 181. He calls a 'tranquillizer', a special chair into which he put the unruly insane, finding it preferable to the 'straitwaistcoat'. Rush, George Washington's physician, belongs among the precursors of the views of this chapter in that he took insanity (disordered emotion) to be an affection of the blood.

[2] See de Ropp, R. S., *Drugs and the Mind*, N.Y., 1957, for a good account of the many varieties of such 'psychopharmaceutics'.

[3] Fabing, H. D., 'The Dimensions of Neurology' (Pres. Address), Am. Acad. Neurol., 1955.

[4] 'In America . . . in 1956 30,000 million tablets of one popular tranquillizer alone were sold.'—*The Times* (London) July 17, 1957, p. 6.

[5] Himwich, H. E., 'Prospects in Psychopharmacology', *J. Nerv. Ment. Dis.*, 1955, p. 422.

[6] Gold, H., 'How to Evaluate a New Drug', *Am. J. Med.*, 17, 1954, p. 722-7.

[7] Lasagna, L., von Felsinger, J., Beecher, H., 'Drug Induced Mood Changes in Man, I and II', *J.A.M.A.*, *157*, 1955, pp. 1006-20, 1113-19.

[8] Sabshin, M., and Ramot, J., 'Pharmacotherapeutic Evaluations and the Psychiatric Setting', *Arch. Neurol. Psychiat.* 1956, pp. 362-70.

Tranquilizing Drugs, and their Influence on Affect', *Research in Affects* (Psychiatric Research Reports, 8, 1957), p. 164.

And again we find that in explaining the relation of drugs and emotions the theories must rely upon such basic kinds of hypotheses as situation, meaning, the unconscious, genetic constitution or upon emotion itself as mood, suggestibility or personal idiosyncrasy.

Recent research into the organic component in the psychoses leads no further in solving the problem of the relation of chemical substances and emotions. Experiment establishes that certain substances (LSD and indole compounds) produce emotional patterns of behaviour, just as other substances 'tranquillize'. But, unless we are willing to say that these substances are emotions crystallized out in the form of protein molecules, we are left trying to figure out this connection of substance and behaviour in terms of one of the basic hypotheses already mentioned. As a help here the model of Aristotelian causes can be useful. On this model, these substances can be causes of one type, e.g. efficient or material, and as such are components of emotional behaviour. Precision of this component, valuable as it might be, can never circumscribe the entire event of which the purpose (final cause) and the specific pattern (formal cause) are also components of the personality disorder, the emotion, or the psychosis.

Therefore, chemical ataraxia as well as chemical ecstasy (mescalin visions,[1] going berserk on bufotenine[2]) is an attempt to reduce a complex to a simple. The whole emotion, the whole personality, is treated in terms of its chemical component. And even in the extreme case, e.g. where an emotional state is considered due only and directly to a chemical toxin, such therapy neglects the complexity of the event. Chemical therapy treats the living body as a retort in which substances work on one another.[3] But is it not by now well known that nothing happens in that retort without the catalyzing activities of the retort itself? A substance outside a living body is not the same as a substance inside a living body of which it forms a partial component. Once assimilated, it is no longer independent and therefore no longer rightly a substance, but becomes an aspect of the body's life. Toxic conditions may well be emotional; but it does not follow that emotional conditions must be toxic. To think like this is to be caught

---

[1] Huxley, A., *The Doors of Perception*, N Y., 1954.

[2] Fabing, H. D., 'Toads, Mushrooms, and Schizophrenia', *Harper's Magazine* 214, May ,1957, N.Y. Further references available in de Ropp, *op. cit. sup.*

[3] 'All diseases are caused by chemicals, and all diseases can be cured by chemicals. All the chemicals used by the body—except for the oxygen which we breathe and the water which we drink—are taken in through food. If we only knew enough, all disease could be prevented, and could be cured through proper nutrition.'—T. D. Spies (Recipient of the A.M.A. Distinguished Service Award), quoted in *Newsweek* (Internat. edn.), XLIX, 24 June 1957, p. 41.

in that ancient rationalistic cobweb—which we shall try to take apart in later chapters—that entangles emotion with disease.

The fundamental conclusion of this section is a paradox. Emotion as a physical, corporal, material event cannot be explained directly by these events. Bodily location is not the same as, nor does it necessarily entail, bodily explanation. There are two different things being said in this section: 'Emotion consists of bodily demonstrations' and 'Emotion is produced by bodily activities'. By not keeping separate these two ideas, various muddles develop, such as taking a location as explanatory, or an explanation as a concrete localization. Dunlap's pain-in-the-toe is a statement of location not explanation. When others explain emotion through chemical substances it does not mean that emotion is located in those substances.

The first idea, 'Emotion consists of bodily demonstrations', strictly locates the emotion in the place where it appears. The manifest peripheral events are the emotion. Emotion is located, here and now, in these visceral, glandular, vascular changes. It is not somewhere else in a psychic state, a hidden system, an external situation, a buried complex, or a chemical substance.

The second idea, 'Emotion is produced by bodily activities', reduces the manifest to something else. This something else in the body has ranged through an incredible number of postulates in the history of theory-forming.[1] Every gland, region, organ, system, fluid, tissue and chemical substance has been mentioned at one time or another. The difference between these various postulates depends in part upon empirical techniques. But it depends even more upon which level of abstraction is considered to provide the necessary and sufficient conditions for explanation. These levels range from specific organs, to more complicated systems (vasomotor, endocrine, autonomic), to higher and more central abstractions such as we saw in the last section (X A). In all one idea is dominant: the gross and general bodily events are produced by higher, subtler, and partial events. The higher operates the lower. This approach, where scientifically conventional in proceeding from the many, particular and concrete to the one, general and abstract, also betrays an attitude towards the body.[2] The body's dramatic demonstrations are reduced to symptoms, toxic states, expressions or discharges. Action is called reaction.

[1] Duprat, G. L. ('La Psycho-physiologie des passions dans la philosophie ancienne', *Arch. f. d. Gesch. der Phil. XI* (N.F.), 1905, pp. 395–412) gives many examples from the ancients.

[2] A beautiful example of this devaluation of the body can be found in the seldom quoted last paragraphs of Lange's famous monograph: 'The goal of all education . . . is to lead the individual towards the mastery, subjugation and destruction of the instinctual impulses (*Triebe*). . . . Taken physiologically, one can see education as a training of the ability of resolving or mastering reflexes of a simpler or more primitive

All the theories of this second, central kind cannot stand alone as bodily theories. As we have seen they rest upon other main hypotheses which must be called in to deal with the relations of chemical substances and behaviour, between body and mind, and also to deal with the problem of this third factor which complicates the relations. Therefore, these theories are not body theories, but ultimately theories of situation, isomorphism, energy-balance, etc.

We are left then with the first, peripheral kind—emotion consists of bodily demonstrations. But this statement is encrusted with disputable corollaries which must be stripped away, e.g. the bodily demonstrations cause mental events like feelings; the bodily demonstrations are caused by other bodily events, mental events, external events; the demonstrations are significant or meaningless; they are disordered or ordered; emotion is only bodily demonstrations— (God having no body has no emotion).

So that now if we ask what this section has told us about emotion, there remains the one striking fact which these theories each have pointed to: *emotion is physical. It consists of gross demonstrations of the body.* This statement must be qualified in two ways. First, the bodily demonstrations are not identical with the emotion, nor even can they be predicted for or correlated to specific emotions. Fear, for example, can be demonstrated by shaking, by running, by motionless paralysis, by vomiting and urinating, by excitement and thrill and screaming. One cannot say that each emotion has its own specific demonstration. One can only say that for an emotion to be an emotion there must be some bodily demonstration—and this holds true for those rare and saintly states of beatitude, not just the turmoils of fright, rage or lust. This leads to a second qualification: all emotion must be judged by this criterion. When hope, awe, boredom or gladness do not transfuse the body, we have only feelings, sensations, attitudes, or what you will. But we do not have emotion. As Darwin put it: 'So a man may intensely hate another, but until his bodily frame is affected he cannot be said to be enraged.' [1]

C. THE MUSCLES

In the last section the vegetative and visceral events were presented

kind through higher reflexes. . . . In the course of the years, the vascular nerve centre loses, through the influence of control and the lack of use, more and more its emotional activity and this developmental result . . . is carried over through heredity to successive generations. . . . So that finally is reached indeed Kant's ideal of the man of pure reason to whom every affect, every joy or sorrow, anxiety or fright—providing such attacks are still experienced—is taken as an illness, a mental derangement, which is unfitting for him.'—*Op. cit.*, pp. 79–80.

[1] Darwin, C., *The Expression of the Emotions in Man and Animals* (pop. edn.), London, 1904, p. 248 (Chapter X).

as primary to the muscular ones. A statement from Sherrington puts the matter slightly differently. It implies the visceral events serve the muscular ones:

> There is a strong bond between emotion and muscular action. Emotion 'moves' us, hence the word itself. . . . Every vigorous movement of the body, though its more obvious instrument be the skeletal musculature of the limbs and trunk, involves also the less noticeable cooperation of the viscera, especially of the circulatory and respiratory. The extra demand made upon the muscles that move the frame involves a heightened action of the nutrient organs which supply to the muscles the material for their energy. This increased action of the viscera is colligate with this activity of the muscles. We should expect visceral action to occur along with the muscular expression of emotion.—Sir C. Sherrington, *The Integrative Action of the Nervous System*, 1947 edn., Cambridge, p. 266.

The 'strong bond between emotion and muscular action' is the theme in these views. The work of Tuke in the last century gives much space to this idea.[1] This muscular action through its connection to the voluntary motor system is not remote from 'willing' as were those vegetative, autonomic and chemical activities of the blood, glands and gut. Furthermore, this muscular action as motion involves the positions or postures of the musculo-skeletal system, conceived as *attitudes*, which the dictionary meaning of the word brings out: 'posture of the body proper to or implying some mental state'. And so emotion in this section is also presented as an attitude.

Kennard[2] differentiates three aspects of emotion—cortical, autonomic, muscular—like these three parts of this chapter we have devoted to physiological location. For her, the muscles play their part in serving emotional expression. Allport, too, does not confine his explanation all to the muscles. The primary division of emotions into pleasant and unpleasant is based upon the activation of one or the other of the two divisions of the autonomic nervous system. Besides, in his view, emotion is to be understood in terms of conditioned and innate responses. But the qualitative differentiation of one emotion from another depends upon 'the proprioceptors in the muscles, tendons and joints'.[3]

Washburn interprets emotion in terms of muscular movements:

> An emotion occurs in a situation of vital significance to the organism; primitively, perhaps, the flight, fighting, or mating situations. In such a situation, the possibilities of response may be divided into several classes. First, there may occur adaptive movements of the striped muscles,

[1] Tuke, D. H., *Illustrations of the Influence of the Mind upon the Body*, London, 1872.
[2] Kennard, M. A., 'Autonomic Interrelation with the Somatic Nervous System', *Psychsom. Med.*, 1947, p. 29 f.
[3] Allport, F. H., *Social Psychology*, Cambridge, U.S.A., 1924, p. 92.

adequately meeting the situation: movements of flight, fighting, or mating. Secondly, there may be non-adaptive movements of the striped muscles. Some of these, like human facial expressions, are survivals. . . . But the most striking instance of non-adaptive movements is constituted by what may be called the motor explosion: the kicks and screams of the baffled child, the curses and furniture abuse of the baffled adult, the wild expansive movements of extreme joy. A motor explosion tends to happen when adaptive response is impossible.—M. Washburn, 'Emotion and Thought: A Motor Theory of their Relations', FE 28, p. 106.

On the motor theory here suggested, emotion, then, interferes with thought only when the movements made in emotion are incompatible with the movements and attitudes essential to thinking. . . . Emotion will aid thought when conditions favor the discharge of . . . energy into the maintenance of a steady innervation of the trunk muscles, which is the basis of introspectively reported feelings of will, determination, activity, or effort . . . (p. 111).

Her theory brings in various hypotheses: the three basic reaction patterns of Watson (Chapter XII), the notion of phylogenetic survival, the notion that emotion is a failure, and a notion of energy. The main hypothesis, however, is that emotion is a muscular event.

Jacobson, who did extensive experimentation on muscular events, finds an essential part of emotion to consist of 'neuro-muscular patterns'. This goes beyond the notion put by Kennard, for example, that the muscles merely serve the expression aspect of emotion. For Jacobson, as for Washburn, the muscular patterns are essential.

Evidence has been given in the preceding pages which suggests that an essential part of mental and emotional activities consists of neuro-muscular patterns; the latter are not just 'expressions' of emotion . . . in physical terms, the energy expended in a neuromuscular pattern is identical with, and not a transformation of, the energy of the corresponding mental and emotional activity. If this is true, it follows that the extreme relaxation of a muscular pattern essential to a particular mental or emotional process must bring with it the diminution of that process.
—E. Jacobson, *Progressive Relaxation*, Univ. of Chicago, 1929, p. 295.

Finley's theory emphasizes the striped and unstriped muscles. Like Jacobson, he holds that a change in muscle patterns can change emotional behaviour. He suggests this as a therapeutic procedure.

The psychiatrist who holds many long interviews analyzing the patient's thoughts and alleged environmental stresses in an attempt to cure him of his emotional illness too often fails to reach the root of his problem, the unhealthy emotion. His unhealthy emotional behavior can be corrected through explaining in simple terms the mechanism of muscle relaxation. . . .—K. H. Finley, 'Emotional Physiology and its Influence on Thought Content', *J. Nerv. Ment. Dis.*, 1953, p. 445.

Emotion, when conceived as identical with muscular patterns (Jacobson), i.e. located in the muscles, can be re-ordered by re-ordering these patterns. This can be done in a multitude of ways. Following Finley, the therapy of emotional disorders consists in becoming conscious of muscular tensions. Other techniques are physical shock treatments with their tonic and clonic muscular effects, muscle-relaxant drugs, or such old-fashioned therapeutic and pedagogic measures as the hot bath, the walk-around-the-block, drill and marching in military organization, and games and exercises to correct school-children's 'unhealthy emotions'. More refined are the meditative techniques of Autogene Training[1] and Hatha Yoga. The prerequisite for Hatha Yoga is posture (*āsana*). A prodigious number of them have been described, but 'there is not a single *āsana* that is not intended directly or indirectly to quiet the mind . . .' [2] The dominant hypothesis in all these measures is that emotion is the postural set of the person; change it and emotion is changed, or even done away with.

The work of Nina Bull and her collaborators has produced a theory of emotion which is based upon this idea of postural set.

> Actually emotion is conceived as a sequence of neuromuscular events in which postural set or preparatory motor attitude is the initial step. This preparatory attitude is both involuntary and instinctive, and is the end result of a slight tentative movement which gives a new orientation to the individual, but does not go immediately into the consummatory stage of action. . . .
>
> The attitudinal factor is necessarily present (as postural preparation) in every bodily action whether emotional or not. When the behavior is impulsive and there is no delay between the preparatory and consummatory phases of the process, the sequence

> ATTITUDE————————————————➤ACTION

> proceeds without a break. In the course of the delay (not a delay of *reaction*, it should be noted, but of *action*) the process can be represented thus:

> ATTITUDE———— ————————————————————➤ACTION

> And since under these conditions of delay, *and these alone*, it is possible for feeling to arise, we can represent the double issue of the activated motor attitude in the following manner:

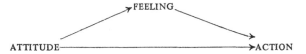

> ➤FEELING
>
> ATTITUDE————————————————➤ACTION

[1] Schulz, J. H., *Das Autogene Training*, 3rd edn., Leipzig, 1937.
[2] Bernard, T., *Hatha Yoga* (Ph.D. Thesis), Col. Univ., N.Y., 1944, pp. 1–6.

In this arrangement the attitude-plus-feeling combination, considered apart from the final-action stage, is equivalent to an *affective state.* . . . N. Bull, 'The Attitude Theory of Emotion', *Arch. di Psicol. Neurol. e Psichiat.*, 1951, pp. 108–9.[1]

She supports her theory with hypotheses drawn from two different areas of study: the neuro-anatomic mechanisms described by Papez and elaborated by MacLean and others, and her own experiments in hypnosis. The latter has bearing on her theory in the following way:

> A series of hypnotic sessions was conducted in which a specific postural set (emotional attitude) was first induced and then locked (hypnotically fixed), after which a contrasting affect was suggested. *There was repeated demonstration of the dependence of affect on bodily changes, those in the realm of postural set being particularly marked.* Without somatic changes of some kind no new affect of any kind was obtained. . . .— B. Pasquarelli and N. Bull, 'Experimental Investigations of the Body-Mind Continuum in Affective States', *J. Nerv. Ment. Dis.*, 1951, p. 521.

(The same sort of experiments resulting in the same sort of conclusions were made a century before by James Braid, the Manchester physician and coiner of the term 'hypnotism' (1843). 'Braid found that passions can be produced by putting hypnotized people in appropriate attitudes.' [2]) Bull further supports her view with a statement from Coghill: 'Emotion is a psycho-organismic posture charged with feeling, or motivated feeling toward an object.' [3] Gemelli[4] identifies what he calls an instinctive or biological nucleus, a kind of inborn complex pattern, with this motor attitude of Bull. Gesell[5] also follows Bull in calling emotion 'the feeling of a motor attitude'.

In connection here, several papers by other writers bring into significant relationship emotion and motor activity. Ferrari[6] and

---

[1] See also, Bull, N., *J. Nerv. Ment. Dis. Monograph Series No.* 81, 1951; N. Bull, *Psychosom. Med.*, 1945; N. Bull and E. Strongin, *J. Nerv. Ment. Dis.*, 1956. However, long before Bull's concept of the postural set became concretized into the muscles, the same sort of conceptual model was being used as the explanation of emotion. Aristotle's *orexis* literally means 'a stretching out; as of the hands, in entreaty'. This faculty was different from the faculty of movement, just as Bull's affective states are different from actions. Other examples of this postural set are such concepts as appetite (*appeto* = I seek, attack) and desire (*desidero* = I look eagerly towards) which have been given as the traditional equivalents of *orexis* and as the ground of emotion. (Definitions in this paragraph from C. Spearman, *Psychology Down the Ages*, London, 1937, Vol. I, p. 172.)

[2] Darwin, C., *The Expression of the Emotions in Man and Animals* (pop. edn.), London, 1904, p. 388, fn. 6 (Chapter XIV).

[3] Quoted by Pasquarelli and Bull, *op. cit.*, p. 520, from C. J. Herrick, *George Elliott Coghill*, Univ. of Chicago, 1947.

[4] Gemelli, A., 'Orienting Concepts in the Study of Affective States', *J. Nerv. Ment. Dis.*, 1949, pp. 306–7.

[5] Gesell, A., 'Emotion from the Standpoint of a Developmental Morphology', FE 50, p. 393.

[6] Ferrari, G., 'Psicologia dei Moribundi', *Riv. di Psicol.*, 1920, pp. 101–7.

130

Gualino[1] have described the behaviour of several military deserters condemned to be shot. Evidence of disintegration of their behaviour appeared earliest in postural reflexes, mental control usually being maintained until the last. Blatz[2] observes that his subjects, whose organic reactions during the fear of falling were under investigation, called their emotion 'fear' only in the first experience, when they tried to escape, i.e. when they made motor movements.

There seem to be two different ways in which the muscles and the voluntary motor system are used in this section to ground emotion. Kennard, Washburn, Sherrington, and Blatz take emotion as *motion*, while Bull and co-workers and Finley interpret emotion as *delay*, as motion delayed in the muscles, still in the tension of the postural set. But whether it is taken as motion or as delay, the basis of explanation is the striped muscles and voluntary motor system, i.e. a system amenable to the will.

Emotion and will have a long history of conceptual involvement. Such concepts as *orexis*, desire, conation, *horme* have been given as the common basis of both. (Such common bases in modern terms are instinct, drive, motivation, sub-cortical levels, endothymic ground.) Augustine[3] best represents those who reduce emotion to will, while Hobbes[4] stands for those who place emotion first. Maine de Biran[5] presents the classic argument for a basic separation of emotion and will. But Bain, Rehmke, Ribot, Heymans, Wiersma and Jordan group will and emotion together.[6] In Losskij's 'voluntarism', emotion is a 'rudimentary' kind of willing.[7] This conative theory of emotion is still current, e.g. Ewing states: 'I shall in fact contend . . . that the central feature in emotion is not feeling but conation'[8] and 'I certainly . . . do not wish to reduce emotions to bodily actions, but I do wish to insist that the essential point for their valuation is the conative side, the mental counterpart of bodily action'.[9] The attempt of Harms[10] to differentiate emotion and affect from feeling and willing through the idea of ego-control is also based on a psychology of

[1] Gualino, L., 'Psicofisiologia dei Fucilandi', *Riv. di Psicol.*, 1920, pp. 42–60.

[2] Blatz, W., 'The Cardiac, Respiratory and Electrical Phenomena Involved in The Emotion of Fear', *J. Exper. Psychol.*, 1925, pp. 109–32.

[3] Augustine, *De Civitate Dei*, XIV, 5 f.

[4] Hobbes, *De Homine*, II, 11, 2.

[5] Maine de Biran, F. P. G., 'Essai sur les fondements de la Psychologie' (1812), Chapters I and II, *Œuvres inédites*, Paris, 1859.

[6] Spearman, C., *Psychology Down the Ages*, London, 1937, Vol. I, p. 175.

[7] K.B., pp. 253 ff.

[8] Ewing, A. C., 'The Justification of Emotions', (Symposium) *The Aristotelian Society, Suppl. Vol. XXXI*, London, 1957, p. 62.

[9] *Ibid.*, p. 71.

[10] Harms, E., 'A Differential Concept of Feelings and Emotions', FE 50, p. 153.

conation. For him feeling, willing and thinking are ego-controlled, that is, voluntary; emotion, affect and day-dreaming are their uncontrolled or involuntary counterparts. (We might recall Plato's discussion of the passions in terms of the 'voluntary' and 'involuntary' (*Laws*, IX).—With all this, what then is the relation of emotion and will?

This entanglement of the two concepts has to do with two ways of conceiving that primary fact of life—motion. When this motion is conceived as a being-moved, as a *passio*, it is linked with the *autonomic* nervous system, the sub-cortical brain, the irrational instincts, the unruly horse, archaic autonomous images, or any set of explanatory hypotheses which posit this motion as *uncontrolled*, contrary and inferior to the conscious will.[1] Such motion is always conceived as *disorder*. When the motion is taken to be an *action* in accordance with, or of the same kind as, the conscious will, then emotion tends to be formulated as an intentional, creatively purposeful attitude, posture or set, served by or located in the *voluntary* nervous system. In the views of this section, this division does not quite hold since emotion is taken as a disorder or *passio* (delayed action—Bull; motor explosion—Washburn; disintegration of postural reflexes—Ferrari and Gualino), yet it is in the *voluntary* system. How can we account for involuntary events in a voluntary system?

Conceptual analysis may lead us to an answer better than physiological analysis, since we are dealing with the concept of voluntary as an interpretation of physiological facts, not with the neural facts themselves. Only a cursory glance at the concept of will reveals a fundamental division. From Plato's two horses, rational and irrational and Thomas Aquinas' division of appetite into sensitive and intellectual, to the division of the will in modern philosophy (natural determinism *vs.* individual free-will) exemplified on the one hand by Schopenhauer's objective, natural will and on the other by Keller's[2] subjective, directed activity of the ego, we find *the will is two wills*. But only one of these wills is considered conscious (Plato's white horse, Thomas Aquinas' intellectual appetite, Keller's directed ego activity). The dictionary meanings of both 'will' and 'voluntary' bring this out. The first group of meanings is: desire, wish, inclination, carnal appetite; impulse, without constraint or prompting, spontaneous. The second set of meanings is: action of choosing, attitude of mind directed with conscious intention, determination; deliberate intent, designed. We find a concept of will associated with conscious deliberate action and a concept of will associated with

---

[1] See Chapter XI, p. 138, for Abelard's statement: 'Nusquam enim passio esse potest, nisi ubi contra voluntatem aliquid fit.'
[2] Keller, W., *Psychologie und Philosophie des Wollens*, München/Basel, 1954.

spontaneous non-conscious action. The concept of disorder does not enter unless we judge the spontaneous will from the standpoint of the deliberate will. Therefore, we have not so much to do with involuntary events in a voluntary system, but with *two different kinds of voluntary events*. The muscles and the voluntary motor system serve both kinds equally.

This has bearing on the conclusion of this section in the following way. When the motor system serves the second kind of willing we get those disintegrations, explosions and expressions which Washburn, Kennard and Blatz call emotion. When the motor system serves both wills simultaneously we get the delays and muscular tensions which Bull and Finley describe as emotion. In both views emotion is conceived as *disorder* and as *conflict*. We are told: In the muscles the two wills contend. (These tension patterns are the emotion—Jacobson. The proprioceptions of these muscular patterns are the differentia of emotion—Allport. These delayed actions still in the muscles are the ground of emotion—Bull.) We are simply being given the usual view of emotion as a conflict of two forces, here concretized into muscular behaviour.

This concretization, however, is just the positive *advantage* of these theories. Once emotion is explained through the muscles, it can be dealt with practically through the conscious will. (This is not so much the case when it is explained in terms of outer stimuli, universal energy, phylogenetic reaction patterns, autonomous complexes, erogenous zones, dream images, or the autonomic nervous system.) Therapy seeks to re-order the muscular patterns which are the emotion in conformity with the habitual, conscious will. This restoration can be brought about on a physiological level through shock or muscle-relaxants, or it can be done through the various disciplines and postural techniques mentioned above.[1] The aim is always to dominate the second kind of willing through the first kind, by not allowing it access to the motor system.

The question then arises: What happens to the vanquished willing of the second kind? According to the views in this section, when emotion is no longer in the muscles it is gone. Here is the *disadvantage*

---

[1] Choisy, M. ('Recherches expérimentales des émotions', *Arch. di Psicol. Neurol. e Psichiat.*, 1953, pp. 214 ff.) presents evidence for the amazing efficacy of such rational will techniques in overcoming emotion in exceptional cases. 109 Indian yogins were subjected to experimentally produced emotional situations (exposure to scorpions, cobras, etc.) and their physiological reactions (EEG, ECG, basal metabolism, psychogalvanic reflex, etc.) were recorded by a team with modern equipment. Choisy concludes: 'We are confronted with a human physiology that is other than simple animal physiology. The will seems to operate in a way . . . that hints at an infinite power of regulation and order for our higher faculties. . . . This rigorous discipline (yoga) . . . results in an almost complete mastery of vegetative life, which it robs of its designation "autonomous" . . .'

133

of such concretistic thinking, for it is very possible that this defeated and repressed emotion, since it is a kind of willing and therefore not without purpose, has been displaced or has regressed to other levels where it is no longer so accessible, e.g. autonomic symptom formation, dream images, projections on to outer events. In other words, when emotion is no longer muscular behaviour, it might very well be conceived to appear in other segments of the personality. Thus, the rigours and relaxations mentioned in this chapter—the walks and baths and drills, the postures of Yoga and Autogene Training—are in no way therapy in depth. They merely chase away the problem temporarily from its physical manifestations. It is, in fact, to be questioned whether these physical measures *alone* are therapeutic at all, in that under the guise of relaxation they foster repression.

The view of emotion as a bodily set, posture or attitude leads us to the next group of views because the motor system, the will, the muscles are all connected with activity in the world. Posture means a position vis-a-vis the world, or put another way, *posture is the embodied situation.*

XI

EMOTION AND SITUATION

THESE THEORIES still come under the rubric of location, i.e. *situs* = site. In the preceding two groups of location theories, emotion has been presented in terms of intra-personal events, psychological (Chapter IX) and physiological (Chapter X). Ideas of structures, attitudes, qualities and environment which will be appearing in this chapter have already been presented in the chapters previous. But there, when emotion was conceived as an attitude (Bull), this attitude belonged to the subject and could be initiated without regard to the situation. Or when emotion was conceived as a quality (Krueger), the quality belonged to subjective experience, not to the situation. Or when emotion was conceived through structures (Papez), topological centres (Hess), or environment (Braceland), these concepts referred to intra-subjective locations.

This way of thinking is in accord with the main stream of thought about emotion since at least the time of the Stoics, who held that the seat and cause of emotion lay completely within man's reason.[1] MacCurdy puts this position in our times very concisely: '. . . *in no case is it thought to be a quality of the stimulus, except in relation to the subject.*'[2]

But the views here will bring in a new idea. Intra-subjective location is not enough. Emotion cannot be understood or explained without taking into account the total situation in which it occurs. Lund puts it like this:

> . . . fear, horror, disgust, repulsion, aversion, dislike, annoyance, anger, sadness, sorrow, despair, hopelessness, pity, sympathy, hunger. . . . It should be apparent that these terms are not descriptive of so many internal or organic states. They are descriptive, in most cases, of objective situations and of accepted modes of handling and dealing with these.
> —F. H. Lund, *Emotions*, N.Y., 1939, pp. 113–14.

Landis writes: '*For an emotion to be an emotion it must be part of an*

[1] Zeller, E., *The Stoics, Epicureans and Sceptics*, London, 1892, p. 244.
[2] MacCurdy, J. T., *The Psychology of Emotion*, London, 1925, p. 44.

entire integrated situation.'[1] Landis bases his view upon experiments in recognizing emotions from photographs of faces. He concludes from these experiments:

> ... any description of an emotion was incomplete when it dealt only with the reaction of the organism itself, that an emotion was an emotion not because of any particular pattern of bodily reactions or temporal relationships but because of certain relationships existing between the reacting organism and its environment.—C. Landis, 'The Interpretation of Facial Expression in Emotion', *J. General Psychol.* 1929, p. 69.

The psychology of the Russian, Rubinshtein, as presented by London, also explains emotion in terms of situation, a situation taken sociologically.[2] The forms of emotion can be accounted for socially and historically and, rather than searching for causes in phylogenetic reaction patterns, one looks to socio-historical conditioning processes. For man's essence 'derives more from his society than from his bodily apparatus'.[3]

On this view, emotion is the resultant of socially determined forces which make up a situation. It is a reflection of social man's adjustment to social milieu and it forms part of the conditioning process itself, informing the individual of the success or failure of his adjustment. Emotion is but a reflection, a concomitant, in the same way that all psychic events are secondary reflections, as set forth by the postulate '... of the primacy of matter and the derived nature of the psyche as a reflection of it ...'[4]

Unlike this determined, sociological and materialistic concept of situation presented by Rubinshtein, is the situation understood phenomenologically (Nuttin) or psychologically (Prescott), where the emphasis falls on *meaning*.

> The psychological content of feeling and emotion originates in the behavioral contact—or lack of contact—of the individual with the *meaningful* situations of life. Emotional experience in general may be conceived as a *repercussion sui generis*, which the contact with a real or imagined situation evokes in a definite dynamical structure of the subject.—J. Nuttin, 'Intimacy and Shame in the Dynamic Structure of Personality', FE 50, p. 343.

> It is worth reiterating that an adequate insight into the causes of strong emotions cannot be achieved by thinking in terms of a simple, automatic, inciting stimulus. It is rare that emotions are aroused in this

---

[1] Landis, C., 'Emotion', in *Psychology*, by Boring, Langfeld and Weld, N.Y., 1935, p. 398; and also pp. 418–19.

[2] London, I. D., 'Theory of Emotions in Soviet Dialectic Psychology', FE 50. Since 1950, Soviet psychology has changed its tack back to the reflexology of Pavlov and Bekhterev (Chapter XII). (See G. Razran, 'Soviet Psychology since 1950', *Science*, 126 (1957), 3283).

[3] *Ibid.*, p. 85. [4] *Ibid.*, p. 88.

manner. Something more akin to the psychiatric analysis of the meaning of the situation for the individual, in terms of his own needs, wishes, and purposes is needed to gain an understanding of the real causes of emotion.—D. A. Prescott, *Emotion and the Educative Process*, Washington, 1938, p. 27.

Buytendijk also conceives of emotion in terms of situation:

> The phenomenological approach to feelings and emotions starts from the undeniable fact that consciousness is always a being conscious of something else and that we are conscious of our existing, that means our being physically subjected to a given situation. This 'being subjected' is not a causal relation, but it means that the situation must be responded to. . . . Feeling and emotion are the affirmations of our attitudes toward situations. . . .—F. J. Buytendijk, 'The Phenomenological Approach to the Problem of Feelings and Emotions', FE 50, pp. 129–30.

Like Nuttin's 'repercussion', Buytendijk speaks of emotion as a 'rebound'. But this is not the same as the 'reflection' in London. The repercussion or rebound is not an epiphenomenon, concomitant, or causal result of material conditions. It must be grasped in and through itself, as an irreducible phenomenon, in the phenomenological situation in which it occurs. This is how Buytendijk proceeds:

> *Emotion is not an intentional act,* but allied to sensation, irritation, and excitation. We may come to understand this fact in the following way: we have only consciousness of ourselves (regaining ourselves in the vision of things). When I admire something or hate someone, I, in *one* intentional act of feeling, project both myself as admiring or hating and the qualitative structure of the object or person . . . . there is in the act of feeling a *closed* reciprocal relation between the subject and its intentional object. Consciousness is shut up with something and isolated from the rest of the world. The *rebound* of my projection of feeling against the created intentional experience has the character of being moved, i.e. of emotion (possibly in the modality of excitation, excitement, or irritation). The result is penetration of feeling with emotion, of emotion with feeling, a stabilization, a continuity of affected relation, with a certain analogy to the standing vibrations in a closed resonator or the standing waves on a limited surface of water. Thus we conclude that there is no emotion without the act of feeling, but the emotion itself is not an intentional act. It is the specific quality of our own existence, revealed in the regaining of ourselves in the act of feeling.—*Ibid.*, p. 132.

With the statement: 'Emotion is not an intentional act', we come directly into the problem of the relation of emotion to the subject. As we have already said, in those theories where spatial language was used there is an intimate connection between emotion and the subject. It is located intra-subjectively in Chapters IX and X. Here, however, there is an apparent split between the subject and emotion because phenomenologists, following Brentano and Husserl, characterize the subject by intentionality. This separation of emotion from intention was formulated by the Scholastics as follows: *'subitus motus, cui ex ratione non consentitur'*—Bonaventura;[1] *'Nusquam enim passio esse potest, nisi ubi contra voluntatem aliquid fit'*—Abelard,[2] (there can be no emotion unless something is done against the will). Buytendijk does not take up such a radical position. For him even if emotion is non-intentional, it is nevertheless subjective, since through it 'we encounter a specific quality of our own existence'. It is not an action, an intention; rather it is a reaction, a being moved, a *passio*, which is presented on that familiar hydrostatic model: the sensitive or irritable fluid in a closed container.

Allport goes further in separating emotion and the 'proprium' (as he calls what others might call the ego, the self, or the intentional, willing subject).

> Propriate states are by no means always agitated states. A sense of worthwhileness, of interest, of importance is not what we ordinarily call emotion. Each lasting sentiment in personality is a propriate state, but only on occasion does a sentiment erupt into emotion. . . .
>
> There is considerable experimental evidence that bears on this matter. In the course of learning, for example, we know that high intensities of emotional excitement tend to narrow the field of learning, to reduce effectiveness of cues, and to diminish the range of similarity and transfer. Propriate involvement, on the other hand, increases the breadth of learning, of transfer effects. . . . Thus the experimental effects of emotionality and of propriate involvement may be precisely opposite. . . .
>
> The distinction is apparent in yet another way. We sometimes experience emotions without viewing them as having appreciable personal significance. A loud noise may evoke a startle and bring in its train widespread visceral disturbance, without at the same time engaging to any appreciable extent our propriate functions. . . . Even if we doubt that intense emotional experience can ever be totally devoid of a sense of self-involvement, we must at least concede that there is far from perfect correlation between them, and that therefore we should regard emotionality and the proprium as separable phenomena.—G. W. Allport, *Becoming* (The Terry Lectures), Yale Univ., 1955, pp. 58–60.

The separation of emotion from the intentional will we have already discussed in the last section. There the involuntary events were still intra-subjective, and in the views of Buytendijk and Allport the separation of emotion from the intentional subject does not mean its exclusion from the subject altogether. It is simply located in another subjective field—ego-alien or involuntary—but still intra-subjective. That this field can be extra-subjective, that emotion can

---

[1] Bonaventura, *Sententiae, Opera*, III, 342d, 4.
[2] Abelard, *Ethica, scito te ipsum*, III.

exist independent of the subject, is one of the radical contributions of Gestalt psychology. Here emotion is 'outside'. No subject is required.

Let us begin with the emotions, which have been adduced so often in the past as examples *par excellence* for 'subjective', i.e. Ego-related, experiences. And yet we may see a gloomy landscape, even when we ourselves are perfectly cheerful; may not a poplar look proud, a young birch shy, and has not Wordsworth immortalized the glee of daffodils! . . . Therefore it seems much more natural to say that emotions may be carried by (behavioural) objects as well as by myself. . . .—K. Koffka, *Principles of Gestalt Psychology*, 1935, London, pp. 326—7.

Katz denies that these emotional qualities are projected from the subject to the environment:

A landscape may appear cheerful, mountains may seem majestic . . . but in such instances it cannot be said that the emotions are transferred from the self in accordance with Lipps' theory of empathy.—D. Katz, *Gestalt Psychology*, London, 1951, p. 146.

And Köhler definitely places these emotional qualities outside in the environment:

All physical events or states which send similar constellations of stimuli to our eyes and ears, as issue from the physical body of another person, will look or sound 'emotional', 'restless', . . . and so forth, just as a living person does. . . .—W. Köhler, *Gestalt Psychology*, London, 1930 (3rd U.S. edn., 1929), p. 203.

After sitting for half an hour in a restaurant which is full of smoke and talk, I feel restless and ready to leave. Clearly, this restlessness refers to the given situation.—Köhler, *op. cit.*, N.Y., 1947 edn., p. 327.

Hartshorne argues to the same effect.[1]

Before we take up the explanation of how these emotions exist 'in the field', that is, how we can account for their location outside in a landscape, restaurant, thunderstorm, or some other situation, it is necessary to present the general Gestalt theory of emotion:

The general attitude to be taken by this theory is this: the total field is permeated by forces which either hold it in equilibrium or produce change and action. This interplay of forces applies to the Ego as a subsystem of the total field. Emotional behaviour will, in our theory, be considered as the dynamics of these intra-Ego forces, conscious emotion as the manifest aspect of these dynamics. The dynamics of the intra-Ego forces will often transcend the limits of the Ego, the emotions being directed towards objects in the field, and of course we must include these object-Ego dynamics in our definition of the emotion.—K. Koffka, *Principles of Gestalt Psychology*, London, 1935, p. 405.

[1] Hartshorne, C., *The Philosophy and Psychology of Sensation*, Univ. of Chicago, 1934, p. 124 and elsewhere.

What about emotions in the field? It will be admitted that emotions that are not Ego emotions are experienced most frequently and most intensely in other human beings and next to that in higher animals. . . . For other human beings, and next to them the higher animals, are the most complex objects within our behavioural environment. At the same time . . . they are more than any other objects centres of force, and surrounded by fields of force. In these objects qua behavioural objects, there may then arise an intra-object and an object-object or even an object-Ego dynamics, comparable to the intra-Ego and the Ego-object dynamics which we have treated as the real basis of emotions. In this way our theory can be easily generalized so as to account for non-Ego emotional experiences. . . . Our generalization must, however, be broad enough to include emotions in non-living behavioural objects, the sad landscape, for example. Our whole problem has a great deal to do with the problem of the physiognomic characters. . . .—*Ibid.*, p. 407.

The physiognomic characters which are the key for understanding how emotions are 'in the field' are to be understood as qualities, as meanings.[1] They are ultimately referable to the interplay of psychological tensions.[2] So too are the special types of emotional behaviour which Koffka interprets from the investigations of Dembo[3] on anger and Karsten[4] on saturation. And so too the physiological changes which occur during emotions. However, unlike other theories where the interplay of tensions between subject and object is important, emotion on this view does not depend upon the presence of the subject (that is, a landscape can be sad without any observer), but rather upon the *presence of tensions in the situation.—(Ibid.*, p. 406.)

The concept of situation which Lewin uses is similar to that of Koffka. He analyses psychological events in terms of field dynamics and tensions. He further limits the tensions to those which are present. Emotions are not to be attributed to future goals or to past reaction patterns, but take rise only in the immediate situation.[5]

An examination of this present situation is made in terms of forces, tensions, energy, etc., so that the language is like the language in Chapter VI (Energy). Here, however, these terms are to be understood within a *psychical* field, distinct from physical energy. The field is so organized that a stimulus can release energy due to a reorganization of the field; that is to say, a stimulus changes the situation. Emotion is like latent energy released by the psychological meanings of perceptual stimuli:

> The stimulus itself may perhaps be considered in many perceptual

[1] Koffka, K., *Principles of Gestalt Psychology*, London, 1935, pp. 656–9.
[2] *Ibid.*, p. 362.
[3] Dembo, T., 'Der Aerger als Dynamisches Problem', *Psychol. Forsch.*, 1931, pp. 1–144.
[4] Karsten, A., 'Psychische Sättigung', *Psychol. Forsch.*, 1928, pp. 142–254.
[5] Lewin, K., *Principles of Topological Psychology*, N.Y., 1936, p. 34.

processes as being at the same time and to a certain degree the source of energy for the process in the sensory sector (e.g., in the field of vision). In actual behavior and emotions, however, as when one undertakes a journey upon the receipt of a telegram or becomes furious at a question, the physical intensity of the stimulus obviously plays no essential role. Hence it has been customary to speak of a 'release', of a process which has been represented by the analogy of the explosion of a keg of powder by the discharging spark.

That conclusion will nevertheless have to be fundamentally changed in two directions.

. . . the stimulus to perception . . . must be assessed not according to its physical intensity but according to its psychological reality. This sort of perceptual experience may carry with it immediately certain purposes or create certain needs which were not before present . . . there may occur reorganization (*Umschichtungen*, literally 'restratifications') through which available (*arbeitsfähig*) energy becomes free; in other words tense psychical systems may arise which were not present before, at least in this form.—K. Lewin, *A Dynamic Theory of Personality*, N.Y., 1935, p. 47.

Not only does a perception release latent energy, but it also can cause the formation of new, tense psychical systems which—as with Koffka —are the basis of emotion (*ibid.*, p. 51). Furthermore, if there is no response due to a 'satiation' of these tensions, or if there is no response because the tension systems are not connected to the perceptual stimulus, there is no affective process. And so it becomes clearer that Lewin's theory depends upon the relation of a perceptual stimulus to a set of tensions, which in turn depends upon the organization of the total field, or situation.

In summing up these views, we find all turns upon the concept of situation which can be used in many ways: as social environment (Landis), socio-historical conditions (London), geographical or physical location (Köhler), the immediate present (Lewin), a closed subject-object circuit (Buytendijk), an abstract system of field dynamics (Koffka, Lewin), a pattern of meanings (Prescott, Nuttin). Furthermore, the concept of situation plays a dominant role in theories of psychosomatic medicine where correlations are made between life-situations and emotional syndromes. In a recent review[1] of some basic concepts in this field we find that a situation can be understood as socio-cultural patterns (Halliday and Mead), as regressions from maturation (Margolin), as environmental stimuli (Wolff), as a field of communications (Ruesch). Also the 'stress' theory of Selye[2] can be taken as specification of the term situation. The term is also variously interpreted in the writings of existentialism,

[1] 'Basic Concepts of Psychosomatic Medicine', Chapter I in RDPM.
[2] Selye, H., *Stress*, Montreal, 1950.

'Dasein' analysis, and phenomenology. And, as it is a holistic concept, it fits in among the newer ways of approaching diseases in terms of something larger (the situation) rather than something smaller (toxins). A brief and excellent review of the ideas of a score of eminent workers in this field is presented by Mayer.[1]

From the foregoing it is evident that in spite of the unity of the views in this section in relying upon a concept of situation to account for emotion, we cannot possibly have here a unified theory of emotion until we specify this term situation. Depending upon how it is understood, the theory of emotions which follows from it can be typed, for example, as formal (when the situation is taken as a total Gestalt), as efficient (when the stimulating perception is stressed), as material (physical environmental conditions), or as final (meanings and purposes). The term situation and the theory of situation is even more ambiguous and muddled than the term and the theory of emotion. We have one of those cases of explaining the obscure by the still more obscure. The problem is really one of trying to grasp a special concept by means of a generic one. Emotion is a special kind or aspect of a situation, just as an apple is a special kind of fruit. But what exactly makes an apple an apple, and an emotion an emotion, requires differentia more specific and more immediate to the phenomena in question. Where the theories in the last section tried to pinpoint emotion within too narrow a frame of physiological location, these theories use a frame too large and vague—situation. A situation, no matter how spoken of—as total field, or as 'Existenz' —is after all nothing else than life itself. Without life, there can hardly be emotion, yet life hardly provides an adequate theory.

But it is not enough to leave these theories with such a negative dismissal and on looking again we can find that they make one significant distinction: emotion and the subject are not necessarily bound up together. They are in fact separable phenomena (Allport). Not only is emotion not a part of subjective intentionality (Buytendijk), but it can exist independent of the subject (Koffka, Katz) as a set of meanings, qualities or tensions. Yet, emotion so conceived is not to be confused with physical tensions physically located in physical objects. It is an objective event, but a *psychological* objective event. This realm of the psychologically objective, or objective psyche, we have encountered before in the explanation of emotion.

For example, in Chapter V where emotion was attributed to the unconscious, it was accounted for by a region separate from the subject where it existed in a latent state (Freud) without being experienced. And when this non-subjective psyche was no longer limited to intra-personal location, we had hypotheses about emotions

[1] Mayer, C. F., 'Metaphysical Trends in Modern Pathology', *Bull. Hist. Med.*, 1952.

and para-psychological events, that is, emotions were said to be attached to what are here called behavioural objects. In Chapter IX, where emotion was accounted for by the 'inner', we saw that the inner and the subject were not to be identified. Other such pertinent formulations are explanations of emotion in terms of transpersonal energy (Chapter VI), the objective will (Chapter X C), and inherited, objective reaction patterns (Chapters XII and XIII).

Here in this section, the non-subjective psyche is placed 'without' in a landscape or restaurant, in a pattern of social, environmental forces or meanings, or, to use the general term, in a situation. *A situation can be taken as the objective psychological field, or as the field of the objective psyche.*[1] The organization of this field can be described in the language of field dynamics of Gestalt psychology, or in the language of Existential phenomenology when the concern is with ontological meanings. Or this field can be described in the language used to describe the collective unconscious, where the field is presented as organized in typical forms. In each case, a situation is not only material conditions and emotion is not to be accounted for only by physical events, but rather by the momentary constellation or organization of the psychological patterns which compose the situation. The existence of these patterns and meanings, of emotion-in-the-field, is only in potentia, unless the field includes an intentional subject. Individually experienced emotions are reflections, rebounds, repercussions of these constellations.

If, as these views have told us, experienced emotion is only the subjective reflection of the objective psychic situation without which it cannot be accounted for, then any adequate theory of emotion must take this realm into account. This leads beyond emotion as a behavioural act; it leads to an inquiry into the nature of this realm which is objective and yet psychic, emotional and yet not subjective. Such an inquiry involving metaphysical or ontological hypotheses becomes a necessary adjunct to a theory of emotion of this kind, just as emotion in terms of physiological location requires minute inquiries and speculative hypotheses about the nature of life, or emotion as energy requires the same sort of inquiry into the nature of the physical universe.

And so the conclusion to this section becomes: Emotion is grounded (located) in the existential situation, the momentary constellations of the objective psyche, the nature of which can be charted in the language of Existential phenomenology, Gestalt psychology, or Jung's analytical psychology.

---

[1] See M. Geiger's classic paper on objective (i.e. independent of subjective experience) psychic reality: 'Fragment üeber den Begriff des Unbewussten und die psychische Realität', *Jbch f. Phil. u. phänomen. Forsch.* IV (ed. E. Husserl), 1921, pp. 1–137.

XII

EMOTION AND THE
SUBJECT-OBJECT RELATION

THESE THEORIES form a separate group because they define the total situation, the interaction of man and world, in terms of a specific pair of opposites: subject and object. This relationship can be conceived on a more simple and mechanical model as stimulus-response, and even more simply as the conditioned reflex. This simplicity provides an answer to our complaint that the 'situational' view of emotion is too ambiguous and too wide. These theories set out a specific framework so that the specific criteria of emotion can be defined. Webb, for example, proposes a definition of emotion which would mark out the kind of situation in which it is justifiable to use the term:

> ... emotion or emotions, would be inferred in a situation in which responses occurred that are not directly definable in terms of the existent conceptual properties of habit or drive. Emotions would be defined when the responses were lawfully related to some measureable property of the stimulus (either antecedent to or existent with the response situation).— W. B. Webb, 'A Motivational Theory of Emotions . . .', *Psychol. Rev.*, 1948, p. 332.

On this view, emotion refers to actions which other concepts do not cover, and it would be defined in terms of the laws of the stimulus-response relationship. Weiss puts the same sort of view, except that he specifies this relationship and these laws in the terms of physical mechanics. In the last chapter, Lewin made clear the difference between a psychological stimulus and a physical stimulus. The question-which-makes-us-furious is not to be understood as a physical stimulus, he pointed out, except as a 'source of energy in the sensory sector'. Weiss, however, conceives the emotional process within this 'sensory sector'. The interaction of man and society for him is really between two physical systems and the situation is one of physical energy.

144

Feeling and emotion should be regarded as categories of behavior resulting from the interaction between physical stimulating conditions and the sensorimotor system.—A. P. Weiss, 'Feeling and Emotion as Forms of Behavior', FE 28, p. 190.

Tolman, who also uses the stimulus-response framework, qualifies it. He links this pair of coordinates not just mechanically, but with an idea of intention.

It is not a response, *as such*, nor a stimulus situation, *as such*, that constitutes the behavior definition of an emotion, but rather the response as affecting or calculated to affect the stimulus situation.—E. C. Tolman, 'A Behavioristic Account of the Emotions' (reprinted from the *Psychol. Rev.*, 1923), in *Collected Papers in Psychology*, E. C. Tolman, Univ. of Calif., 1951, p. 27.

Bekhterev's theory is first of all based upon an implicit concept of isomorphism as we showed in Chapter IV. Also, the theory brings in ideas which are central to theories of other groups. For example, the ultimate physiological source of emotion are the glands of internal secretion; emotions serve the general needs of the organism today and are not phylogenetic remnants. These ideas are not as central to his theory as is the fundamental hypothesis of the conditioned reflex.

Emotions, as they are called, consist of these external mimetic movements together with the above-mentioned somatic and conditioned reflex changes. Reflexology regards them as specialized somato-mimetic reflexes.—V. M. Bekhterev, 'Emotions as Somato-Mimetic Reflexes', FE 28, p. 273.

He examines the genesis of emotion both biologically and socially and finds that perceptions are conditioned reflexes, that the three 'innate' emotions of Watson can be conditioned reflexes, and that the visceral phenomena of emotion are also conditioned reflexes. He concludes, then:

These investigations supply experimental proof that somato-mimetic states originate as conditioned reflexes.—*Ibid.*, p. 282.

Against the notion of the conditioned reflex as the basis of emotion we might marshal some of the classic arguments: (1) it reduces complex behaviour to simple units; (2) it assumes a materialistic and causally mechanistic universe to which the psyche is an insubstantial appendix; (3) it claims validity for human emotion based on animal experiments; (4) it claims validity for fluid emotional life situations based upon rigid laboratory techniques (for example, a dog in harness is reduced to a passive state, deprived of his capacity to act on the environment, his intentionality); (5) it is only a reformulation of associationist theories whose outmoded approach can be traced back through Locke and La Mettrie to Democritus; (6) it does not come to terms with such 'higher' emotions as, say, awe, hope or dread; (7) it neglects or denies the problem of meaningful integration into a significant relation—that set of qualitative factors between the stimulus and the response; (8) it fails to take into account an independent source of emotion (the primal patterns of unconditioned responses) which can both enhance conditioning and also overcome it. Witness to these primal patterns which can overcome conditioning is given, for instance, in the well-known anecdote of the dogs in Pavlov's Leningrad laboratory which lost their conditioned responses during the great Leningrad flood.

It is just upon these primal patterns or innate responses of fear, rage and love that Watson's theory lays stress. And not only is the response end of the relation widened by this emphasis on inheritance, but the stimulus aspect is widened to include the whole general setting or situation beyond mere exciting objects. The framework is stretched out of the mechanistic reflex concept to imply the interaction of biology and sociology, or man and world.

> *An emotion is an hereditary 'pattern-reaction' involving profound changes of the bodily mechanism as a whole, but particularly of the visceral and glandular systems.* By pattern reactions we mean that the separate details of response appear with some constancy, with some regularity and in approximately the same sequential order each time the exciting stimulus is presented. It is obvious that if the formulation is to fit the facts, the general condition of the organism must be such that the stimulus can produce its effect. . . . Stimulus then in this sense is used in a broad way to refer not only to the exciting object but also to the general setting.— J. B. Watson, *Psychology from the Standpoint of a Behaviorist*, Philadelphia and London, 3rd edn., 1929 (first edn., 1919).
>
> We may express our formulation in convenient terms somewhat as follows: when the adjustments called out by the stimulus are internal and confined to the subject's body, we have emotion, for example, blushing; when the stimulus leads to adjustment of the organism as a whole to objects, we have instinct, for example, defense responses, grasping, etc. Emotions seldom appear alone. The stimulus usually calls out emotional instinctive and habit factors simultaneously.
>
> The above formulation fits only the more stereotyped forms of emotional response. . . . When we take into account the whole group of phenomena in which we see emotional manifestations in adults, a pronounced modification is necessary. Apparently the hereditary pattern as a whole gets broken up . . . and there *can be noted only a reinforcement or inhibition of the habit and instinctive . . . activities taking place at the moment.—Ibid.*, p. 227.

From this we can see that Watson views emotion in three different ways: (1) as a kind of innate response, (2) as a kind of stimulus-response correlation, and (3) as an accompaniment (reinforcement or inhibition). The main difference between the theory of Watson and the theory of Bekhterev lies in how each regards the nature of the response. For Watson it is innate; for Bekhterev it is conditioned. The view of Harlow and Stagner brings these two ideas together by making the *basis of emotion* unconditioned, but the *emotion itself* conditioned.

> The theory which we wish to advance is to the effect that: uncon-ditioned affective responses form a basis for the emotions . . . and that emotions themselves are conditioned responses subsequently formed (pp. 189–90).
> . . . there are no innate emotions. The advantage of our theory, how-ever, is that *it suggests a group of unconditioned responses as a basis from which emotions may develop.* Although the number of emotions . . . is without limit, we agree . . . that certain fundamental emotional classes are delimited by the underlying feelings.
> The innate components of the emotional experience are the four funda-mental feeling-tones, pleasure, unpleasantness, excitement and depres-sion. These feelings represent the only identifiable conscious elements in an emotion, aside from sensations and cognition of the stimulating situation; . . .—H. F. Harlow and R. Stagner, 'Psychology of Feelings and Emotions, II, Theory of Emotions', *Psychol. Rev.*, 1933, p. 191.

Babkin presents essentially the same point of view with the addition of supportive phylogenetic and physiological hypotheses—such as we have seen before. He constructs his theory on the model of two systems of mental functioning: (*a*) cortical, conditioned, civilized and (*b*) sub-cortical, unconditioned, primitive. The former is more recent and higher and built upon the latter. '. . . a conditioned reflex is based on an unconditioned one.' [1]

There is no need to detail other behaviorist views (Skinner, Estes, Dollard, Mowrer, Miller, etc.) which are reviewed by Beebe-Center,[2] since they present nothing fundamentally different, but are rather refinements and complex variations of what we have just seen. All attempt to solve the problem of emotion theory within the S-R system of operations. The same holds for J. Hunt *et al.*[3]

The main problem in all the theories here is the *nature of the relation* between stimulus and response. Emotion does not occur with just any stimulus and any response, nor can it be accounted for only through study of responses or of stimuli. The concept of the reflex

---

[1] Babkin, B., 'The Conditioning of Emotions', FE 50, p. 36.
[2] Beebe-Center, J. G., 'Feeling and Emotion', in *Theoretical Foundations of Psy-chology*, ed. H. Helsen, N.Y., 1951, with bibliography.
[3] Hunt, J. McV., *et al.*, 'Situational Cues Distinguishing Anger, Fear, and Sorrow', *Am. J. Psychol.*, 1958, pp. 136–51.

itself brings out the importance of the relation, for it means some measurable, lawful, significant or predictable relation between the stimulus and the response. The *meaning* of the relation is expressed by the authors in this chapter in various ways: Watson says: 'the general condition of the organism must be such that the stimulus can produce its effect.' Tolman says: 'It is not response as such, nor a stimulus situation as such . . . but rather the response as affecting . . . the stimulus . . .'. And Webb would express the meaning of the relation in terms of laws: 'Emotions would be defined when the responses were lawfully related to some measureable property of the stimulus.' A quotation from Allport nicely brings out the importance of meaning in the stimulus-response relation:

> The pure conditioned reflex readily dies out unless the secondary stimulus is occasionally reinforced by the primary stimulus. The dog does not continue to salivate whenever it hears a bell unless sometimes at least an edible offering accompanies the bell. But there are innumerable instances in human life where a single association, *never* reinforced, results in the establishment of a life-long dynamic system. An experience associated only once with a bereavement, an accident, or a battle, may become the center of a permanent phobia or complex, not in the least dependent on a recurrence of the original shock.—G. W. Allport, *Personality*, London, 1951—reprint of 1937, U.S.A. edition, pp. 198-9.

In other words, reflex functioning is meaningful functioning, not mere mechanical functioning. To put it in a nutshell, emotion in the S-R theory really depends on the enigmatic hyphen in the S-R. When the bell no longer means food, the dog quits salivating; yet as long as this curve on the road where I had the accident means death I shall have an emotional reaction.[1] It would seem from this that the relation between stimulus and response depends not only on such quantitative, mechanical principles as repetition and physical intensities, or on the laws of association, but also upon values, signs and meanings. Without them the stimulus-response pair do not hold together; they lose the lawful inner connection represented by the hyphen.

An investigation of that hyphen, however, is an enormous job. Upon inspection it shows itself to be no simple, single stroke, but rather a tangled gap (the Greek word *chaos* might be better!) of infinite interdependent variables, involving all the problems of

---

[1] Szasz' theory is in the same vein; again we have emotion discussed in terms of the subject-object relation (T. Szasz, in 'Discussion of Symposium', *Research in Affects*, Psychiatric Research Reports, 8, 1957), p. 80. When he says '. . . *affect is an indicator of the nature of the relationship between ego and object*', he does not mean the object as such, as a bare sensory stimulus datum. Rather he speaks of the 'internal object', or what we might call its meaning to the ego. When this changes, says Szasz, then the affect will change also. Again, when the curve in the road no longer means something fearful and dangerous, then my affect changes. What gives 'internal objects' their emotional character we shall come to in Chapter XIV on Representations.

psychology: sense data, perception, representations, memory, body-mind relation, motion, etc. In other words, the real problems of a theory of emotion arise as soon as one steps through the façade of the simple S-R formula. Taking it on face value we are given only a mechanical account which cannot even be supported from the physiologists' concept of the simple reflex which Sherrington[1]—the pioneering master in this field—says 'is a convenient, if not a probable fiction'.[2]

The hyphen, the relation between stimulus and response, conceived meaningfully leads to the dissolution of the mechanistic framework of conditioned reflex and stimulus-response, and the substitution of the more fundamental category of subject-object, a traditional explanatory model with traditional philosophical riddles. The following theories which use this conceptual pair to account for emotion agree in their interpretation of the relation between the poles of the pair. The relation is *motion*. And again we find as we press forward from chapter to chapter that the same ideas come up in new ways. The subject-object pair has appeared often before; so too, the idea of motion, especially when emotion is presented as action, as behaviour, as expression, as muscular motoric will, as dynamic force, or, in the old way as a 'motion of the soul', as opposed to an entity, a quality, or a 'state of the soul'. What is new in the position here is that emotion is fundamentally explicable as a motion between subject and object.

The evident example of this position is the historically long and widely held view that emotion is a *passio* of the subject. The subject is *moved* by an object or the idea of an object. In the last chapter, Buytendijk gave us this in the complicated situational frame. Minkowski[3] takes emotion as 'to be moved' ('ému'). It is the result of *'heurts extérieurs'* which particularly concern us on the somatic level. Affectivity, however, is 'to be touched' and concerns the human, the psychic level.

Kafka[4] also takes emotion as a *passio* of the subject, a being moved or affected by objects. But he gives this being moved a different interpretation from the usual. Objects are not just mechanical stimuli printing impressions. They present demands and problems; they call for activity. They have 'intentions' on the subject—to put the

[1] Sherrington, C., *The Integrative Action of the Nervous System*, Cambridge, 1952, p. 7.

[2] According to T. H. Bullock ('Neuron Doctrine and Electrophysiology', *Science*, 129 (1959) pp. 997 ff.) nerve cell behaviour can no longer be taken as simply as it once was conceived; it is now thought that there is 'an enormous range of possible complexity within this single cellular unit'.

[3] Minkowski, E., 'L'Affectivité', *L'Evolution psychiatrique*, 1947, pp. 47–70.

[4] Kafka, G., 'Ueber Uraffekte', *Acta Psychologica*, 1950, p. 256 ff.

matter in the scholastic language of Henry of Ghent. The subject's response to the demand can be charted in four basic movements (*'Uraffekte'*) of the organism, expressed through actual physical motions. Such a concept of basic movements as the root of emotion is similar to the reaction patterns of Watson, the two basic movements of the protoplasm of Reich, and the three basic movements of Horney.[1] De la Chambre in the late Renaissance, like Kafka today, postulates four basic movements as a then up-to-date improvement of the older Stoic-Scholastic movements of *accessum* and *recessum*.[2]

For Michotte there are two basic motions: toward and away from, called integrative and segregative. Emotions can be regarded as functional connections—integrative or segregative—between two things. In the eyes of the observer, the motions between two objects performed slowly and hesitantly, or rapidly with jerks and rushes, or in rhythmical parallels, etc., become described in the language used for human behaviour, e.g. A approaches and embraces B, A runs after B and B is afraid and withdraws. A feels attracted by B and goes gently towards B, etc. The effectiveness in evoking emotional descriptions from such experiments in motion between two abstract perceptual objects (rectangles called A and B), Michotte says,

> ... proves that it is the kinetic structure as such, the combinations of movements, which are above all effective; and it proves that the nature of the moving object is quite secondary *from this point of view*. How could one otherwise explain the fact that experiments with little inert rectangles could suggest the idea of emotional reactions?—A. E. Michotte, 'The Emotions Regarded as Functional Connections', FE 50, p. 121.

In other words, we recognize emotion by the kind of motion obtaining in the relation between any two objects, one of which is interpreted as a subject. This view of emotion as a motion also holds for the subjective experience of emotion.

> It is evident that an emotion toward a thing, animal or person establishes some form of liaison between the object and the subject whom it affects. Emotion is a modification of the subject *in regard to* these objects. Joy, sorrow, fear, and anger are undoubtedly states belonging to the person who experiences them, but they are states with a characteristic type of connection with their cause, a connection which differs qualitatively according to the kind of emotion experienced.
>
> If we look at the emotions from this point of view . . . they can be classed in the same group of phenomena as the visual kinetic structures. —*Ibid.*, p. 123.

[1] Horney, K., *Neurosis and Human Growth*, London, 1951.
[2] FE 37, p. 147.

Where Michotte proceeds from studies of perception, causality and *Gestalten* and arrives at a theory of emotion as motion between subject and object, Jonas comes to the same conclusion from the viewpoint of 'philosophical biology'.

> Three characteristics distinguish animal from plant life: motility, perception, emotion. The necessary connection of locomotion with perception is obvious: that with emotion calls for closer scrutiny, which will show that all three proceed from a common principle.
> Locomotion is towards or away from an object, i.e. pursuit or flight. A protracted pursuit, in which the animal matches its motile powers against those of the intended prey, bespeaks not only developed motor and sensor faculties but also distinct powers of emotion. It is safe to assume that the number of intermediate steps over which the purpose can extend itself is a measure of the stage of emotional development. The very span between start and attainment which such a series represents must be bridged by continuous emotional intent. The appearance of directed long-range motility (as exhibited by the vertebrates) thus signifies the emergence of emotional life. Greed is at the bottom of the chase, fear at the bottom of flight.—H. Jonas, 'Motility and Emotion', *Actes du XIème Congrès International de Philosophie*, VII (Bruxelles, 1953), Amsterdam-Louvain, p. 117.

Animal life, unlike plant life, is mediate. There is a distance between 'start and attainment'.

> Without the tension of distance and the deferment necessitated by it there would be no occasion for desire or emotion generally. . . .
> Of this principle of mediacy, sentience, emotion and motility are different manifestations. If emotion implies distance between need and satisfaction, then it is grounded in the basic separation between subject and object. . . . 'Distance' in all these respects involves the subject-object split. This is at the bottom of the whole phenomenon of animality. . . .
> —*Ibid.*, p. 118.
> The mediacy of animal existence . . . creates the isolated individual pitted against the world. . . . This precarious and exposed mode of living commits to wakefulness and effort, whereas plant life can be dormant. . . . the indirectness of animal existence holds in its wakefulness the twin possibilities of enjoyment and suffering. . . . The suffering intrinsic in animal existence is thus primarily not that of pain . . . but that of want and fear, i.e. an aspect of appetitive nature as such. Appetition is the form which the basic self-concern of all life assumes under the conditions of animal mediacy, where it emancipates itself from its immersion in blind organic function and takes over an office of its own: its functions are the emotions. Animal being is thus essentially passionate being.— *Ibid.*, pp. 120–1.

This last sentence of Jonas restates splendidly the conclusion to Chapter IX—'emotion is the essence of life'. But Jonas comes to this conclusion on other grounds which we might examine since they are the same for all the theories in this chapter. All depend on the subject-object split. This concept has several difficulties.

In the first place, arguments from other theories contest that both members of the pair are necessary for emotion. Michotte shows two objects are needed, but no subject. The same was said in Chapter XI by the Gestalt psychologists. Others say only the subject is needed (Chapter IX). Emotion is not object-directed, object-connected, nor is the object needed to provoke emotion. It can be brought about by images which do not necessarily take rise in or result from objects.

In the second place, the subject-object duality, like isomorphic unity is not so much a fundamental fact as it is a fundamental attitude which 'creates the isolated individual pitted against the world' (Jonas). It is an attitude of a consciousness closed in on itself separated from objects. There are many ways around this supposedly fundamental duality. One way is reducing one member of the pair to the other, e.g. the subject is only another physical object, or objects depend on the consciousness of a subject. Another way is embracing the duality in a higher unity, such as the older monist arguments or the newer concepts of situation, *Dasein*, organism-plus-environment, and objective psyche. There is the Hindu concept of *Maya* which presents the duality as illusion. There is the approach through semantics which finds the duality only grammatical, due to an ontologizing of the subject-predicate construction of statements. Then there is the resolution provided in the scholastic notions of subject and object themselves. The object was taken as in these theories: something 'put before' the mind. But the subject was not apart from the object. It referred to the thing-in-itself which 'underlies' the object.[1] The most radical solution (both historically and conceptually) of this split is presented by the Eleatics (Parmenides, Zeno, Melissos) who denied space, plurality and motion. Here we come to the root metaphor of this section.

It has been said all along that emotion does not depend upon the stimulus as such or upon the response as such (Tolman) or upon the nature of the moving objects (Michotte), but it depends upon the motion between them, the functional connection, or what we have called the hyphen. Now *all the motion concepts in this chapter—* somato-mimetic reflex movements (Bekhterev), pattern-reactions (Watson), basic movements (Kafka), conditioned and unconditioned responses (Harlow and Stagner, Babkin), etc.—*require a gap between the subject and object*. This position is the Eleatic position: motion requires a void. Applied to our theories this means: the motion of

---

[1] See Spearman, C., *Psychology Down the Ages*, London 1937, Vol. II, p. 305.

emotion is due to a gap between subject and object, stimulus and response, between external situation and internal reaction, between man and world. Emotion is the locomotive result of distance.

If, however, following Aristotle[1] we allow for *two other kinds of motion* (qualitative alteration and quantitative increase or decrease) there can be motion that is not locomotion. Such motion would have nothing to do with the void represented in the subject-object gap, and such motion might be wholly conceivable without the subject-object category. Emotion, then, could be accounted for without this extraverted attitude which limits motion to spatial models.

The same distinction in kinds of 'motions of the soul' can be found in a Chinese book of life. There is a movement based on the subject-object split, that is upon our animal condition as Jonas would put it. External objects excite instinctual responses. But a second kind of motion which starts from the 'heart' is objectless. The text runs as follows:

> Therefore it is said: If, when stimulated by external things, one is moved, it is the instinct of the being. If, when not stimulated by external things, one is moved, it is the movement of Heaven. . . . The instincts are based upon the fact that there are external things. They are thoughts that go beyond their own position. Then movement leads to movement. But, when no idea arises, the right ideas come. . . . If things are quiet and one is quite firm, the release of Heaven suddenly moves.[2]

This distinction in kinds of motion gives two conclusions. (1) That aspect of our life which we can call our 'animal being' is passionate because its motion is locomotion, its life mediate, its subject pitted against a world of objects. Emotion is the hyphen, the functional connection between subject and object. It is the Eros (flow of relation) across the Chaos (gap). (2) But another aspect of ourselves, that which we might say is particularly our 'human being' is passionate not only because its motion is locomotion, but also because its motion and emotion are part of the process of alteration, growth and decay. It comes from 'Heaven' or the 'Heart' according to our Chinese text; or as we might put it: *the objectless movement of self-actualization is also the ground of emotion.*

Further, for clinical practice this conclusion means that emotions and their disturbances cannot be conceived as due only to subject-object or inter-personal relations, but can just as well be *due to intra-personal processes of qualitative alteration, growth and decay.*

[1] Aristotle, *Physica*, Bk. II, 192b; Bk. V, 225b.
[2] Wilhelm, R., and Jung, C. G., *The Secret of the Golden Flower*, London, 1931, p. 65.

XIII

EMOTION AND GENESIS

THE THEORIES of Watson, of Babkin, and of Harlow and Stagner posit some sort of innate emotional factor. The theories of this group take up this problem and explain emotion through reference to its origins in the subjective response. This concern with origins leads beyond the immediate problems of the nature of the response to the wider problems of explanation through origin-hypotheses in general. It is the aim of all the theories in the group to show *the starting point* of emotion.

Such a starting point can be the 'startle pattern' as described by Landis and Hunt.[1] It is a concept similar to the 'unconditioned affective response' (Harlow and Stagner) out of which emotions develop. Bridges calls the initial state out of which emotions develop 'excitement'.

> The genetic theory of the emotions is thus that excitement, the undifferentiated emotion present at birth, becomes differentiated and associated with certain situations and certain motor responses to form the separate emotions of later life. This process . . . takes place gradually, so that at different age levels different emotions are distinguishable. The first two emotions to be thus differentiated . . . are . . . distress and delight. These are distinguished by slight differences in visceral reactions, by the accompanying overt behaviour, and by differences in the provoking situation.—K. M. B. Bridges, 'A Genetic Theory of the Emotions', Chapter XV, *The Social and Emotional Development of the Pre-School Child*, London, 1931, p. 201.

Wallon[2] presents a usual situational view like those in Chapter XI. But he bases emotion on a primary state in the infant called 'spasm'. There is a curious eighteenth-century parallel to the view of Bridges and Wallon about the undifferentiated emotion present at birth and its development.

[1] Landis, C., and Hunt, W., *The Startle Pattern*, N.Y., 1939, p. 153. 'It seems best to us to define startle as pre-emotional . . . it is a rapid, transitory response much more simple in its organization and expression than the so-called "emotions". It may or may not be followed by emotion proper.'

[2] Wallon, H., *L'Evolution psychologique de l'enfant*, Paris, 1950, pp. 129–39.

We have taken notice that children on their first entrance into the world have a general notion of action, though they know not what manner to apply it: therefore when anything affects them strongly they strain every nerve and exert all their little powers of motion. But as they grow acquainted with the uses of those powers they confine their efforts to some particular quarter: yet their knowledge for a long while being very imperfect, they still employ more exertion than necessary. . . . These efforts . . . widen the passages communicating with the vital circulation, which thereby more readily admit the animal spirits and take in a larger flow. . . . Whence proceeds the violence and obstancy of passion. . . .—
A. Tucker ('Ed. Search'), *The Light of Nature Pursued*, Vol. II, Chapter XXI, 'Passions', pp. 48–9, London, 1768.

We are told in these excerpts that emotion is a complex pattern which starts in a relatively simple one. Also implied is that the simple is quantitative out of which the qualitative complex develops. The primary state has been called spasm, excitement, startle, and also *étonnement* (Condillac)[1] and *choc* (Dumas).[2] It is always genetic explanation, and only ontogenetic when the growth of the emotional complexity is explained in terms of maturation of the individual.

Bousfield and Orbison[3] propose a theory of emotion based on a concept of maturation of cerebral and endocrine functions. They notice 'increase in the vigour of emotional states with increasing age'. They associate the slower and later development of the frontal lobes and the adrenal glands with the relatively retarded emotions of the infant. K. Bühler[4] also treats emotion in terms of maturation. In the emotional development (*Affektentwicklung*) of a child there is a 'deutlichen Umschlag vom Negativen zum Positiven', a change which begins in the middle of the first year of life. Bühler explains this in the same way as do Bridges and Tucker, i.e. in terms of the child's control of his body and surroundings. This means that positive emotions go hand in hand with the control of the situation and negative ones with lack of control. This implies the judgment that negative emotions are disorder, a fundamental attitude we shall take up in Chapter XVII. So far, the ontogeny of emotion begins in infancy. Gesell, however, traces the origins of emotion back to the embryo. For him, 'the genesis of emotion may be sought in the fetal period' when as early as the twentieth week after conception certain postural patterns of behaviour appear which form the basis for the progressive development of emotion, subject to the laws of 'developmental morphology'. (Gesell, as we saw in Chapter X C, conceives

[1] de Condillac, E. B., *Traité des Sensations*, II, Paris, 1754.
[2] Dumas, G., *Nouveau Traité de Psychologie*, II, 3; III, 2, Paris, 1932–3.
[3] Bousfield, W., and Orbison, W., 'Ontogenesis of Emotional Behavior', *Psychol. Rev.*, 1952, p. 6.
[4] Bühler, K., *Die geistige Entwicklung des Kindes*, 6th edn., Jena, 1930, pp. 103 ff.

emotion as a postural attitude.) This development does not depend upon surroundings, but upon the genes, which 'engender the sequences of ontogenesis . . . operating in a self-limited time-cycle'.[1]

The importance of internal factors prior to the earliest stimuli—in other words the role of heredity in emotion—is particularly stressed by Williams.[2] The work of Lacey *et al.*[3] shows that the patterns of response are individually specifically different. Richmond and Lustman,[4] in examining new-born infants, show qualitative and quantitative differences in autonomic functioning which they call 'autonomic endowment'. Mall's[5] work brings out the differences in affective reactions according to constitutional types. All these accounts of emotion stress the individually different, constitutionally given factors.

Emotion in terms of genes and constitution leads from ontogeny to phylogeny, when the constitutional given factors are taken to be the results of racial inheritance. This was the theory of emotional expression presented by Sir Charles Bell and by Darwin in the last century. Crile, a pioneer medical investigator of emotional phenomena, presents this phylogenetic view:

> By both the positive and negative evidence we are forced to believe that the emotions are primitive instinctive reactions which represent ancestral acts. . . . The mechanism by which the motor acts are performed and the mechanism by which the emotions are expressed are one and the same. These acts in their infinite complexity are suggested by association —phylogenetic association. When our progenitors came in contact with any exciting element in their environment, action ensued then and there. There was much action—little restraint or emotion. Civilized man is in auto-captivity. He is subjected to innumerable stimulations, but custom and convention frequently prevent physical action. When these stimulations are sufficiently strong but no action ensues, the reaction constitutes an emotion. A phylogenetic fight is anger; a phylogenetic flight is fear; a phylogenetic copulation is sexual love, and so one finds in this conception an underlying principle which may be the key to an understanding of the emotions and of certain diseases.—G. W. Crile, *The Origin and Nature of the Emotions*, Philadelphia, 1915, pp. 75–6.

Crile adds a bit to Darwin. The notion that emotion is an *action manquée* and due to restraint is a view that we shall take up in the section on the conflict theories. Much in this phylogenetic theory

---

[1] Gesell, A., 'Emotion from the Standpoint of a Developmental Morphology', FE 50, p. 394.
[2] Williams, R. J., 'Some Implications of Physiological Individuality', FE 50, p. 268.
[3] Lacey, J., Bateman, D., Van Lehn, R., 'Autonomic Response Specificity', *Psychosom. Med.*, 1953, pp. 8–21.
[4] Richmond, J., and Lustman, S., 'Autonomic Function in the Neonate: 1. Implications for Psychosomatic Theory', *Psychosom. Med.*, 1955, pp. 269–75.
[5] Mall, G., *Konstitution und Affekt*, Leipzig, 1936.

depends on romantic fictions about our primitive ancestors—like 'the happy savage' and 'the primal horde'—who according to Crile must have led a life of instant and emotionless action. So too, the phylogenetic view which sees emotion as a primitive trace serves very well such modern rejections of emotion as, say that of A. Meyer, who says: 'Emotion is a gradually evolved and hereditarily transmitted action-tendency, hardly ever, or hardly any longer, suited as such to form a solution.' 'An emotional note presents something quite elemental, often crudely fitted to ... modern life.' [1]

Cobb's phylogenetic theory rests less upon the *interpretation of expressions* as with Crile, Bell and Darwin than upon an idea we have already seen (Chapter X A, pp. 89–90): the *similarity of brain structure* in animals and man.

> The old brain seems to have much to do with emotions and emotional expression. It comprises a much larger proportion of the brain of lower animals, such as carnivora, than of primates. It is not a vestigial organ in man; it is large and important. It seems to set the emotional background on which man functions intellectually.
>
> Men with understanding ... have always known that ... decisions were made on a background of emotion. ... During the last century psychologists and physiologists have talked of levels of nervous function, reflexes, instincts, the learning process. Recently psychoanalysts have seen functions as at different levels—'deep' and 'superficial understanding', the 'id, ego and super-ego' concept. They have considered the relation of mouth to love and to passivity as a deep infantile relationship, founded in the first few months of life. The neurologist now comes out with experiments on animals, showing that these relationships are far deeper. They are laid down in the anatomy of the simple mammalian brain. These roots go farther down than individual or racial experience. They are embedded in the phylogenesis of the brains of all mammals.— S. Cobb, *Emotions and Clinical Medicine*, N.Y., 1950, pp. 87–8.

Ruckmick's phylogenetic theory traces the origin of emotion back yet farther. Before the ontogenetic basis of startle or excitement, before the autonomic endowment, before human genes, before the actions of our progenitors, before even the mammalian brain existed in the evolutionary scale, there was the single living cell. Here Ruckmick begins:

> 1. The affective life begins with consciousness itself in the lowest forms of animal life. The simple or elementary feelings, or the affective processes, are to be identified with this early form of experience. In other words, consciousness is nothing more than feeling in the technical sense of the word.
>
> 2. As the mental life develops, this elementary phase of consciousness

[1] Meyer, A., 'Discontent', *Collected Papers of Adolf Meyer, IV. Mental Hygiene,* Baltimore, 1952, p. 388.

spreads from whole to part in the sense that it becomes attached to, that it permeates through, every succeeding phase of developing conscious processes. . . .—C. A. Ruckmick, *The Psychology of Feeling and Emotion*, N.Y. and London, 1936, p. 214. (Entire passage in italics in original.)

Landauer integrates a phylogenetic view with the psychoanalytic system:

> Affects are typical responses to typical demands, responses handed down from one generation to another in the form of potentialities. That is to say, they do not belong to the personal ego which comes into existence in every individual life, but are an important part of the impersonal ego.—K. Landauer, 'Affects, Passions and Temperament', *Int. J. Psycho-Anal.*, 1938, p. 388.

Following Darwin, these ancestral traces need no longer be useful. For Crile they are only vestigial representations of actions, useless remnants of a gloriously active past. What then is their value today? The many answers to this fundamental question will be collected in the chapter on 'final cause'. Landauer's interesting suggestion is that emotions have the function of making man whole:

> Are we then to conclude that an affective attack is a storm of instinct, in which every zone pursues the aim determined for it by its structure, regardless of the body as a whole . . .?
>
> In the case of moderately strong stimuli we see that single groups of organs seem to aim at producing a uniform result but that different groups seem to aim at producing different and often contrary results. An affective attack is precisely a conflict of this kind within the human being, upon whom demands are made from every side but who is not a homogeneous whole. Through the fact that as a practical event he functions with all his organs and is sensible of this functioning, he becomes more or less conscious of himself as a whole. Thus affects tend toward integration . . . they are sought after, even when consciously experienced as unpleasurable.—*Ibid.*, p. 408.

Up to this point, the variety of emotional life is a secondary development of a primary root. This root has been given a biological description and the views have been ontogenetic or phylogenetic. There is a second way of describing this root, this genesis of emotion, without a biological interpretation, yet which retains the main idea of evolution as pronounced by Herbert Spencer, 'Evolution is a change from an indefinite, incoherent homogeneity to a definite, coherent heterogeneity through continuous integration and differentiation.' Such an approach, for example, would be Dumas' notion of *choc* or the startle pattern or excitement were these to be taken as root *principles*. Shifting the interpretation in this way we arrive at psychogenetic views rather than biogenetic ones. Such psychogenetic views differ from others which are more complex like 'situation', 'unconscious', 'distinct entities', 'conflict', etc., which can also explain emotion psychogenetically. There the explanation requires a complex interacting system; here it only requires a single, simple root. Examples of such roots are: pleasure/unpleasure,[1] *ira* and *cupiditas*,[2] *amour-propre*,[3] sympathy,[4] anxiety,[5] thrill.[6] The theory of Suttie is of the same kind:

> I consider that the most true and useful way of regarding the infinitely varied forms of human emotion is as *interconvertible forms of one and the same social feeling*.
>
> . . . but why should we hesitate to draw the inference that in the social emotions we are dealing *not with a number* of hypothetically abstracted primary emotions blended together in an endless variety of ways, but with one and the same love-urge expressed under the stimulus of *different relationships to the loved object*.
>
> . . . it seems to me better to suppose that we are dealing with a single 'fund' of love-energy capable of endless transformations of quality or aim, even into the apparent opposite of love—hate.—I. D. Suttie, *The Origins of Love and Hate*, London, 1935, pp. 60–1.

Senault, in the 1600's, wrote to just the same effect:

> Reason therefore will have us to believe that there is but one Passion; and that hope and fear, sorrow and joy are the motions or properties of love; and to paint her in all her colours, we must term her, when longing after what is loved, Desire. . . . Or to express the same thing more clearly, desire and eschewing, hope and fear are the motions of Love . . .
>
> But if it be true that Love causeth all our Passion, it follows that she must sometimes transform herself into her contrary; and that by a Metamorphosis . . . she converts herself into Hatred. . . .

---

[1] According to A. Wreschner (*Das Gefühl*, Leipzig, 1931, p. 187), Lehmann, Titchener, Külpe, Ebbinghaus, Hoffding and Wreschner all follow the same view that emotion is a kind of feeling and feeling originates in the basic pair of opposites, *Lust-Unlust*. K. Bernecker (*Kritische Darstellung der Geschichte des Affektbegriffes*, Berlin, 1915, pp. 256–7) concurs that the classic basis for theory of affect is the *Lust-Unlust* pair. Kant, we remember from Chapter VI, held that pain or unpleasure was primary.

[2] The *ira* and *cupiditas* of the Schoolmen as the two basic categories of the passions finds its echo, so to speak, in modern depth psychology. The two basic emotions of man according to Adler and Freud are the emotions arising from power and those arising from desire.

[3] 'Les passions ne sont que les divers goûts de l'amour propre', La Rochefoucauld, *Maxims posth.*, No. 531, (also Delisle de Sales). See Chapter X A, Rof Carballo, for a modern interpretation of *amour-propre*; also Sergi, p. 99 above.

[4] 'Adam Smith . . . finds the foundation of all our sentiments in sympathy.'— FE 37, p. 211–12.

[5] 'At the core of the problem of emotions and the very many ways in which these are expressed and encountered in clinical practice lies anxiety.'—Rome, H. P., 'The Dynamics of Emotions', *Minn. Med.*, 1953, p. 1232.

[6] '. . . "a craving for thrill" is the fundamental instinct; all varieties of activity are the results of this fundamental instinct'. Kaiser, I. R., 'The Psychology of Thrill', *Ped. Sem.*, 1920, pp. 243–80.

... if there be diverse Passions, Love is the Sovraign thereof....
She is the *primum Mobile*. ...—J. F. Senault, *The Use of the Passions*
(transl. by Henry, Earl of Monmouth), London, 1649; quoted from the
1671 edition, pp. 27–9.[1]

Shand's 'laws of character', which are principally concerned with
the interaction of the emotions, number 144. The last of these laws
reveals the special place that desire holds in the system:

> *Every emotion, when its end is obstructed, tends to develop its impulse*
> *into desire, and so give rise to the prospective emotions: the system of every*
> *emotion potentially contains desire with its prospective emotions.*—A. F.
> Shand, *The Foundations of Character*, 2nd edn., 1920, p. 519.

For him 'desire is not an independent system'. It is not emotion like
other emotions; it is a potential, a *primum mobile* in all emotions. A
concept of love or desire has been put forward time and again as the
single root of all emotions. Examples are: the *amor* or *dilectio* of
Augustine,[2] Spinoza's[3] *cupiditas*, Freud's[4] libido, as well as the notion
of *Maya* in Hindu thought which, as a kind of desire,[5] is the ground
of the multitude of illusions, errors and passions. In recent times,
Binswanger's[6] concept of *liebende Miteinandersein* also takes love as
a unique and fundamental phenomenon, ontologically different from
all other emotions.

Gregory of Nyssa also presents a single source of all passions. It
is not desire as love, but desire as animal sexuality.

> For I think that from this beginning all our passions issue as from a
> spring, and pour their flood over man's life; and an evidence of my words
> is the kinship of passions which appear alike in ourselves and in the
> brutes; for it is not allowable to ascribe the first beginnings of the con-
> stitutional liability to passion to that human nature which was fashioned
> in the Divine likeness; but as brute life first entered into the world, and
> man, for the reason already mentioned, took something of their nature
> (I mean the mode of generation) he accordingly took at the same time
> a share of the other attributes contemplated in that nature; for the like-
> ness of man is not found in anger, nor is pleasure the mark of the superior
> nature; . . .
> These attributes, then, human nature took to itself from the side of the

---

[1] Belouino, P., (*Des Passions dans leurs rapports avec la religion* . . ., Paris, 1873,
2 vols., Vol. I, pp. 29–31), quotes Senault and agrees with him, but qualifies the term
'love' as 'love of happiness'. 'L'amour du bonheur est donc, suivant nous, la source
unique de nos passions.'

[2] Augustine, *De Trinitate*, IX, 7, 8, 10; X, 12; XII.

[3] Spinoza, *Ethica*, III, 59, Def. 1 and 48; 57.

[4] See Chapter VI, p. 76 fn. 3 on the libido concept.

[5] Das, B., *The Science of the Emotions*, Madras, 1924. Das defines emotion in terms
of desire thereby following the classical Hindu approach.

[6] Binswanger, L., *Grundformen und Erkenntnis menschlichen Daseins*, 2nd edn.,
Zürich, 1953.

brutes; for these qualities with which brute life was armed for self-preservation, when transferred to human life, became passions. . . . All these and the like affections entered man's composition by reason of the animal mode of generation.[1]

This fourth-century statement is a clear prefiguration of the view of Darwin and Crile. The qualities with which brute life was armed for self-preservation, in other words the actions of our primitive ancestors, when transferred to human life become passions. The difference lies in the word 'transferred'. For Gregory, man and beast shared qualities or participated in an essence. In the view of nineteenth-century evolutionists, 'transferred' means inheritance or genetic development. Gregory's view can also be taken as a precursor of two other sets of modern views about emotion. The first, as Gardiner[2] has pointed out, is the vasomotor theory (Chapter X B), which Gregory presents (*op. cit.*, xii, xxx). The second needs some more careful exposition.

As we have seen, Gregory derives all passions from a single source —the animal mode of generation. This mode was devised by God because in His foreknowledge He knew man would fall into sin from his original state.[3] Thus sexuality and sin are posited together. Nevertheless, the source of the passions in the inferior, material and irrational[4] part of man is only evil if there occurs a 'rupture'[5] between it and the mind which mirrors God. Such a break in the order of things perverts and alienates the natural relation of God, rational mind and the material part of man.[6] This withdrawal of God and the rational mind from matter is the origin of evil. Evil (vice) is thus described as an absence, a shadow, 'a thing that has no inherent existence'.[7]

Let us turn now to Kierkegaard where a similar view finds expression. Sexuality, sin and an alienation from the innocent, ignorant, natural state result in the fundamental emotion of existential ontology: *Angst*.

[1] Gregory of Nyssa, 'On the Making of Man', XVIII, *Select Works and Letters* (Library of Nicene and Post-Nicene Fathers of the Christian Church, Vol. V), Oxford and N.Y., 1893, pp. 407–8. The selection of Gregory of Nyssa to represent the views of the Ancient Church is deliberate. As Ueberweg says of him: 'The first who sought to establish by rational considerations the whole complex of orthodox doctrines.' Gilson says his treatise 'On the Making of Man' was widely known in the Middle Ages (E. Gilson, *History of Christian Philosophy in the Middle Ages*, London, 1955, p. 55). Thus his influence is of central importance to all later pathematologies. It is a classic attitude deeply rooted in the history of thought about emotion.
[2] FE 37, pp. 95–6.
[3] Gregory, *ibid.*, XVII, 4.
[4] *Ibid.*, XX.
[5] The term 'rupture' is used in the 'Prolegomena' (*op. cit.*, p. 9) by W. Moore and H. A. Wilson.
[6] 'On the Making of Man', XII, 9–14.
[7] Gregory, 'The Great Catechism', V, *op. cit.*, p. 480.

With sinfulness was posited sexuality. That same instant the history of the race begins. Since sinfulness moves by quantitative increments, so does dread also. The consequence of original sin or of its presence in the individual is dread. . . .—S. Kierkegaard, *The Concept of Dread* (transl. by W. Lowrie), Princeton, 1946, p. 47.

Freud, too, gives every indication of considering *Angst* the fundamental emotion. He writes: '. . . all affects are capable of being changed into anxiety'.[1] And in his essay on the uncanny he says that 'psychoanalytic theory' would maintain 'that every emotional affect, whatever its quality, is transformed by repression into morbid anxiety . . .'[2] Also he admits truth in the statement that '. . . anxiety would be the fundamental phenomenon and main problem of neurosis'.[3] There are two *Angst* hypotheses in Freud's work,[4] an earlier and a later one, yet each has its own conceptual involvement with a notion of severance or alienation and with a notion of primordial not-being. On the first view, id-anxiety is the result of libido (sexual) repression. One is no longer in the natural state of the pleasure principle. Repression, a reflection of reality, has intervened. Anxiety is due to a rupture in the natural order of things, an alienation of the Ego (compare Gregory's rational mind) from the primordial Id (compare Gregory's irrational matter, described by him as a 'shapeless unorganized thing'.)[5] On the second view, ego-anxiety is the result of situations of danger, of which the event of birth is the prototype.[6] Anxiety reflects man's separate existence, his exposure to danger, the prototype of which (birth) is the instant when the history of the individual begins (compare Kierkegaard above).

With Heidegger we find again the central role of *Angst*. Again it is a primary phenomenon. As Bollnow says about Heidegger's system: 'All other emotional dispositions are from the outset referable to *Angst*.'[7] Bollnow even claims: 'Thus the entire structure of the philosophy of Heidegger rests on the meagre ground of a single emotional disposition, *Angst*.'[8] Although the theological notions of

---

[1] Freud, S., 'Analysis of a Phobia in a Five-Year Old Boy' (1909), *Coll. Papers*, Vol. III, p. 178. ('Analyse der Phobie eines fünfjährigen Knaben', *Ges. Schr.* VIII, Leipzig/Wien/Zürich, p. 156).

[2] 'The "Uncanny" ' (1919), *Coll. Papers*, IV, p. 394. (*Ges. Schr.*, X, p. 394).

[3] *Inhibitions, Symptoms and Anxiety* (1926), Intern. Psycho-Analytic Library No. 28. p. 119 (*Ges. Schr.* XI, p. 85).

[4] *Ibid.*, pp. 150–4 (pp. 103–5).

[5] Gregory, Prolegomena, *op. cit. sup.*, p. 9.

[6] *Inhibitions, Symptoms and Anxiety*, pp. 104–5 (pp. 151–3).

[7] Bollnow, O. F., *Das Wesen der Stimmungen*, Frankfurt a/M., 1941, p. 38. 'Alle anderen Stimmungen sind von vornherein auf die Angst bezogen.'

[8] *Ibid.*, p. 39: 'So ruht bei Heidegger der ganze Bau seiner Philosophie auf dem schmalen Grund einer einzigen Stimmung, der Angst.' See also L. Binswanger (*Grundformen und Erkenntnis menschlichen Daseins*, 2nd edn., Zürich, 1953), p. 635, where Binswanger considers 'Angst' the central concept of Heidegger's '*Seinsauffassung*'.

sin and the biological notions of sex are not overtly present in Heidegger's concept of *Angst*, we find again that it is linked with a concept of separation, 'thrown-ness' (*Geworfenheit*) and with a concept of not-being ('Dread reveals Nothing' [1]).

The conclusion to all this is: In spite of completely different centuries and nationalities, and even more, completely different systematic approaches, and also in spite of certain missing links in the chains of arguments, there is such a striking parallel that we take the model of thinking to be similar in all, *in one respect—emotions can ultimately be traced to a root concept of not-being*. To make it clearer we can schematize it as follows:

GREGORY:	passions		animal mode of generation	sin	'rupture'	non-existence
KIERKEGAARD:		Angst	sex	sin	the Fall	
FREUD:	affects and neuroses	Angst—	sex	danger	repression → / birth →	Primordial / Id
HEIDEGGER:	all emotional dispositions	Angst			'Thrown-ness'	Das Nichts

The theory of Lacroze serves as example of a theory of emotion based upon a root concept of *Angst* which he presents as the *a priori* essence of all emotions:

> The conclusion which emerges from this study is that all emotion, normal or pathological, in man as well as in animal, in the primitive as in civilized man, in the child as in the adult, has its source in a specific anxiety which represents, consequently, the primary affective fact.— R. Lacroze, *L'Angoisse et l'émotion*, Paris, 1938, p. 247 (my translation).

The elevation of anxiety to such a metaphysical position reminds one of the role of fear in Buddhist thought:

> Fear is innate, not only in man, but in everything which exists. The birds, animals of every sort, men, the sun, the moon, the worlds are continually in dread. . . . It is this that one calls 'World filled with fear and dread'. M. Horiou Toki, 'Si-do-in-dzou, Gestes de l'Officiant', *Ann. Musée Guimet, Bibl. d'Etudes*, Paris, 1899, p. 42.[2]

There, too, as with Kierkegaard and Gregory, dread is a sign of

---

[1] Heidegger, M., 'What is Metaphysics', in *Essence and Being*, London, 1949, p. 366.
[2] I am indebted to Prof. Dale Saunders, Univ. of Pennsylvania, for this reference.

actuality and imperfection. The Divine (Gregory's God, the Buddha) is without dread and without imperfection.

Lacroze finds the origin of *Angst* in the basic metaphysical conditions of life: the opposition between static being and dynamic becoming. The individual seeks to hold back change and the flow of life. Thus: 'All affectivity . . . marks the protestation of the individual against the movement of life . . .' (p. 255).

Again there is a parallel in Gregory who also holds change to be the law of created life.[1] He and Lacroze differ, however, in relating it to emotion. Lacroze opts for dynamic becoming as the preferable principle, and so emotions as negative events are against change. Gregory opts for the perfect changelessness of the creator, thus the emotions as negative events are changes. In both cases, emotions are viewed negatively.

It is just this *negativism* that we have sought to bring out by this exposition of the model underlying these theories. Their root is called in the language of metaphysics, matter; of theology, sin; of moral philosophy, evil; of ontology, the void; of biology, sex. And though Kierkegaard and Heidegger both give *Angst* value and a positive prospect in terms of the possibilities of freedom, responsibility and salvation,[2] and though Gregory says God 'gave scope to evil for a nobler end',[3] it remains problematic if this model in which anxiety, sin and nothingness play such a central role does not taint all emotion with the curse of negativity.

It appears we have shifted from one kind of ground to another as we went along. At first the accounts were in terms of genetic roots, while at last we were exposing ontological roots. But the principle of explanation has in fact remained the same. The account of emotion is given in terms of a single origin, root or ground. And *the fundamental problem of this section is consequently the relation of the many and the one*, a riddle treated classically by Plato in the *Parmenides*. Here, we have seen a variety of solutions. According to Shand, the one is a potential in each of the many. For Suttie, the one *transforms* itself into one or another of the many. For Lacroze, the one is the *source* (as *essence*) of the many. Ruckmick says the one *spreads* into the many, while for Bridges, Williams, Gesell and Wallon, the one *develops* (matures, evolves, unfolds) into the many. For Crile, Cobb and Landauer, the many are *inherited* from the one. However, in spite of these solutions, it remains problematic if the qualitative variety of the emotions, or the multiplicity of their number, or their complexity, or their novelty can be accounted for

---

[1] Prolegomena, *op. cit.*, p. 9.   [2] Kierkegaard, *op. cit.*, Chapter V.
[3] Prolegomena, p. 10.

by reference to a single, simple source. Even if the one single source were agreed upon—which is definitely not the case—there would yet remain the relation of it to the emotions themselves. And so we can conclude with this paradox: although these theories go to the root of emotions, there is more to emotion than its root.

This has the following bearing on therapy. If emotion is explained through a definite first premise—ontological or biological—i.e. laid down in the genes, part of animal inheritance, grounded in unicellular life, Original Sin or primary not-being, etc., then it becomes on this model a fixed constitutional stigma, an immutable essence, which can only be stoically accepted or puritanically fought. But such 'givens' are of course not simply static facts. As these theories have pointed out, they are processes of development and maturation. Therefore, as with all 'givens', therapy will depend upon what is done with this endowment, what will be the nature of the development of the one into the many. Therapy then can be seen as a process of development towards the differentiation of the emotions and away from their single, simple root or essence. For the extraordinary thing about emotion is not its highly dubious single root, but its actual phenomenology, its incredible range and shifting variety. And so the direction of therapy would not be downward and backward towards the extraction of some root, the extinction of some evil essence; instead it would aim towards the full play and free flowering of emotional life, still the mark of heroes in human culture.

XIV

EMOTION AND REPRESENTATIONS

'REPRESENTATIONS' as used here refers wholly to intra-psychic events. In particular, the concept refers to sensations, perceptions, ideas and images. There will be three ways in which these theories link emotion with representations: (1) Emotion consists of representations; (2) emotion arises from representations; (3) representations arise from emotion. Although these theories qualify the concept of representations in terms of phylogeny, or the unconscious, or in terms of significance, these qualifications are incidental to the main hypothesis which holds that emotion can be accounted for through the intra-psychic events of sensations, perceptions, ideas and images.

The first view says, in short, emotions are made up of the stuff of sensation elements. Federn (Chapter V) said this in terms of sensations developing on *ego-boundaries*; Finley and F. Allport (Chapter X C spoke of *muscular* sensations. James (Chapter IV, p. 49) wrote that emotions are 'sensational processes', or a 'sum of elements'. Those who follow James stress *visceral* sensations (Chapter X B). Aveling[1] and Beck[2] emphasize the *molar* nature of the sensations.

Furthermore, sensation is also presented as the stuff of emotion wherever emotion is not differentiated from feeling and feeling is muddled with sensation. This comes about in the following ways: (*a*) when pain and pleasure as sensations are confused with pleasure and unpleasure as feelings; (*b*) when a single faculty, level, field, etc., is posited as a common pool of sensations, feelings, drives, impulses, needs, and the like; (*c*) when difficulties in language lead to conceptual contaminations, e.g. the use of *sensible*, sentimental, sensitive to describe feeling, or the use of feeling to describe touching, sensing, proprioception, etc.; (*d*) when feeling is reduced to sensation or sensation to feeling in a hierarchical schema. The confusion of these terms is a standard problem in psychology. The ground of it may lie

---

[1] Aveling, F., 'Emotion, Conation and Will', FE 28, p. 57: 'An emotion is the massive and generally wholly unclear experience of coenaesthesio-kinaesthetic sensation.'   [2] Beck, see Chapter VIII above.

less in the facts or concepts than in the psychology of the individual who observes the facts or formulates the concepts and in whom these two functions of sensation and feeling may not be at all clearly differentiated.[1]

But to the theories themselves; Russell describes the stuff of emotion as sensations:

> An emotion—rage, for example—will be a certain kind of process, consisting of perceptions and (in general) bodily movements. The desires and pleasures and pains involved are properties of this process, not separate items in the stuff of which emotion is composed. The dynamic elements in an emotion, if we are right in our analysis, contain, from our point of view, no ingredients beyond those contained in the processes considered in Lecture III.[2] The ingredients of an emotion are only sensations and images and bodily movements succeeding each other according to a certain pattern. With this conclusion we may leave the emotions and pass to the consideration of the will.—B. Russell, *The Analysis of Mind*, London, 1921, p. 284.

The view that emotion is an association of sensations is essentially the same as presented by David Hartley (1749) who wrote: 'Here we may observe, First that our Passions or Affections can be no more than Aggregates of simple Ideas united by Association.' [3]

Heller proposes two kinds of representations. The first he calls sensuous, comprising both organic sensations and the primary sensation-feeling of pleasure/unpleasure. This is emotion in its simple, primary and immediately given aspect; the basis of all higher feelings.[4] But for an emotion to be anything more specific and differentiated it must include another kind of representation—a memory image. The analysis of every affect shows that there is no affect without experience, that is, 'recollection of something lived.' 'Affect must have experience previous to it: only the "burnt child dreads the fire".' [5]

---

[1] See Jung, C. G., *Psychological Types*, London, 1923, pp. 543–7; 585–8, for a treatment of Sensation and Feeling as psychological functions. See also C. Hartshorne's excellent discussion, *The Philosophy and Psychology of Sensation*, pp. 107–36.

[2] These ingredients are, according to Lecture III, described by Russell as follows: 'I do not myself believe that there is any value in this threefold division of the contents of the mind. I believe that sensations (including images) supply all the "stuff" of the mind, and that everything else can be analysed into groups of sensations related in various ways, or characteristic of sensations or of groups of sensations.'—*Ibid.*, p. 69.

[3] Hartley, D., *Observations on Man*, I, III, 89, London, 1749.

[4] Heller, R., *Das Wesen der 'Affekte'*, 2nd edn., Wien/Leipzig, 1946, p. 21: '. . . alle höheren Gefühle entweder direkt oder durch Bindeglieder auf diese elementaren Gefühle zurückgehen.'

[5] *Ibid.*, p. 7: 'Wir konstatieren hier gleich, was die Analyse jedes "Affekts" ergibt, dass *keiner von ihnen ohne Erfahrung*, also Erinnerung an Erlebtes und demgemäss etwa Vorstellung eines ähnlichen entstehen kann. Dies unterscheidet den "Affekt" deutlich vom "präsenten" sinnlichen Gefühl: präsenter sinnlicher Schmerz und sinnliche Lust werden vom Kleinkind einmal als Erstes erlebt, *der "Affekt" muss Erlebtes hinter sich haben*: erst das "gebrannte Kind fürchtet das Feuer".'

These memory images, or re-presentations of past experiences, work also as phantasy anticipations of the future. They not only constitute emotion,[1] but they actively develop and create the 'higher' forms of emotion out of past experiences. Thus, for Heller, the memory-image is the intellectual (*geistig*) element which uses the sensuous element as material (p. 64).

This concept of the memory image as playing the main role in the active development of emotion leads over to the second kind of theory in this section where emotion is said to result from representations. In the last century, Wundt[2] said: 'Where an emotion appears we may assume the presence of memorial ideas . . .'; and Stanley,[3] '. . . we make representations the basis of emotion . . .' Brun's criterion of emotion is also based on a mnemic factor:

> There are secondary feelings, already equipped with an experiential component, for which I should like to reserve the name 'Affects'. But feelings which are released not through an initial outer stimulus, but through purely mnemic ways should according to my suggestion be described as 'Emotions'.[4]

What is the nature of these memorial representations? For Heller, Wundt and Stanley—and of course for Russell too—memory representations are ultimately nothing but sensations, or as Hobbes puts it, 'decaying sense'.[5] On the bare wax tablet of the mind sensations leave impressions, or after-images, which are memory representations. Brun, however, indicates another kind of memory in connection with emotion. This is a kind of biological memory, a kind of inherited, instinctual memory like the pattern reaction of Watson and the phylogenetic theories of Chapter XIII. Such a notion of a biological memory factor has been elaborated particularly in the works of Semon[6], Rignano[7], and Bleuler.[8] A passage from Freud connects a concept of inherited memory to emotion:

[1] Heller, R., *Das Wesen der 'Affekte'*, 2nd edn., Wien/Leipzig, 1946 p. 20: 'Phantasievorstellungen zu erwartender sinnlicher Gefühle konstituieren die "Affekte" . . .'

[2] Wundt, W., *Lectures on Human and Animal Psychology* (transl. from 2nd German edn. by Creighton and Titchener), London and N.Y., 1894, p. 375.

[3] Stanley, H. M., *Studies in the Evolutionary Psychology of Feeling*, London, 1895, p. 89.

[4] Brun, R., *Allgemeine Neurosenlehre*, 3rd edn., Basel, 1954, p. 194: 'Es entstehen so sekundäre, bereits mit einer Erfahrungskomponente ausgestattete Gefühle, für welche ich den Namen "Affekte" reservieren möchte; Gefühle dagegen, die nicht durch eine originale äussere Reizsituation, sondern auf rein mnemischen Wege ausgelöst werden, sollten nach meinem Vorschlag als "Emotionen" bezeichnet werden.'

[5] Hobbes, T., *Leviathan*.

[6] Semon, R., *Die Mneme*, 3rd edn., Leipzig, 1911.

[7] Rignano, E., *Biological Memory*, London, 1926 (La *Memoria Biologica*, Bologna, 1922). Also *De l'origine et de la nature mnémonique des tendances affectives*, Bologna, 1911.

[8] Bleuler, E., *Die Psychoide als Prinzip der organischen Entwicklung*, Berlin, 1925.

An affect comprises first of all certain motor innervations or discharges; and, secondly, certain sensations, which moreover are of two kinds—namely, the perceptions of the motor actions which have been performed, and the directly pleasurable or painful sensations which give the affect what we call its dominant note. But I do not think that this description penetrates to the essence of an affect. With certain affects one seems to be able to see deeper, and to recognize that the core of it, binding the whole complex structure together, is of the nature of a *repetition* of some particular very significant previous experience. This experience could only have been an exceedingly early impression of a universal type, to be found in the previous history of the species rather than of the individual. In order to be better understood I might say that an affective state is constructed like an hysterical attack, i.e. is the precipitate of a reminiscence. An hysterical attack is therefore comparable to a newly formed individual affect, and the normal affect to a universal hysteria which has become a heritage.—S. Freud, *A General Introduction to Psychoanalysis*, Lecture XXV, N.Y., 1953.

With this statement from Freud we are led beyond a theory based only upon representations experienced in the life of the individual. And so the problem now becomes one of accounting for the relation of three things: (*a*) emotion, (*b*) the individually experienced representations (present images and ideas, or after-images), and (*c*) the biological mnemic factor. This problem is worked out by Gemelli. He offers a way of bridging the two sets of views we have seen so far: emotion as the result of individually experienced representations; emotion as the result of a biological mnemic factor.

Gemelli's system of affective life has four fundamental elements. The first two are comparable to Heller's, i.e. a sensuous element ('organic sensations') and a cognitive element which can be 'a memory . . . an idea or even a perception or an image'. The third element is the motions (attraction-repulsion, etc., such as we saw in Chapter XII) which accompany the organic sensations. The fourth element Gemelli calls instinct and he identifies it with the motor attitude described by Bull (Chapter X C, pp. 129 ff). This biological nucleus, or instinct, at the root of emotion is what makes the cognitive element, the representations, effective. He writes:

It is through the operation of this fourth element that we can understand how a state of consciousness (an idea, a memory or a perception) produces an affective state, and a particular affective state in a particular case. Every instinct is a biological complex, and any particular affective state is caused only when the preceding cognitive element evokes the biological complex that is necessary to its existence. Let us take an example: a knife seen by the subject does not by itself alone awaken any biological complex; it is purely an object of perception. But if the subject in perceiving such an object, has also knowledge that it has a dark significance, because of the special circumstances in which he sees it, so

169

that it constitutes a menace, immediately there will occur in him a movement of repulsion, with a general feeling of disgust, resulting in the still more general feeling known as fear. The perception of the object, seen in those particular circumstances, has evoked in him a very basic biological complex which is at the core of the instinct of self-preservation, and which causes the reaction known as fear.

Thus the biological complex constitutes the instinct, and is the actual cause of the affective state; without it, feeling would remain unintelligible. . . .

Whenever an inadequate stimulus touches off an affective state, we can be sure it has some element in common with the biological complex which constitutes the instinct at the basis of that particular affective state. These elements, common to the stimulus and the biological complex, are the occasion for the production of the particular affective state which has its origin in that particular biological foundation.—A. Gemelli, 'Orienting Concepts in the Study of Affective States', *J. Nerv. Ment. Dis.*, 1949, pp. 305-6.[1]

Just the same thing is said by Lindworsky; stimuli, inadequate in themselves, release emotion because they share common characteristics with a basic biological complex.[2]

Let us review the ground we have covered so far. Firstly, we were told that emotion is made up of sensations which can be qualified in many ways (visceral, muscular, molar, etc.) but which fall into two main classes: those which arise from the inner organic field and those which arise from the field of outer perceptions. Secondly, we were told by Heller that in addition to these sensations, emotions are made up of—in fact created by—memory images. These memory images are the results of past sensations, e.g. 'only the burnt child fears the fire'. Freud concurs, finding the memory factor more fundamental in emotion than the bundle of sensations arising from the inner and outer fields. However, he does not limit this memory to the life of the individual. It is a nonpersonal reminiscence, belonging to 'the previous history of the species'. Brun, too, relies on a phylogenetic

---

[1] Gemelli would reduce the biological complex to a *single* instinctive root—self-preservation—which might seem to make his theory belong among those of Chapter XIII. However, it is the interplay of this single force with the 'cognitive element' (representations) which is the main contribution of his view.

[2] Lindworsky, J., 'Orientierende Untersuchungen über höhere Gefühle', *Arch. f. d. ges. Psychol.*, 1928, p. 232.

'. . . *warum können die inadäquaten Reize Reproduktionsmotiv für biologische Komplexe sein*, mit denen sie an sich nichts zu tun haben? . . . Damit scheint die Lösung gegeben zu sein: der inadäquate Reiz hat mit dem biologischen Grundkomplex gewisse allgemeine Züge gemeinsam, und darum können diese allgemeinen Züge den biologischen Grundkomplex reproduzieren.'

'Der Grundgedanke unserer Arbeitshypothese ist sonach der: *bei komplexen Gefühlen erleben wir jene biologischen Grundkomplexe—ganz oder teilweise—die mit der gegenwärtigen Situation gemeinsame Züge teilen und zurzeit in genügender Bereitschaft sind.*'

memory factor to account for emotion. And lastly, Gemelli says that a biological, instinctual complex 'is the actual cause of the affective state'. He and Lindworsky say further that the sensations, memories, ideas and images are only effective in giving rise to emotion when they are in some meaningful relation to the biological complex at the root. It would seem with this that we have the usual view of emotion as an accompaniment of instinct, or a phylogenetic behaviour pattern. However, what is different and new here is the implication that this instinctual component is not mere force or action-pattern, but has a memory or *representational* aspect. Further, the explanation of emotion now depends upon the 'elements' common to both the stimulating representations and the biological memory factor.

A theory which links these two factors of instinct and representations is presented by MacCurdy. According to his view, the linking elements are *unconscious complexes* which are both instinctively impelled and consist of representations.

> A given stimulus, if it be productive of emotion, does not merely arouse conscious perceptions and overt behaviour but activates unconscious mental processes as well. These are associated instinctive tendencies incorporated with what can be spoken of for the time being as ideas. These instinctively impelled ideas or 'complexes' tend to come into consciousness but are blocked by an inhibition, not engendered for the first time in this situation, but pre-existent. . . . Being activated the complexes are now co-conscious. . . . There are thus two different systems of thinking going on, a conscious system with one content and a co-conscious with another content. Repression prevents the co-conscious series from emerging as such but the latter does reach expression in two ways, as emotional expression and as affect, i.e., objectively and subjectively. . . .
> —J. T. MacCurdy, *The Psychology of Emotion*, London, 1925, p. 86.

MacCurdy differentiates three concepts: affect, emotional expression and emotion. Affect is the subjective 'feeling' side; emotional expressions are the objective behavioural phenomena. 'A complete emotion is a combination of affect and emotional expression' (p. 44). All, however, stand on the hypothesis that emotion is 'the product of unconscious images':

> Emotional expression is the product of unconscious images which stimulate involuntary behaviour, either overt or visceral, accessory to purposive actions. Affect is the impression made on consciousness by active unconscious imaginal processes, which do not gain any other outlet.—*Ibid.*, p. 567 (original in italics).

Does the 'unconscious image' then provide the element in common to both instinct and representation? It does not because in MacCurdy's view these unconscious images, although instinctively impelled and bound up with instinct in a complex, *remain separable from instinct.* The images are like a stuff pushed along by a force, or the complex is like a structural system through which runs instinctual energy. Fundamentally, the image—even when qualified as an unconscious image—is separate from instinct, and we are still no wiser about why certain images have something in common with instinct, a connection out of which emotion results. Gemelli, too, cannot make this connection, while Lindworsky tries it through the concept of memory association. In all views so far they remain separable phenomena. Emotion stands on the two legs of instinctual force and representational content, but the connection between the two, and therefore the explanation of emotion in terms of the two, remains unclear, What is the relation of instinct and image?

Fouillée[1] unites the two in his concept of 'idées-forces'. Lévy-Bruhl says that in primitive psychology there are certain kinds of representations (*représentations collectives*) which are inseparable from their dynamic aspects, 'où les éléments émotionnels et moteurs sont des *parties intégrantes* des représentations.' [2] Onians, on the basis of an analysis of the earliest Greek concepts, presents a similar theory of 'the primal unity of mind in which perception or cognition is associated with or immediately followed by an emotion and a tendency to action . . . a unity whose survival in our own processes is stressed by the "ideo-motor" theory of modern psychology which asserts that "every 'idea' is not only a state or act of knowing but also a tendency to movement".' [3,4] 'Animals, says Seneca, have images from which arise impetuous movements... violent, obscure, and fleeting'.[5] Cuvier, the early nineteenth-century naturalist, brings the force and the image even closer together by holding the view that 'instinct consists in images, or innate and constant sensations, which determine to action in the same manner as ordinary sensations; it is "a sort of vision, a dream, analogous to somnambulism" '.[6] Today, Jung takes up the same point of view in further elaboration of his earlier complex theory upon which MacCurdy's view is based.

Jung writes: 'There are in fact no amorphous instincts, as every instinct bears in itself the pattern of its situation. Always it fulfils an image, and the image has fixed qualities.' [7] These images are an

[1] Fouillée, A., *L'Évolutionisme des idées-forces*, 5th edn., Paris, 1911.

[2] Lévy-Bruhl, L., *Les Fonctions mentales dans les sociétés inférieures*, 2nd edn., Paris, 1912, pp. 28 ff.

[3] McDougall, W., *An Outline of Psychology*, 12th edn., London, 1948, pp. 290–1 (McDougall criticizes the theory).   [4] OET, pp. 16–17.

[5] SS, p. 54. *Cf.* H. Hediger, 'Der Traum der Tiere', *Ciba Ztschft.*, 99, 1945.

[6] Quoted from T. Ribot, *The Psychology of the Emotions*, London, 1897, p. 252.

[7] Jung, C. G., 'The Spirit of Psychology', in *Spirit and Nature, Papers from the Eranos Yearbooks*, N.Y. and London, 1954, p. 411.

integral part of instinct; they represent the *'meaning* of instinct'.[1] They are in fact instincts, not as dynamic impulses and overt actions, but as the forms, patterns or significations of action. The concept 'pattern of behaviour' unites the two concepts of image and instinct, without identifying the two as with Cuvier or separating the two as with MacCurdy. This double aspect of the same phenomenon can also be grasped by an analogy to the spectrum: 'The dynamism of instinct is lodged as it were in the infrared part of the spectrum, whereas the instinctual image lies in the ultraviolet part.'[2] Just as the dynamism of instinct has a meaningful image, so too the image is dynamic. It stimulates to action and gives rises to emotion.[3]

In this view, the unconscious images of MacCurdy would be re-interpreted as instinctual images. The complex would consist not of two separate elements—stuff and force—but the stuff is the specific pattern of the force. Emotion would result when the stimulus-image (individually experienced representation) and the instinctual representation resemble each other, or 'click' in such a way that the stimulus image represents the instinctual image.

To return to the example of Gemelli, the image of the knife raises fear only when that image has elements in common with instinct. According to MacCurdy, as we understand him, the image of the knife gives rise to emotion when it is part of an unconscious (repressed) complex impelled by instinctual forces. While for Jung, the complex to which the image of the knife is associated has a specific archetypal core which is the energetic drawing power of the complex and which makes the association, from an energetic point of view, possible. It is this instinctual image, this archetypal core of the complex which would give to the image of the knife its 'dark significance . . . so that it constitutes a menace' (Gemelli) giving rise to fear. *The image of the knife thus becomes a symbol.*[4] It has a partly conscious and presented aspect and also a partly unconscious, non-presented and undefined aspect. Therefore, at the root of emotion is not just the image of the knife, but an instinctual, memorial image which resembles, or has assimilated, the knife image, turning the relatively simple conscious representation into a symbol. (In German, it has given the *Bild* a *Sinn*.) Or, in other terms, the conscious image is a *causa efficiens*, the unconscious image a *causa formalis* which unite in the symbol giving rise to emotion.

[1] *Op. cit.*, p. 412.
[2] *Op. cit.*, p. 421–2. (MacCurdy also uses the analogy of the spectrum in terms of the physiological and mental aspects of emotion, *op. cit.*, p. 574.)
[3] *Op. cit.*, p. 416.
[4] For clarification of Jung's use of the concepts 'archetype', 'complex', 'instinct', 'symbol', etc., see, in addition to 'The Spirit of Psychology', J. Jacobi's *Complex, Archetype, Symbol*, London and N.Y., 1959, and L. Stein's 'What is a Symbol supposed to be?', *J. Analyt. Psychol.*, 1957.

This in turn ties in with the views of emotion as energy (Chapter VI). The symbol, for Jung, because of its mediating function between the known and the unknown (conscious and unconscious) acts as an energy transformer. Portmann, who hesitates identifying the images which unlock instinctual behaviour with the archetypal images of Jung, nevertheless shows how certain images act as energy transformers in animals.[1] (The concept of 'symbolization' plays a further role in this chapter at the end where we take up the therapeutic methods consequent on these theories.)

So it becomes clearer in this view why casual images, sensations and ideas in themselves gentle and tepid enough can give rise to gigantic seizures of emotion. Such images have been associated to, or resemble, instinctual dynamisms; they have been symbolized and perceived *sub specie aeternitatis*—or better *instinctus*—in their archaic and symbolic form. So too it becomes clearer why emotion can arise even without the gentle and tepid provokers.[2] As the Stoics noted the origin of emotion is in man's reason alone, not in some separate extraneous force: 'Imagination . . . alone calls it into being . . .'[3] It arises from the *phantasiae* (representational impressions) in the soul.[4] Depression, irritability, joy and dread can occur spontaneously, without conscious stimulating images, without special situations, without observable physiological ground. This could be accounted for in this view by the continual changing constellation of individually experienced *phantasiae* collected in complexes around instinctual images. They remain subliminal, perhaps revealing themselves occasionally in dreams and in new ideas and schemes, but acting as the continually changing ground of emotion.

We can pass now to the third kind of theory in this section: *representations result from emotion*. A view of this kind is given by Plotinus[5] who held that emotions could arise out of ideas and that

---

[1] Portmann, A., 'Die Bedeutung der Bilder in der lebendigen Energiewandlung' *Eranos Jahrbuch*, XXI, Zurich, 1953, pp. 325–57. His own view of emotion as expressed in this paper is an energetic one. The energetic aspect of behaviour brought about by 'Bilder' (images) is only one aspect, whose other side is experienced as emotion. ('. . . die im Verhalten beobachteten Transformationen dieser Energien nur der eine Aspekt eines Geschehens sind, welches seine andere Seite in der Innerlichkeit des Organismus hat und dort als Emotion einen besonderen Spannungszustand des Erlebens schafft, den wir aus unserer Erlebnisweise kennen, dessen Erforschung aber beim höheren Tier mit ausserordentlichen Schwierigkeiten verbunden ist' (p. 331).)

[2] See D. O. Hebb ('The Problem of Consciousness and Introspection', *Brain Mechanisms and Consciousness*, ed. by J. F. Delafresnaye, Oxford, 1954) who describes experiments in which highly emotional reactions occurred as a result of spontaneous 'visual hallucinations' in subjects placed in isolation with a minimum of visual and tactual stimuli. 'Sensory deprivation' is not emotion deprivation, again indicating that emotion does not need outer stimuli.

[3] Zeller, E., *The Stoics, Epicureans and Sceptics*, London, 1892, p. 245.

[4] FE 37, p. 71.   [5] Plotinus, *Enneads*, III, 6, 4.

they could also arise independently of ideas, developing ideas out of themselves. Onians suggests the same: 'Emotion may precede the idea, may be vaguely felt before taking definite shape in consciousness and being 'intellectualized'.[1] Bleuler[2] makes affect prior to representations in the realm of autistic thinking, where affects facilitate or inhibit associations and direct the representational content of dreams, fantasies, hallucinations, etc. Emotion can also be said to control memory. Rapaport's[3] extensive report on this field gives a great deal of evidence for a theory of the 'emotional organization of memory'. The selection, retention, forgetting and confusion of memory representations are the result of emotion. Wundt makes the essential criterion of emotion to be the results it has upon ideas.

> This twofold relation of emotion to feeling and ideation has led to a diversity of view as to its nature. It has been regarded both as an intensive feeling, and as a feeling originating from the train of ideas. Neither of these definitions does it full justice. The typical emotion has three stages: an initial feeling; a subsequent change in the train of ideas, intensifying and qualitatively modifying the initial feeling; and (always supposing that the emotion is distinct and well defined) a final feeling, of greater or less duration, which may possibly give rise to a new emotion of which it forms the initial feeling. The principal difference between feeling and emotion, that is, consists in the second stage: the alteration in the train of ideas.—W. Wundt, *Lectures on Human and Animal Psychology* (transl. from 2nd German edn. by Creighton and Titchener), London and N.Y., 1894.[4]

What has been said so far amounts to this: *Emotion is prior to representations* since it precedes (Onians), directs (Bleuler), organizes (Rapaport) and alters (Wundt) them.

Evaluations of the psychological results of psychosurgery can also be taken to mean that emotion might be the ground of images, imagination and thought. Costello's[5] investigation 'suggests that the operation lessens the vitality of . . . images and makes them easier to control'. McFie, *et al.*[6] suggest that a 'flatness of affect rather

---

[1] OET, p. 17. See also Bergson (Chapter XVIII, p. 226) for this view in connection with creativity.

[2] Bleuler, E., 'Das autistische Denken', *Jhb. f. Psychoanal. Psychopath. Forsch.*, 1912, pp. 1–39.

[3] EM.

[4] Compare A. Lehmann (*Die Hauptgesetze des menschlichen Gefühlslebens*, 2nd edn., Leipzig, 1914, pp. 310–16) who also makes the main criterion of emotion to be an *alteration*, not just of the train of ideas, but of the whole self, or ego-personality.

[5] Costello, C., 'The Effects of Pre-frontal Leucotomy upon Visual Imagery and the Ability to Perform Complex Operations', *J. Ment. Sci.*, 1956, pp. 507–16.

[6] McFie, J., Piercy, M. F., and Zangwill, O., 'The Rorschach Test in Obsessional Neurosis with Special Reference to the Effects of Pre-frontal Leucotomy', *Brit. J. Med. Psychol.*, 1951, p. 178.

than intellectual loss' accounts for the occasional autobiographically reported loss of imagination after the operation. Petrie writes:

> It is also of interest that Brain attaches so much importance to the part which emotion and imagery play in human achievement because emotion provides the motive power which sustains our course of action, and if action is to take time the object to which it is directed must be constantly represented to us by means of mental imagery. Our results suggest that a leucotomy patient has diminished emotion and there is also some evidence to suggest that he has less vivid mental imagery.—A. Petrie, *Personality and the Frontal Lobes*, London, 1952, p. 105.

Leucotomy 'is said to "decrease emotional tension" and "remove anxiety".'[1] In addition to this aim, Tow sums up its results as follows: 'Possibly the truest and most accurate way of describing the net effect on the total personality is to say that he is more simple . . .'[2] The impoverishment of imagination is a significant contributing factor to this post-operative simplicity.[3] The literature gives many examples confirming this observation. Freeman and Watts write: 'Creative capacity in artistic, literary, musical, theatrical and other fields undergoes a decided reduction after prefrontal lobotomy.'[4] This operation

---

[1] Cobb, S., *Emotions and Clinical Medicine*, N.Y., 1950, p. 114. Also H. W. and S. G. Allison, 'Personality changes following transorbital Lobotomy', *J. Abn. Soc. Psychol.*, 1954, pp. 219–23.

[2] Tow, P. MacD., *Personality Changes Following Frontal Leucotomy*, London, 1955, p. 235.

[3] Tow, *op. cit.*, pp. 222 ff.

[4] Freeman, W., and Watts, J. W., *Psychosurgery*, Oxford and Springfield, Ill., 2nd edn., 1950, p. 256. The same authors are said by Tow (*op. cit. sup.*, p. 235) to 'affirm that the need for creative expression has gone after leucotomy'. Freeman, however, in a later report ('Frontal Lobotomy, 1936–56: A follow-up study of 3,000 patients from one to twenty years', *Am. J. Psychiat.*, 1957, p. 877) writes: 'High level performance is possible after major pre-frontal lobotomy, and especially so after transorbital lobotomy. This is indicated by the competence of lobotomized patients in such professional fields as medicine, law, teaching, nursing, etc.' What is decisive is not *what* jobs people hold but *how* they perform these jobs. Many professional tasks can be performed regularly with flattened affect and impaired imagination. The debate in this field of psychosurgery continues, e.g. A. Smith and E. F. Kinder ('Changes in Psychological Test Performances of Brain-Operated Schizophrenics after 8 Years', *Science*, 129, pp. 149–50, 1959) report 'marked and definitive losses by operated subjects after a post-operative interval of eight years . . .' Further, Freeman's report can be brought to task because he does not present any descriptions or personality evaluations of these subjects, with an adequate comparison of their post-operative and pre-operative personality. In all this we can see that conclusions in this field are not conclusive; progress is too rapid and refinements of technique outdate previous methods both of surgery and of evaluation. At least the following variables must be kept in mind when assessing the literature: (1) the kind of operation; (2) the amount of area involved and the size and location of the cut; (3) the prior personality of the patient, e.g. level of deterioration; (4) the 'spiritual quality' of the patient; (5) the prognostic role of emotional tension in the case; (6) the method of evaluation of results (tests, statistics, autobiographies, clinical findings, etc.); (7) length of time after the operation the evaluation is made and 'follow-ups'. And finally, the attitude of the observer to what is 'good', 'healthy', 'normal', 'improvement' and to emotion plays the decisive role.

both flattens emotion and reduces imagination. The role of imagination for creative and higher forms of mental functioning would here seem to depend upon the emotional vitality or vividness with which the reprsentational content of imagination is 'charged'. This does not mean that emotion is the ground of imagination or imagery on the model of levels (Schichtentheorie), but that it is *emotion which makes imagery effective*, and is, in that sense, prior to it.

Tow, however, takes pains to point out that the basic changes following surgery are not primarily emotional:

> It is not, however, suggested at any point in this discussion that the basic or essential changes underlying the syndrome demonstrated are emotional. Intellectual and affective changes may well both be primary, and both due to interruption of the same or neighbouring pathways. But the intellectual changes cannot be explained solely as effects secondary to the emotional. . . .—P. MacDonald Tow, *Personality Changes Following Frontal Leucotomy*, London, 1955, p. 234.

This would appear to contradict our thesis in this section. However, Tow hypothesizes that the basic change is due to an 'over-all lack in motivation'. His use of that concept is equivalent to the way Petrie uses the concept of emotion above: 'emotion provides the motive power which sustains our course of action'. Therefore, Tow's statement that the 'intellectual changes cannot be explained solely as effects secondary to the emotional' depends upon a more restricted way in which he uses the concept of emotion. Emotion as 'motive power', as that which makes imagery effective, would still remain primary.

The theory of Nahm elaborates the role of emotion in the development of imagery and the higher forms of thought. First he distinguishes instinct and emotion in terms of images:

> . . . there is implied in emotional reactions the 'awareness' (i.e. the effectiveness) of alternative stimuli or alternative modes of action. Epistemologically there is not only as in instinct a reproductive image allying a present stimulus to the *appercepzionsmass* but imagination in the true sense of the word—the presentation by the organism to itself of an alternative stimulus offering possible modes of action. The individual carried over into instinctive behaviour is blind to alternative stimuli.—M. Nahm, 'The Philosophical Implications of Some Theories of Emotion', *Phil. of Sci.*, 1939, p. 482.
>
> . . . in the emotional-instinctive continuum both reactions involve reproductive 'images' (i.e. effective stimuli). In instinct, however, the organism's activity is governed by . . . one productive image, or . . . stimulus. In emotion the organism's activity indicates the awareness . . . of more than one . . . image or stimulus (p. 483).

This view that emotion evolves an awareness of alternative images, i.e. imagination, would accord with the views of Costello and Tow that poverty of imagination, inability to deal with two things at once (abstract, complex and synthesizing operations), and reduction of emotional life go together. According to Nahm, emotions are important because of their flexible and imaginative function.

> They are important epistemologically through their alliance to contemplation. Practically they function to allow increased flexibility into otherwise reflex action and involve an emphasis upon the individual's increasing freedom from the control by nature . . . The end process, that portion of the continuum known as 'mood' presents at once the antithesis to the instincts and the development of the factors of 'imagination' apparent in the emotions.—*Ibid.*, pp. 485—6.

As Thomas Aquinas observed: 'Human contemplation at present cannot function without images . . .'[1] 'The image is the principle of our knowledge. It is that from which our intellectual activity begins . . .'.[2] What Nahm adds to this is that it is emotion which makes images effective. Contemplation and imagination cannot rely upon a heap of sense-perceptions alone (Thomas' source of images), but these 'higher' activities require emotion for their elaboration.

Bartlett's explanation for the production of images out of emotion is based upon the idea of conflict: images arise when emotion is hindered.

> . . . we can see at once a biological reason for two commonly noted facts: the very close connection between affect and image, and the tendency for images to arise when some normal reaction is hindered. The image method of solving a conflict really represents a new start in mental development. It is the beginning of the growing dominance of cognitive reactions. . . . In one respect it is undoubtedly a very great step forward. . . . But in another respect the image method is even more inefficient than the affective mode. The affect . . . seems normally to carry with it . . . a tendency to hasten its own end. The image does nothing of the kind. Hence, though the image may show *how* a practical dilemma may be overcome it provides no sort of drive for making the necessary effort. Thus, although the image method is now acquired the affect method cannot be wholly dropped.—F. C. Bartlett, 'Feeling, Imaging and Thinking', *Brit. J. Psychol.*, 1925-6, p. 26.

In this view, impulse (or action) and image are distinct and perhaps opposed phenomena, which implies the impotence of imagery and a frustration theory of consciousness. The higher forms of mental life only come into being when the more emotional forms are blocked. This is not of course the case on the model of the continuum used by MacCurdy, Jung and Nahm where emotion and imagery were not dissociated.

[1] *Summa Theologica*, II, II, clxxx, 5, ad 2.
[2] Opusc. xvi, Exposition, *de Trinitate*, vi, 2, ad 5.

To conclude: the hypothesis put in these last views is *without emotion there is no imagination.* Without imagination there is no higher thought and creativity. (The relation of emotion to creativity we shall come to in Chapter XVIII.) The model of this hypothesis is not one of levels, e.g. 1 = emotion, 2 = imagery, 3 = thought. Rather the model is ontological. Emotion is the condition *sine qua non,* the *a priori* essence of imagery, giving it its strength and variety. Emotion makes such representations possible and effective.

We come now to the therapeutic implications of these theories. If representations are bound up with emotions, either as their very stuff, or as their ground, or as their consequent, then the therapy of emotional disorders might well lead through representations. Such a notion in its simplest form is *thought-control,* e.g. 'changing one's ideas', 'not thinking bad thoughts', avoiding wishful fantasy and those life situations evoking stimulating images and sensations. Another way of approaching emotion through representation might be *psychosurgery* which can be interpreted as an attempt to sever the connections between the brain areas which serve representations from those serving emotion. There is also the method of verbalization or intellectualization, or the 'talking-cure' as Freud called *psychoanalysis* in its beginnings. Here the idea is to bring to conscious expression the representational content which is either the stuff or ground of emotion. That free association, confession—even cursing, wit or the use of taboo words and thoughts—alters an emotional condition is a banal fact.

But it is also just as evident that such methods, where they might provide temporary results in terms of avoidance or relief, do little or nothing about the fundamental problem in ethics and therapy: the *transformation* of emotion from an inferior and unadapted mode of behaviour to a form which is serviceable and creative. They do not meet this problem because they do not conceive the problem in this way. Fundamentally, they are all—thought-control, psychosurgery, psychoanalysis—attempts to dissolve the complex of emotion and representations. Thought-control tries to keep ideas clean of emotional contamination. Psychosurgery severs the connections so that ideas lose their emotional values. Psychoanalysis frees ideas and images from their associated affects by abreaction, i.e. releasing or getting rid of the emotion. It treats emotion as a primitive instinctual energy which gets attached ('cathected') to representations, forming complexes and thus distorting them. The union of representation and emotion in a complex is an unholy mixture. The aim is separation (analysis) of the elements, a rational method having for its result dispassionate ideas and images on one side and motor discharge of emotion on the other. It is an ethic for the sake of intellect and will, where action, decision, peaceful order and rational planning are the goals. It is a therapy of representations, curing representations of their emotional attachments. It is not a therapy of emotion, curing emotions of their fixated images. We might sketch a hypothetical contrast of the two methods as follows: the first, 'rational' method aims at freeing the image of Mother or Father from the emotion of hatred; the second, 'emotional' therapeutic method aims rather at developing the emotion of hatred by freeing it from such infantile representations.

The problem as we have put it is not the relief of ordered behaviour from emotion, but the reorganization of the inferior behaviour itself, that is, the transformation of emotion. The theories of this chapter are instructive here. In presenting what they offer to therapy we follow the old hypothesis given by Vives[1] and by Spinoza[2] that *only through emotion can emotion be cured*. The rational methods mentioned above do not deal with the emotion itself. They do not seek to cure emotion, but to cure one *of* emotion. That this is not possible by voluntary and intellectual means has long been observed—were it possible emotion would long ago have been got rid of since the best minds and wills for centuries have been turned against it. Even the Stoics, whose aims and attitudes are much like those in the preceding paragraph, noted that rational methods failed to subdue the passions. Even the ideal man, although not consenting to them, still suffered them.[3] Luria (whose theory we come to in Chapter XVI) states a fundamental law about the control of emotion: '*Direct attempts to control his behaviour always lead to negative results; its mastery is achieved only by indirect means.*' He proposes 'indirect' methods of control which he calls 'symbolic circuition'. The aim is the organization of affective behaviour, transforming the primitive into the complex and organized.

> In the control of behaviour the chief role is played by the mechanism of circuition, the mechanism of coupling-up the impulse and the motor appearance of some intervening link regulating the process of excitation. Experiments with children and hysterics showed that this process overcomes the primitive diffusion of the reaction, transforming it into organized, complex forms. Speech is a preeminent factor as an auto-regulator of behaviour, and helps to bring about the above transformation. . . . Conditioned optical symbols should play the same organizing role as the activity of speech does.
>
> The symbolic application included in this system of behaviour, diverts the reaction, in the same way as does speech, separates the excitation

---

[1] FE 37, p. 131. (Cf. Maass, FE 37, p. 273: To cure passion, reason must become *leidentlich*, impassioned). [2] *Ethica*, IV, 7.

[3] Augustine's account of the Stoic tale of Aulus Gellius, *De Civitate Dei*, IX, 4.

from the direct transfer to the motor system, and leads to a complex organized structure of the reactive process.

Every symbolic system may be a powerful means in organizing affect. This can be proved by the part that symbolic systems as images have played in the history of culture; they are connected with emotions and are widely employed in art, in the theatre, etc., to organize affect. We shall try to show how the control of affect is brought about by symbolic measures.—A. R. Luria, *The Nature of Human Conflicts, or Emotion, Conflict and Will*, N.Y., 1932, pp. 422–3.

He finds in experiments with hypnosis that the symbol can overcome the affect (p. 426), and that the motor disturbances which marked the unadapted behaviour could be controlled—in that they disappeared—through symbolization.

The organization of affect through symbols is a therapeutic method used by Jungian psychologists and is called 'active imagination'.[1] The method consists essentially in a confrontation with the mood or emotion in an open, contemplative frame of mind, allowing it to take full expression in words, visual images, plastic forms, etc.[2] Once this material is presented, the ego's role is to react to it as if it were real, and not 'just an emotion' or 'just a fantasy'. Through conscious questioning, interpretation and elaboration, a dialectical relation is established between the emotional fantasy product and the attentive ego. The aim is to get to the meaning (the representational content or instinctual image) of the mood or emotion and to effect a joint transformation of it and of the ego's attitude through the dialectical interchange. Similar methods used in therapy are discussed by Kretschmer;[3] religious and Asian meditation techniques are also on the same lines. From the religious point of view, the ultimate curative agent is the central image of the personality, the image of God. It is with this image that the most intense and important emotions are bound and which—still from the religious point of

---

[1] Jung, C. G., *The Transcendent Function* (1916), C. G. Jung Institute Zurich, 1957; 'The Psychological Aspects of the Kore', *Coll. Works*, IX, 1, p. 190; v. Franz, M.-L., 'Die Aktive Imagination in der Psychologie von C. G. Jung', in W. Bitter (ed.), *Meditation in Religion und Psychotherapie*, Stuttgart, 1958.

[2] Goldberger, E., 'Simple method of producing dreamlike visual images in the waking state', *Psychosom. Med.*, 1957, pp. 127–33, reports a similar method and refers to H. Silberer, 'Bericht über eine Methode, gewisse symbolische Halluzinations-Erscheinungen hervorzurufen und zu beobachten', *Jhrb. f. Psychoanal. Psychopath. Forsch.*, 1, 1909, p. 513. Goldberger calls his paper 'a preliminary report', indicating the novelty of his 'finding', although it has been used by Jung and his school for at least forty years and is a part of traditional meditation techniques since centuries. Goldberger, however, misses the real value of what he describes since for him the images are only screens for thought and reducible to it. Thus therapy through them is only a substitute for verbalization, while for Jung it is prior to such 'higher' functions.

[3] Kretschmer, W. E., Jr., 'Die meditativen Verfahren in der Psychotherapie', *Ztschft. f. Psychotherapie u. med. Psychol.*, I, 3, 1951; 'Meditation in der Psychologie und Psychiatrie der Gegenwart', *Ztschft. f. Rel. u. Geistesges.*, X, 1958, pp. 231–9.

view—is the ultimate source of all emotion. The Hindu psychology of Akhilananda makes this point emphatically: 'The most outstanding urge in people is the search after the abiding spirit or God'; 'the primitive instincts are reduced to the master urge for bliss'. When the central image of God is not recognized there is no end to emotional confusion, for it is this God image which integrates the other emotions.[1] It is in this light we can recall a little-known, mid-nineteenth century work by the English physician Cooke[2] who considered religion a medical agent in treating the emotions, and the medical man as a kind of religious practitioner. His job, on the view we are elaborating here, would be to lead the patient towards relating his emotions to the God image. Cooke, in fact, analyses each emotion and makes a religious connection.

In these various meditative and imaginative techniques, expression, abreaction and separation are *not* the aim. Rather the image and the emotion are aspects of the same complex, so that confrontation with the fantasy image, or symbol, is the very stuff and ground of emotion. It is the emotion in its formal aspect.The development of such symbolic forms is thus the development of emotion. So is emotion 'tamed'. Thus the arts, religious ceremonies and practices, meditation techniques and active imagination transform the emotions Sechehaye's work with schizophrenics is an excellent example of this method of therapy. The transformation achieved through symbolization is of the whole personality.[3] (That imaginational techniques go beyond the transformation of the subject, but have an actual effect in the world, the objects of images, is certainly an essential hypothesis in a theory of prayer, meditation, ritual and art. Involved here is the idea of a correspondence between innermost and outer.[4]

Symbolic realization works, according to these hypotheses, because it fulfils the maxim: only through emotion can emotion be cured.

---

[1] Akhilananda (Swami), *Hindu Psychology*, London, 1948, Chapter III, 'Emotion', pp. 51–3.

[2] Cooke, W., *Mind and the Emotions in Relation to Health, Disease, and Religion*, London, 1852.

[3] Sechehaye, M. A., *Symbolic Realization* (transl. from French by B. and H. Würsten), N.Y., 1951. It is useful to note that she credits her effects to 'symbolic realization', and not 'mother-love' which others often find the panacea in this field.

[4] Paracelsus writes (Strassburg edition, 1603, Volume I, Section 334): 'All imagining of man comes from the Heart: the Heart is the Sun in the microcosm. And all imagining of man out of the microcosmic Sun goes into the Sun of the great world, into the Heart of the macrocosm. Thus is microcosmic imagination a seed which becomes materialized, etc.' (Quoted by A. Schopenhauer, 'Animalischer Magnetismus und Magie', *Ueber den Willen in der Natur*.) The idea of correspondence of inner and outer here expressed ties in with ideas we have already seen, e.g.: Chapter VI, that emotion is the subjective aspect of objective energy; Chapter IX, that the innermost psyche as ground of emotion is not subjective, but also relatively objective; Chapter XI, that emotion is grounded in a region describable as the objective psyche. See, too, Chapter XV.

The emotion which cures emotion is the upper end which transforms the lower end of the spectrum. The upper end—the mood out of which imagination develops (Nahm) or the meaningful instinctual image (Jung)—is both the same as the lower end and its antithesis. An active confrontation with the image end, developing and refining it, alters the inferior and primitive end by giving it a new meaning, a new pattern of behaviour, and a new object-image of satisfaction. Kubie[1] also conceives of instinctual behaviour and symbolic processes (including learned cultural patterns) as being on the same continuous spectrum in which the upper end alters the lower. The model of the spectrum or continuum is essential here. If symbolic realization were intellectualization, that is, a process which was not on the same continuum with the instinctual energy, it would not satisfy the biological need. The same is true of such substitutes as sublimation. In both, the instinct would remain unsatisfied and fixated. There would be no development and no cure.

These ideas are of leading importance. The transformation of processes which are innate and largely physiological, even to the vegetative level as the report of Choisy shows (Chapter X C, p. 133), through symbolization means much for psychosomatics. It should mean even more for education and ethics. In our society repression has been shown to have failed, it either kills the primitive end or causes a delayed—and so much worse—explosion. The *direct integration* of emotion through emotion as in the orgiastic practices of Frankism in Jewish mysticism, the mystery cults of ancient Greece, or the left-handed sect of Tantric yoga are also not possible since our collective moral standards would no longer tolerate this descent into the dark.

Another alternative of curing emotion through emotion is choosing one emotion to transform and re-order the others. Energetically expressed we tap the sources of all emotions if we live one fully. This is the way of *passion*. The emotion often recommended in the literature is love, but patriotism, racial hatred, ambition, sensual indulgence can serve as well, as long as the one chosen is lived fully and fanatically. Again, however, we find that an elaborate process of symbolization is required in the transformation, since the love (patriotism, ambition, etc.) requires images, rituals and shibboleths in order to work.

Finally, therefore, the therapy of emotion is a process of symbolization. It is a becoming conscious of the symbols which produce affects, and re-ordering the affects through 'symbolic circuition'. Through the careful elaboration and refinement of these symbols, there takes

[1] Kubie, L. S., 'Influence of Symbolic Processes on the Role of Instincts in Human Behaviour', *Psychosom. Med.*, 1956, pp. 189–208.

place an educative, aesthetic and moral process which alters the raw, red end of the spectrum making it serviceable and even creative. But as such symbols and such emotions are part of human inheritance, they cannot be made conscious once and for all and thus the job is done. Rather the process of symbolization, of transformation of emotion, goes on continuously as long as the blood in the red end pulses, so that life becomes the symbolic life.

In conclusion, these views which treat emotion as an intra-psychic event tend to neglect other aspects of the phenomenon such as its relation to the world and to the body. Further, even if representations can be the material stuff of emotion, the efficient stimuli of emotion, and the formal pattern of emotion, these theories do not take up in enough detail the final purpose of emotion. A hint as to this purpose however has been given: if emotion alters the train of ideas, presents choice, is related to creative imagination, and frees us from the blind impulse of instinct, we have the adumbrations of a theory of the development of consciousness. Emotion then would signify the possibility of development. Its purpose would be to make change possible. These notions of signification and purpose lead us to the next chapter, which introduces a new phase of the amplification of our theme.

XV

EMOTION AS SIGNIFICATION

UP TO THIS POINT we have been dealing with theories whose main concern is the nature and origin of emotion. We have been told what emotion is: a distinct entity, energy, a quantity, etc. And we have been told where it comes from: physiological location, situations, phylogenesis, representations, etc. This group of theories asks, and seeks the answer to, another question. What does emotion signify, intend, indicate, mean? What is its purpose?

We have encountered some of these notions before. The concept of intention appeared in Chapter X C in connection with the will and voluntary motor system. The concept of meaning came into Chapter XI, where a situation was described as a pattern of meanings. In Chapter XIV, the image was explained as the meaning of instinct and emotion arose from such meaningful images. And in Chapter III, emotions as accompaniments could be taken as indicators of what they accompanied. But it is not in these few places alone that the signification of emotion is treated. When emotion is presented as energy, as disorder, or in terms of the unconscious, or representations —in short in nearly every view, there is, along with the account of the origin and nature of emotion, a more or less explicit view about its meaning, its functional purpose, its significance. The orientation of this group of theories is to make this aspect of theory-forming primary and to start the inquiry with this question. The view of Adler shows this well:

> Our interest is not that anxiety influences the nervous (*sic*) sympaticus and the parasympaticus, but what is the end and aim?
> We are very interested in where a feeling has arisen, but we mean the psychical rather than the bodily roots, striving towards totality. We do not believe that anxiety arises from suppression of sexuality nor as the result of birth. We are not interested in such explanations, but we know and understand that a child who is accustomed to be accompanied by the mother uses anxiety—whatever its source may be—to arrive at his goal of superiority to control the mother. In this we are not concerned

with a description of anger, but we are experienced enough to see that anger is a means to overcome a person or situation. We believe that only such a view is a psychological one, and not other views such as the description of feelings, emotions, and affects, or such as, for example, that of inherited instincts. It can be taken that every bodily and mental power must have inherited material, but what we see in mind and psyche is the use of this material toward a certain goal.—A. Adler, 'Feelings and Emotions from the Standpoint of Individual Psychology', FE 28, p. 316.

Sartre's method of approach is similar: to understand emotion we must understand what it means:

> One can understand emotion only if he looks for a *signification*. This signification is by nature of a functional order. We are therefore led to speak of a finality of emotion. We grasp this finality in a very concrete way by objective examination of emotional behavior.—J.-P. Sartre, *The Emotions: Outline of a Theory* (transl. from the French by B. Frechtman), N.Y., 1948, p. 41.

'Objective examination of emotional behaviour' reveals for Sartre 'the laws of its appearing and its signification':

> . . . we can conceive of what an emotion is. It is a transformation of the world. When the paths traced out become too difficult, or when we see no path, we can no longer live in so urgent and difficult a world. All the ways are barred. However, we must act. So we try to change the world, that is, to live as if the connection between things and their potentialities were not ruled by deterministic processes, but by magic (p. 58).

He calls this modification of man's being-in-the-world a 'degradation of consciousness':

> Thus the origin of emotion is a spontaneous and lived degradation of consciousness in the face of the world. What it cannot endure in one way it tries to grasp in another by going to sleep, by approaching the consciousness of sleep, dream, and hysteria (p. 77).
>
> We shall call emotion an abrupt drop of consciousness into the magical. Or, if one prefers, there is emotion when the world of instruments abruptly vanishes and the magical world appears in its place. Therefore, it is not necessary to see emotion as a passive disorder of the organism and the mind which comes *from the outside* to disturb the psychic life. On the contrary, it is the return of consciousness to the magical attitude, one of the great attitudes which are essential to it. . . . (p. 90–1).

Sartre's theory has been praised for its originality, but it in turn depends upon such pioneer ideas as 'going out of the field' in Gestalt psychology, 'regression' in depth psychology, 'abaissement du niveau mental' (Janet), 'la mentalité primitive' (Levy-Bruhl), and 'abstract' and 'concrete' behaviour (Goldstein). Again we have the model of two systems, or ways of behaving, which are here called 'deterministic' or 'instrumental' *versus* 'magical'.

For both Adler and Sartre emotion has a functional purpose, which is the key to an understanding of it. For Adler, it might be a means to gain mastery; for Sartre, a means to transform magically the world. It is a specific way of behaving, a kind of attitude or way of looking at things. Burloud says: 'Mais il est bien vrai que l'émotion se caractérise, dès le premier moment, par une manière nouvelle de voir les objets . . .' '*Le phénomène initial n'est pas*, comme le croit James, *une perception qui bouleverse mon organisme, mais un bouleversement affectif de ma perception.*' [1] The new way of looking at things is a manner of adaptation which has meaning.

The view that emotion signifies a kind of adaptation is presented also by Dejean and Britan. Dejean first makes maladaptation the criterion of emotion.[2] It would appear that she presents a view of emotion as disorder such as we shall see in Chapter XVII. But Dejean makes a significant distinction by refusing to judge the maladaptation which occurs in emotional behaviour in terms of adaptation to reality as in other forms of behaviour.[3] The deficient behaviour in emotion has a cognitive function; it reveals the value of an event by means of this being 'affected', 'derailed', and 'over-excited'. As Marañón aphorizes: 'La emoción es la atmósfera de lo excepcional.' [4] Not only does emotion reveal values, but its origin depends upon the scale of values which the subject holds. Therefore, the prophylaxis of emotion depends upon reorganization of the scale of values.[5]

For Dejean and Sartre, 'emotion is the atmosphere of the exceptional'. It is adaptive in a special, magical, over-excited way. Britan,

[1] Burloud, A., *Psychologie de la sensibilité*, Paris, 1954, pp. 67–8.

[2] Dejean, R., *L'Emotion*, Paris, 1933, p. 189: 'Ce qui distingue le sujet émotionné de celui qui n'est pas, c'est que, d'une part il est impuissant à s'adapter à la situation présente, et que, d'autre part il se produit chez lui des phénomènes organiques inopportuns—relevant de l'excitation du système autonome—qui viennent aggraver sa déficience mentale et motrice vis-à-vis du réel.'

[3] *Ibid.*, p. 237: 'Définir le comportement émotionnel par rapport au comportement adapté au réel, c'est postuler, sans preuve, que tout comportement a pour but de nous adapter à ce qui nous entoure, c'est préjuger de la nature réelle du phénomène émotion. . . . C'est négliger, chez le sujet émotionné, ce que sa modalité psychique a de spécifique, à savoir: qu'il est "affecté" et "dérouté" en même temps que "surexcité". . . . En d'autres termes, c'est négliger ce qui distingue l'émotion d'une autre forme de l'activité psycho-physiologique, c'est la considérer comme un comportement du même genre que le comportement adapté au réel, avec une simple différence de degrés—. . .'

[4] Quoted by C. de Nogales Quevedo, *Psiquismo y Secreciones Internas: Emoción Nosógena*, Barcelona, 1950, p. 5.

[5] This idea has a forerunner in French psychology. P. du Moulin, *fils* (*A Treatise on Peace of Soul, and Content of Mind*, transl. by J. Scrope, Salisbury, 1765, Vol. II, Bk. III) writes: 'The great Mistake which causes Passion to be directed towards wrong Objects, or to be applied to right ones in Excess, proceeds from hence, that we are ignorant of the due and undue Value of Things'. 'Thus, the first, or rather the only Way to set our Will free from vicious Passions, is to enlighten our Mind, and banish from it the false Ideas of Infancy'.

however, finds emotion adaptive within a biological view of man.

> The position here maintained then would be that the emotions as an instrument of adaptation are superior to sensory pain and the affective qualities of pleasantness and unpleasantness, in that they enable the organism to adapt its reactions to the object as an object, and not merely in terms of sensory stimulation to which it gives rise. As perception gives us information at a distance, so emotion gives adaptation at a distance.— H. H. Britan, *The Affective Consciousness*, N.Y., 1931, p. 113.

Again, as with Dejean, the adaptive function of emotion is linked with its cognitive function. It gives adaptation because it is an instrument of cognizing objects. Furthermore, this is not mere perception, but a tendency to achieve something. As for Sartre and Adler, emotions have specific purposes. This is Britan's main hypothesis.

> There remains to be discussed another attribute belonging to emotional reactions, that, all things considered, must be regarded as their most characteristic feature. This has been variously denominated, 'drive', 'reaction tendency', 'impulsion', and the like. It calls attention to the fact that the emotions are functionally dynamic leading to some more or less specific end-result. Here from a broad biological view, we find their purpose their *raison d'être*. As conscious states they are essentially extrovertive with a drive toward objective results (p. 137).

Price writes:

> Emotions and conations are directed towards something, whether real or fictitious. They have objects. . . . One cannot be just afraid or surprised. One is afraid *of* something. . . . It follows that cognition is not just an accompaniment of emotion and conation, but an essential constituent of them.—*Thinking and Experience*, London, 1953, p. 152.

A recent paper of Broad's describes emotion along the same lines as a kind of cognition, while Rosenzweig, from another point of view, says, 'the affect system is a predicting device which anticipates the future in terms of the past.' [2]

Reviewing the material we have covered so far we find that emotion signifies the values of objects. As such, it is a way of perceiving, a way of knowing, a way of adapting and a way of being in the world. It intends a specific object, goal, or end-result. In short, there is reason in emotion. 'Le cœur a ses raisons que la raison ne connaît pas.'

The relation of emotion and reason is an ancient problem solved usually by splitting them asunder. The meaning of this breach in our civilization is a subject for itself, but its tragic effects are every-

[1] Broad, C. D., 'Emotion and Sentiment', *J. Aesth. Art. Crit.*, 1954, pp. 203–14.

[2] Rosenzweig, 'The Affect System: Foresight and Fantasy', *J. Nerv. Ment. Dis.*, 1958, p. 113 f.

where present in the violence of emotion unmitigated by reason and the sterility of intellect uninformed by emotion. Woodger,[1] in his short and valuable essay on the methods of physics, psychology and medicine, thinks the split and conflict between emotion and reason unnecessary. Because this split leads to the exclusion of emotion from the sciences, he finds it hinders the development of fruitful hypotheses in medical psychology, and renders inadequate the training of medical psychologists. A general division between emotion and reason appears also in other realms where it does the same harm.[2] In aesthetics, works of art are found to be either emotional or intellectual. In religion, enthusiasm, revivalism and emotionalism are divided from the higher councils of orthodox wisdom. In politics, reason makes 'policy' and 'law' and 'peace' while emotion makes 'lying propaganda' and 'war'. In contemporary philosophy the split takes two significant forms. Statements are said to be verifiable and logical, or they are said to be 'emotive'.[3] Ethical statements have been placed in the 'emotive' category, thereby excluding ethics from the realm of truth and reason. Another form of the split in philosophy is between Continental existentialism and 'Anthropologie' which proceeds from emotional conditions (nausea, dread, etc.) and British logical positivism which proceeds from mathematical logic. Emotive

[1] Woodger, J. H., *Physics, Psychology and Medicine*, Cambridge, 1956. A statement from Reichenbach (*The Rise of Scientific Philosophy*, Univ. of Calif., 1954, p. 312) gives good example of this sort of compartmentalized psychology: 'The scientific philosopher does not want to belittle the value of emotions, nor would he like to live without them. His life may be as rich in passion and sentiment as that of any literary man—but he refuses to muddle emotion and cognition, and likes to breathe the pure air of logical insight and penetration.'

[2] Dewey also notes this split as being fundamental in the modern dilemma: 'The hard and fast impassible line which is supposed by some to exist between "emotive" and "scientific" language is a reflex of the gap which now exists between the intellectual and the emotional in human relations and activities. The split which exists in present social life between ideas that have *scientific* warrant and uncontrolled emotions that dominate practice, the split between the affectional and the cognitive, is probably one of the chief sources of the maladjustments and unendurable strains from which the world is suffering.' J. Dewey, 'Theory of Valuation', *Inter. Enc. of Unified Science*, 2, 4, Chicago, 1939, p. 65. One can, of course, question whether the split is only modern. Compare Pascal's *Pensées*, 412 and 413 also M.-D. Chenu ('Les Catégories affectives dans la langue de l'Ecole', *Le Coeur* (Etudes Carmélitaines), Paris, 1950, p. 126) observes that all the mediaeval theologians 'tried to overcome the irreducible and necessary distinction between cognitive faculties and affective faculties . . .'

[3] The modern dogma of this division was laid down by C. K. Ogden and I. A. Richards in *The Meaning of Meaning*, 1923, London, 7th edn., 1945, pp. 10 and 149–50, in particular. This influential book, designed as a therapy of language, has had a less than healthy effect on the soul of logical positivists, since it has perpetuated by refashioning in extreme style the ancient and academic habit of sundering emotion from reflective reason, calling the former a more primitive, not strictly scientific, disturbance of the latter. (In the same vein is R. H. Thouless, 'The Affective Function of Language', FE 50, pp. 507–15). Richards' ideas are worked over by Collingwood who refuses the split—*The Principles of Art*, Oxford, 1938, pp. 262–7. See further, Richards' second thoughts on this subject: 'Emotive Meaning Again', in *Speculative Instruments*, London, 1955.

propositions, like emotional works of art or emotion in politics, religion and science, are said to be nothing but *expressions of attitudes*. They have to do with subjective states of mind and have nothing to do with reason and objective reality.

The whole fault—and it runs to bed-rock—is the *persistent identification of emotion with subjectivity* (see Chapter IX), and the corollary assumption that the intellect, as the only place of reason, is *not* personal, subjective or an expression of the individual in whom it performs. The divorce of emotion and reason is now so long-standing and has worked so to the benefit of reason that emotion has become by definition in most textbooks[1]—as well as in common speech—a pejorative concept of irrationality bordering on the insane. The exclusion of emotion from the temples of art, science, religion, law, and moral philosophy, leaves it little recourse but to appear where it has been driven, in the market-places and alley-ways of crime, mobs, war and the asylum. The great danger of divorcing reason from emotion (as 'Beat' Bohemia *vs*. the 'Organization Men' in America, the 'Paras' *vs*. Parliamentary Paris in France, the 'Angry Young Men' *vs*. the 'Establishment' in Britain) is such that when bourgeois society chooses only reason it petrifies and leaves to the rebels only the energetic aspect of emotion, violence. A return of emotion to the councils of respectability in state, church and laboratory might relieve the underworld, the asylum and youth of part of their emotional burden.

Now the views in this chapter which hold that emotion signifies deny in one way or another this separation. Beck brings evidence from the Rorschach test, from statements of scientists and psychologists and from other relevant fields to support his conclusion: '. . . we cannot know without the intellect; we do not know until we experience with the emotions. All the current evidence in the study of personality, both integrated and disordered, leads to this conclusion'.[2] McGill also challenges the divorce of emotion and reason, finding in Plato, Aristotle and Spinoza witnesses to their interrelation, and making this the contention of his recommendable little book.[3] In spite of his brief for the reason of emotion, he does not take emotion itself as a kind of reason (magical, overexcited, a means to gain mastery). Thus he does not accept emotion as rational in its own way, but only that it has a rational 'component'. He seeks to find reason *in* emotion, not to find the reason *of* emotion as do Adler,

---

[1] F. Fearing ('Group Behavior and the Concept of Emotion', FE 50, p. 449) examines nine textbooks in social psychology and finds the split between emotion and reason to be general, to the detriment of emotion.

[2] Beck, S. J., 'Emotional Experience as a Necessary Constituent in Knowing', FE 50, p. 106.

[3] McGill, V., *Emotions and Reason*, Springfield, Ill., 1954, p. 62.

Sartre, Britan and Dejean. The same pair of concepts form the title to MacMurray's book. Again the argument is for the union of the two, and again the procedure is similar: an exhibition of the cognitive aspect of emotion. 'Reason reveals itself in emotion by its objectivity, by the way it corresponds to and apprehends reality.'

> Reason—the capacity in us which makes us human—is not in any special sense a capacity of the intellect. It is not our power of thinking, though it expresses itself in our thinking as well as in other ways. It must also express itself in our emotional life, if that is to be human. Emotion is not the Cinderella of our inner life, to be kept in her place among the cinders in the kitchen. Our emotional life is *us* in a way our intellectual life cannot be; in that it alone contains the motives from which our conduct springs. Reason reveals itself in emotion by its objectivity, by the way it corresponds to and apprehends reality. Reason in the emotional life determines our behaviour in terms of the real values of the world in which we live. It discovers and reveals goodness and badness, right and wrong, beauty and ugliness and all the infinite variety of values of which these are only the rough, general, intellectual abstractions.— J. MacMurray, *Reason and Emotion*, London, 1935, pp. 49–50.

MacMurray deals in particular with the education of the reason in emotion. Irrational emotion is subjective—just as the hostile critics of emotion say. This, says MacMurray, is because it is egocentric and does not correspond with objective reality. Rational emotion, however, does. It is best exemplified in art and religion. The whole position depends upon the main hypothesis that emotion cognizes values.

Emotion cognizes values. The point has been variously made by Dejean, by Britan, by Lersch (Chapter IX), by the Gestalt psychologists (Chapter XI), by Jung (Chapter V, XIV). Reid makes this an important part of his view on emotion, which he defines as 'the marked psychical affect arising in certain complex situations' (*op. cit. inf.*, p. 84). These situations are not only instinctual ones, but emotion can arise in connection with 'intrinsic' values:

> Having established that emotion may arise under certain conditions in any situation (and not only in instinctive situations) I may now go on to indicate the significant part which certain non-instinctive emotions . . . play in the higher life of man. I refer to . . . 'emotions of value'. . . . there can arise situations in which the subject is confronted with objects (ideal or actual) which he realizes as revealing 'intrinsic', as opposed to instrumental, value. His reaction to these objects may be emotional, and from the emotional situation may issue the very complex conditions and actions which are typical of the moral, the artistically creative, and the truth-seeking life.—L. A. Reid, 'Instinct, Emotion and the Higher Life', *Brit. J. Psychol.*, 1923, p. 88.

191

Again we find this concept of higher emotions related to the concept of reason:

> There are also 'value' emotions which may occur at the level of 'reason', reason involving, not merely the power to syllogize but also to contemplate and to feel intrinsic values or ends in themselves. Value emotions . . . are not reducible to terms of instinct but are 'new' (p. 93).

And finally such emotions are related to the purpose of life, not in some instinctual way of self-preservation (homeostasis, or emergency) but through revealing the 'Good'.

> If I may speak of 'moral evolution', I might add that it is the existence of the supreme value or end or purpose in human life which is, through its felt apprehension, the 'final cause' of moral evolution from the savage to the saint (p. 91).

The statement that emotion signifies (cognizes) intrinsic values has seemed to entail the statement that *such values exist*, and are powers which draw us onward and upward. The existence of objective values revealed through emotion is the view of Meinong and Scheler. Meinong[1] holds that emotions present qualities—actual, objective, intrinsic values which are, so to speak, in things. Scheler[2] holds that the realm of value is an ontological real world, consisting in a hierarchy of 'fühlbare' phenomena not given to the intellect but presented to feeling. Hartshorne's [3] theory of sensation is of the same kind. Qualities, characters, values, and sense data are all bound together in an 'affective continuum'. Values are objectively given along with sense-data and qualities; and they are grasped by the subject through an affective mode of apprehension, combining sensation and feeling. His ultimate hypothesis is that the affective order is the order of the spirit. A similar view, however complicatedly expressed, is given by Bertrand-Barraud.[4] The spirit presents itself through immediate qualitative facts of concrete reality. These are affective facts or affective values and they are primary to reflection and relational statements about such facts or values. Drever's hypothesis that meaning is affective also presumes a notion of intrinsic values, revealed through the affective order. His theory does not, as with the others, involve idealist metaphysics, because emotion on his view is rooted in instinct which gives affective interest or meaning. Meaning has two aspects—affective and cognitive. 'Our

---

[1] Meinong, A., 'Ueber emotionale Präsentation', *Wien. Sitzungsberichte*, 183, 1917.
[2] Scheler, M., 'Der Formalismus in der Ethik und die materiale Wertethik', II. *Jahrb. f. Phil. u. phänomenologische Forsch.*, I and II, 1916–22.
[3] Hartshorne, C., *The Philosophy and Psychology of Sensation*, Univ. of Chicago, 1934. Compare, F. Hayek, *The Sensory Order*, London, 1952, pp. 99–100.
[4] Bertrand-Barraud, D., *Les Valeurs Affectives*, Paris, 1924.

contention is that this [affective] element is the primary and original factor without which Meaning, as such, could never arise, and which actually . . . converts bare sensation into experience.' [1] Sense-cognition only reveals the 'thatness' of objects, emotion their 'whatness'. (Or as Britan puts it, emotion gives adaptation 'to the object as object, and not merely in terms of sensory stimulation'—p. 188 above.) This corresponds with the two modes of thought which Whitehead calls 'importance' and 'matters-of-fact'. Importance has to do with interest, with the creative impulse, with valuations, and it is revealed by emotion. Emotion, as value-experience, comes before the discrimination of matters-of-fact. Emotion's basic expression is: 'Have a care, here is something that matters!' 'Importance reveals itself as transitions of emotion.' [2] In short, *emotion is the primary mode of cognition.*

It is interesting to see how well this theory of speculative philosophers, like Scheler and Whitehead, fits the experimental facts reported by Klüver. Monkeys submitted to bilateral temporal lobectomy showed the following primary symptoms relevant to this discussion:

(1) We observe, first of all, forms of behavior which appear to indicate a 'psychic blindness' or visual agnosia in the sense that the ability to recognize and detect the meaning of objects on the basis of visual criteria alone seems to be lost although the animal exhibits no or at least no gross defects in the ability to discriminate visually. There is a strong tendency to approach every animate and inanimate object without hesitation, even objects which previous to the operation called forth extreme excitement, avoidance reactions, and other forms of emotional response. . . .

(2) There are strong oral tendencies in the sense that the monkey insists on examining all objects by mouth. . . . The monkey even tends to examine orally objects which have previously acquired 'meaning' through training. . . .

(3) There is an excessive tendency to attend and react to every visual stimulus. The monkey behaves as if forced . . . to contact all objects in sight. . . .

(4) There are profound changes in emotional behaviour, and there may even be a complete loss of emotional responses in the sense that such forms of motor and vocal behaviour as are associated with anger and fear . . . are not exhibited. The very fact that the animal approaches and touches every object, whether it be a stranger, a cat, a dog, a snake, or an inanimate object, must be considered a striking deviation from normal behaviour. . . . All expressions of emotions . . . may be completely lost.

[1] Drever, J., *Instinct in Man*, Cambridge, 1917, p. 258.
[2] Whitehead, A. N., *Modes of Thought*, Cambridge, U.S.A., 1938, pp. 159–60. See also Whitehead's view, Chapter VI above.

(5) There is a striking increase in the amount and diversity of sexual behaviour. . . .

(6) There occurs a remarkable change in dietary habits. . . .—H. Klüver, 'Functional Differences between the Occipital and Temporal Lobes', in *Cerebral Mechanisms in Behavior*, ed. by L. Jeffress, 1951, p. 151

It would seem plain that the meaning, importance and objective recognition of the 'whatness', or value, of things seems to suffer (in these monkeys) a change corresponding to a change in emotion. In spite of the many conceptual and theoretical difficulties in drawing such conclusions, we say: psychic blindness and emotional distortion are inter-related.[1] Perhaps even, emotion is the vision of the psyche which reveals signification in a world of fact.

To sum up briefly: we have been told that emotion signifies objects—and not just objects, but an objective psychic world of qualities and values. It either has a rational component or it is rational in itself and therefore is not to be separated from reason. In fact, it is a primary kind of reason, giving meaning and importance to a world of bare sense cognitions and matters-of-fact. Emotion signifies something as Adler and Sartre said; but more, *it is signification itself.* Where there is emotion, there is meaning; where there is meaning, there is emotion. Emotion also gives ourselves meaning. As Whitehead says: 'My importance is my emotional worth now. . . .'[2] Further, emotion is the only mode of apprehending, cognizing and experiencing certain aspects of existence. Examples would be the *numinosum*[3] or the love-encounter where the other is grasped through the emotions. It is only through emotion that we are led to higher spiritual and aesthetic awareness, and to God.

Practically, this point of view means that there is so much hatred, fear and depression in our lives because there is so much to hate, fear and be sad about. The emotions only cognize the real facts. These real facts are in the social world and not only subjective ideas and images within the personal psyche of the perceiver. And so these emotions are not conditions to be medicated and cured away for the sake of normalcy. Such a therapeutic approach to the negative emotions is, in fact, a perversion of man's relation to his world which is objectively given as evoking hatred, fear and depression. On this

---

[1] Brain and Strauss conclude from these experiments: 'Perhaps the most useful conclusions which can be drawn from these observations for the study of disorders of the human temporal lobe are the two broad generalizations that bilateral temporal lobectomy in monkeys causes a profound disturbance (1) of the appreciation of external reality and (2) of the emotional life.' (Sir Russell Brain and E. B. Strauss, *Recent Advances in Neurology and Neuropsychiatry* (6th edn.), London, 1955, p. 38. H. Terzian and G. Dalle Ore (*Neurology*, 1955, pp. 373–80) present evidence of the reproduction of the same Klüver-Bucy syndrome in man.   [2] *op. cit.*, p. 160.
[3] Otto, R., *The Idea of the Holy* (trans. by J. W. Harvey), Oxford, 1923.

view, normalcy itself takes on another meaning: what is normal and real is what is presented by emotion. The concept of normalcy then becomes based on importance, on meaning, on value and not on collections of data. With this concept of normalcy, or reality, therapy would consist not in the adaptation of the patient's emotion to his (or the therapist's) view of normal reality, but in adaptation of the patient to his emotion which, as the vision of the psyche, tells the truth about the world. Such an adaptation would mean living an emotional life, with all its hatred, fear and depression, which in turn might well lead, as these writers suggest, to the higher life of art and morality and to God.

There is another way in which the signification of emotion can be taken. The functional purpose can be to signify something to others as *communication* and *expression*. For example:

> The direct purpose of the emotional storm is to effect a practical conversion in other minds by communicating feeling. Not only shouts, angry glances, tears and sighs are employed, but outbursts of words, written communications, art products, music, drama, song and poetry.—G. B. Dibblee, *Instinct and Intuition*, London, 1929, p. 217.
> Our most intense feelings are directed toward other human beings . . . always our emotions are toward human beings.—L. J. Saul, *Bases of Human Behavior*, Philadelphia, 1951, p. 91 (see also Chapter II for fuller statement of Saul's view).
> It is true that people will carry out expressive movements, even when alone, but these, too, are aimed at an audience: an imaginary one. Whenever one has the opportunity to observe a major outbreak of desperation or violent affect, one cannot help noticing a communication tendency. In final analysis, every attack of affect is directed to an audience.—P. Schilder, 'Studies concerning the Psychology and Symptomatology of General Paresis', in *Organization and Pathology of Thought* (ed. D. Rapaport), N.Y., 1951, p. 527.

The history of the problem of emotional expression goes back to the *Physiognomonica* attributed to Aristotle. The influence of physiognomy on the study of character and types, upon phrenology, and on the art of painting is a rich field of its own. Important works have been written since the thirteenth century, and Buttkus (1956)[1] carries on the tradition. Allport[2] discusses it interestingly; Jeness[3] and Dumas[4] report on the literature. In addition to facial expression, however, there are the related problems of speech and gesture as emotional

[1] Buttkus, R., *Physiognomik*, München, 1956.

[2] Allport, G. W., *Personality*, N.Y., 1937, pp. 65–78, 481–4.

[3] Jeness, A., 'The Recognition of Facial Expression of Emotion', *Psychol. Bull.*, 1932, pp. 325–50.

[4] Dumas, G., 'Introduction à l'étude de l'expression des émotions', *Rev. Philos.*, 1926, pp. 223–57.

expression which in turn involve theories of language,[1] of hand-writing, of stage acting, and the like.

The basic issue here has been put succinctly, if quaintly, by one of the earliest scientific writers in English on the emotions. Wright observes: 'First, it cannot bee doubted of, but that the passions of our mindes worke diuers effects in our faces . . .'[2] The problem for some is to establish the relationship between the expressions and the emotions, between the 'diuers effects' and the 'passions of our mindes'. According to isomorphism (Ribot and Klages, for example) the expression is an objectification of the emotion. Collingwood contends: 'To whatever level of experience an emotion may belong, it cannot be felt without being expressed. There are no unexpressed emotions'.[3] Inner experience and outer expression are one; such is the thesis of physiognomic studies from Porta and Lavater to the correlations of types in Kretschmer. Duchenne,[4] in one of the most painstaking and elaborate researches on this problem, concluded that each muscle of the face corresponds with an individual passion, a fact which, being the same for all mankind, forms the instinctive facial language of emotion. The expression of terror on the face of an Eskimo would be, on this theory, instinctively grasped by a Boston Brahmin. Whether or not there is instinctive recognition of emotional expression is a debated issue in the literature.[5]

The problem for others is not to understand the relationship between the two different aspects, emotion and expression, but rather to discuss *emotion as expression. Theory of emotion becomes a theory of emotional expression.* Such is the work of Darwin; and also Dugas[6] whose description of emotion over and against passion makes the former concept refer only to what is expressed and acted out. Quite different from the 'innermost' views of Chapter IX!

[1] See E. Cassirer, *The Philosophy of Symbolic Forms*, Vol. I, Yale Univ., 1953, pp. 147–55, 'Language as an Expression of Emotion'; J. Donovan, 'The Festal Origin of Human Speech', *Mind* (O.S.), 16, pp. 498–506; 17, 325–39. Also, Hobbes finds the origin of speech in the passions. See Collingwood's discussion of emotion and language in *Principles of Art*, Oxford, 1938, Chapter XI.

[2] Wright, T., *The Passions of the Minde in generall*, London, 1604, p. 26.

[3] Collingwood, *op. cit. sup.*, p. 238.

[4] Duchenne, G. B., *Méchanisme de la physionomie humaine, ou Analyse électrophysiologique de l'expression des passions*, Paris, 1862. (Eng. summary by E. B. Kaplan, in *Physiology of Motion* (by Duchenne), Philadelphia, 1949).

[5] See C. Landis, 'The Interpretation of Facial Expression in Emotion', *J. General Psychol.*, 1929; P. T. Young, *Emotion in Man and Animal*, N.Y., 1943, pp. 11–27; D. O. Hebb, 'On the Nature of Fear' and 'Emotion in Man and Animal: an Analysis of the Intuitive Processes of Recognition', *Psychol. Rev.*, 1946. Claparède's theory (Chapter IV) would hold for an instinctive or intuitive apprehension of emotional expression. The debate would seem to amount to this: In 'real life' it is evident that we recognize emotion in ourselves and others when it appears; in the laboratory or experimental situation this is hard to prove.

[6] Dugas, L., 'Les Passions', *Nouveau Traité de Psychologie* (ed. G. Dumas), Vol. VI, Paris, 1938.

Dugas follows Kant[1] in imaging passion as a river deepening its bed, and emotion as a river which bursts its dams, which ex-presses itself. Dumas, too, treats emotion as expression:

> . . . we begin to see a conclusion which emerges, we believe, from the facts themselves in the course of all these chapters. It is possible to explain the expression of emotions almost entirely by their biological and social conditions, and the conditions called psychological are subordinated to physiological and social conditions to the point of their being confused most of the time with them.
>
> But if one puts the question of the expression of emotions within this bio-social frame—and we do not believe it could be put otherwise—one cannot be prevented from declaring how much more extensive and more objectively important is the realm of physiological expression than the realm of social expression.—G. Dumas, 'Introduction à l'étude de l'expression des émotions', *Rev. Philos.*, 1926, p. 147.

Nony's approach is similar, even if she prefers to lay more emphasis on the social aspect. Again the concern is not 'with the problem of the *nature* of emotion, we use the term "expression of the emotions" without assuming any particular theory which it may imply'.[2]

Marañón differentiates between the expression (emotional gesture) and the emotion itself, but he holds that these two factors are so closely bound together that the expression can be the source of the emotion, in a way rather similar to the motor-attitude theory of Bull and Gemelli (Chapter X C):

> . . . emotion is not produced in this way only—that is to say, by the perception within our own bodies of the visceral trembling—but also by simply seeing in another individual the expressive phenomena, the gestures of emotion. A gesture of terror or of loathing in a person near us, infects us with the terror or the loathing causing us to execute more or less the same gesture and to experience the same vegetative sensation. . . .
>
> Furthermore, if we ourselves execute the gestures of a given emotion, we can come to experience the corresponding visceral disturbance and to have the idea of it; in short, we can emotionalize ourselves completely. . . .
>
> Gesture is, in short, the expression of a certain emotion; it has in its turn a reverse power over the emotion, and can itself produce the emotion. But this effect, also fundamental to our thesis, does not occur always, but only in favorable conditions of the environment, which we have suggested and which we can define with sufficient precision.—G. Marañón, 'The Psychology of Gesture', *J. Nerv. Ment. Dis.*, 1950, pp. 485–6; (transl. from Spanish by E. Beard and G. Massa).

[1] Kant, I., *Anthropologie*, Section 74.
[2] Nony, C., 'The Biological and Social Significance of the Expression of the Emotions', *Brit. J. Psychol.*, 1922–3, pp. 76–7.

The theories of emotional expression can differ widely as these passages show, but the main hypothesis is the same: 'the passions of our mindes work diuers effects upon our faces' and this basic fact is intrinsic to emotion. These effects are phylogenetic traces for Darwin; part of a universal God-given language for Duchenne. Schilder finds them directed to an audience. For Marañón they can be the origin of emotion; for Dumas and Nony they are the results of heredity and environment. These theories take up the fact that emotion—unlike thought, intuition, memory, feeling, sensation—manifests itself in the face and body. It has a public aspect. The dynamic ex-movere is linked to a formal ex-primere. Yet to identify these two, or reduce one to the other, or even to make expression the criterion of emotion neglects other central hypotheses brought by other theories. For example, those theories which present emotion as unconscious (unexpressed), as in dreams, would seem to deny a necessary connection between emotion and expression. Also, any theory attempting to identify the two—say, Marañón's view that we can emotionalize ourselves completely through expression—must adequately account for 'sham' and 'cold' emotion, and also for the curious disparities in theatrical emotion between actor, role played and audience. Through emotional expressions of pity and terror the audience can be purged, yet the actor can be left singularly unmoved. These issues can be solved by returning to the notion of emotion as a complex phenomenon. Expression is a necessary constituent of the full complex, but in itself expression is only a constituent aspect.

There is yet another way that signification comes into the account of emotion and this is where emotion is described as an *intra-systemic sign*. Its functional purpose is to *communicate* something to the person in whom it occurs. Rapaport (Chapter V) speaks of emotion as 'affect-signals released by the ego'. McDougall (Chapter III) takes the emotions as 'indicators of the motives at work in us'. Different writers interpret the message of emotion differently: for Cannon it is an emergency, a mobilization for action. This idea was foreshadowed by Vives (sixteenth century) in describing the 'felt' side of fear which he explained is 'felt as a warning to the subject . . . to take the requisite measures for defence'.[1] For Nogales Quevedo,[2] too, emotion is an alarm signal indicating human vulnerability. But the upset condition —rather than a mobilization for action—is sign of evasion from a menace. Bartlett suggests it is 'a sign to the organism concerned that

[1] FE 37, pp. 136–7.
[2] de Nogales Quevedo, C., *Psiquismo y Secreciones Internas: Emoción nosógena*, Barcelona, 1950.

there is conflict or that integration and the achievement of a new response is possible'.[1] The theories of Chapter IX take feelings as significations about the innermost regions of the personality. Knapp's communication view can be quoted as follows:

> ... whatever else enters into an emotion, it has some general *meaning*, some overall significance for the organism. Somehow, it 'puts together' elements of experience in a fashion that has relevance for the subject. Insofar, then, as emotion is a conscious experience, it may be regarded as a communication, if only to one's self.[2]

He finds an 'inner syntax of emotion' and views 'emotion as an archaic stream of inner, non-verbal communications'.[3] In cybernetics, 'Wiener has regarded emotions as communications that are not directed to a particular place in the mechanism. They are messages labelled "to whom it may concern", and it is hypothesized that hormones circulating in the blood-stream are their carriers'.[4] One is reminded here of Bishop Berkeley's notion of Animal Spirits that 'are the Messengers, which running to and fro in the Nerves, preserve a Communication between the Soul and outward Objects'.[5]

This catalogue of 'communication views' could be extended to cover every kind of theory. Although such an extension leads back to the main problem of confusion in theory which this work is trying to expose, it nevertheless shows how wide the agreement is that emotion signifies something. Again, to put it in brief, where there is emotion there is a meaning.

In looking back on this chapter two main problems appear. The first is the usual one of *disagreement*. 'Where there is emotion there is a meaning' is a very unspecific conclusion. Each of the ways signification is understood gives a different meaning to emotion. Therefore, only if we make the conclusion fully general can we have a unified result. Thus the conclusion becomes: where there is emotion there is meaning (not *a* meaning), value, importance, or significance—or, *emotion is signification*.

The second problem is the muddle of signification with *teleology*. To ask what does emotion signify is a necessary question to achieve a full understanding of the phenomenon. It is also perhaps the most fruitful question of all, in so far as we assume life to be a search for

---

[1] Bartlett, F. C., 'Feeling, Imaging and Thinking', *Brit. J. Psychol.* 1925-6, pp. 24-5. (See also Chapter XIV, p. 178, for fuller statement of Bartlett's views.)

[2] Knapp, P. H., 'Conscious and Unconscious Affects: A preliminary approach to concepts and methods of study', in *Research in Affects* (Psychiatric Research Reports, 8, 1957), p. 60.

[3] *Ibid.*, pp. 61-2.

[4] Allport, F. H., *Theories of Perception and the Concept of Structure*, N.Y. and London, 1955, p. 496.

[5] Berkeley, *Min. Philos*, IV, IV, 214 (1732).

meanings. Nevertheless, it does not have to lead to a teleological explanation in which the valuable results of a process are taken as having a causative, determining role in the process which yields the valuable results. For example, the question 'what does emotion mean' can well lead—as Sartre says—to speaking of the finality of emotion and to the question 'what is its purpose'. But this does not have to lead to the view that this purpose (to communicate with others, to act as an intrasystemic sign, to master the world in a special way, to cognize values, to reveal the higher life, etc.) determines the process.[1]

Such a view tends to place the situation, the hereditary constitution, the physiological processes, unconscious constellations and flow of energy all at the disposal of, to serve and support, the purpose. And it is well to note how this teleological and vitalistic view of emotion tends to bring in the metaphysics of idealism. In other words, in asserting that emotion has a final cause, we must avoid asserting that this final cause is its only cause, or even its dominant cause. Also, we must avoid attributing to final causes what is by definition reserved to efficient causes, e.g. the initiation of a motion or process.[2]

For therapy, in addition to the comments already made, *there is one overall conclusion*. If emotion is reason, if it signifies, expresses, communicates, the fundamental form of therapy is *education*.[3] This theme is elaborated particularly by MacMurray, and also by Phillips.[4] Education of the emotions, like all education, would aim at refining the modes of expressions, communication and apprehension of the world. In this way, emotion could develop from signifying only the primitive, crucial and radical to signifying also the more subtle events of life. An education of this sort would involve primarily a transformation of values, of meanings, of the sense of importance, as Dejean points out. How this can be put into practice will depend, first of all, upon how emotion itself is valued. The split between emotion and reason gives little hope that the education of the emotions will take place in the recognized seats of learning. This education might well have to begin in the consultation room of the psychologist or psychiatrist—one of the few last places where emotion still is acknowledged to have at least some value.

[1] Compare A. O. Weber and D. Rapaport, 'Teleology and the Emotions', *Phil. of Science*, 1941, pp. 69–82, where a separation is made between asserting that emotion has a functional purpose and asserting that this purpose—realized as goal—causes the functional process leading to the goal.

[2] Aristotle, *Physica*, II, 7. (See Part I, p. 20, above, for quotation of this passage.)

[3] John Haslam of 'Bedlam' Hospital (*Observations on Insanity*, 1798) recommended early education of the emotions as prevention against insanity.

[4] Phillips, M., *The Education of the Emotions through Sentiment Development*, London, 1937.

XVI

EMOTION AS CONFLICT

WE RETURN HERE to a special kind of psychogenesis. As starting point we might say that the next groups of theories can be taken as interpretations of Wundt's apparently simple idea that emotions alter the train of ideas. This event can be seen as conflict. This in turn leads to Chapter XVII where the conflict can signify disorganization or to Chapter XVIII where the conflict can signify a new and creative organization.

We have seen the notion of conflict before, e.g. Federn (conflicts at ego-boundaries), Bartlett (images arise when a normal reaction is hindered), Darrow (intra-cortical conflict). Even more important is the role conflict plays in those theories which propose two systems of psychic functioning held in balance by repression, cortical inhibition, etc. Also, it appears in the energy theories as a damming or blocking of libido. In this chapter, conflict becomes the essential criterion of emotion. This view is credited in modern times to John Dewey;[1] however the notion of arrested tendency in French psychology is similar and has developed independently. Also similar is the notion of 'Hemmung' in German psychology, going back to the psychiatric thought of the Romantic period. If we use the ethical interpretation of conflict (between good and bad, body and spirit, God and Devil) then the relation of the concepts conflict and emotion has a long history—e.g. the conflict between the two horses in Plato's *Phaedrus*.

Angier, based on Dewey, puts the conflict theory as follows:

> Dewey, I feel, is right. But the thesis might be stated somewhat differently, as follows: Whenever a series of reactions required by an organism's total 'set' run their course to the consummatory reaction which will bring 'satisfaction' (i.e. abolish the 'set') unimpeded by other reactions, *that cannot be readily absorbed by (integrated with) them*, there is no emotion. Emotion arises only when these other reactions (implicit or

[1] Dewey, J., 'The Theory of Emotion', *Psychol. Rev.*, 1, 1894, pp. 553–69; 2, 1895, pp. 13–32.

overt) are so irrelevant as to resist ready integration with those already in orderly progress towards fruition. Such resistance means actual tension, checking, interference, inhibition, or conflict—conflict between the intercurrent reactions appropriate to the original 'set' and reactions of other origin threatening the abortion or frustration of the relevant series. Such conflict constitutes the emotion. Whether one says it *is* the emotion or gives rise to a sensory repercussion which *is* the emotion, . . . is not germane to the main issue. *Without* such conflict there is no emotion; *with* it, there is.—R. P. Angier, 'The Conflict Theory of Emotion', *Am. J. Psychol.*, 1927, p. 401.

The conflict theory of Luria uses the notion of a functional barrier operating between higher and lower systems.

That affect basically changes the structure of the reactive processes, destroying the organized behaviour, and converting the reactive process into a diffused one, has been shown already. Experimental tests proved that such a change of structure of the reactive processes occurs each time the behaviour becomes conflicting in its nature; the collision of the opposing tendencies breaks down the 'functional barrier' and transforms the reaction into a diffused state of excitation.—A. R. Luria, *The Nature of Human Conflicts, or Emotion, Conflict and Will* (transl. from Russian by W. H. Gantt), N.Y., 1932, p. 331.

This affect, or diffused state of excitation, is due to a great mass of excitation mobilized 'inadequately' (p. 186). It breaks down the functional barrier and yields behaviour which is regressive and primitive and which is always characterized by 'marked disturbances in the motor system' and 'destruction of higher automatisms' (p. 177). The main hypothesis is that conflict is at the source of affect (p. 187).

This theory of Luria's is strikingly like that of Janet's. Both use a concept of two systems of mental functioning between which operates some sort of barrier or threshold. Both describe the destruction of superior mental functions in emotion. Both speak of emotion as an inadequate mobilization of energy. Luria's 'breakdown of the functional barrier', Janet calls a 'lowering of the mental level' (*abaissement du niveau mental*). Thus emotion appears similar to those semi-normal, semi-pathological states such as intoxications, exhaustions, neuroses, etc.[1] It has a 'dissolving' effect on the higher system.[2] However, where similar to such semi-normal states, emotion differs from them in having different efficient causes. These causes Janet describes as situations of a special sort, e.g. sudden exposures to change in the physical and social milieu when there is neither prior experience nor

[1] Janet, P., *L'Etat mental des hystériques*, 3rd edn., Paris, 1931, p. 93.
[2] 'En un mot, l'émotion a une action dissolvante sur l'esprit, diminue sa synthèse et le rend pour un moment misérable.'—Janet, *Automatisme psychologique*, 1889, p. 457.

the necessary vital force nor enough time to adapt to the present situation.[1] These situations as such are not the explanation of emotion, but only provide the circumstances which prevent an action or a tendency from coming to a proper conclusion. Instead, there is incoordination, useless action, inadequacy which he explains in terms of inhibition. The *action manquée* which is emotion is nothing else than an arrested tendency.

> Emotion is a disorder that seems to arise at the moment a situation is perceived, that seems to develop before action, that seems even to inhibit action; fatigue is a disorder that seems to us to develop later on, after action, and especially after intense and repeated action.—P. Janet, *Principles of Psychotherapy* (transl. from French by H. and E. Guthrie), London, 1925, p. 155.

> Emotivity . . . is just a habit which calls for the regulation of stoppage far too early, at the outset of action, at the very perception of the circumstance that might call for action. There are people who . . . never admit being defeated . . . There are others who fight for a certain time and then quit. Finally, there are those who declare themselves defeated before any beginning of fighting, as soon as they smell an opponent. In the study of these anticipated reactions we find the explanation for emotion.—P. Janet, 'Fear of Action as an Essential Element in the Sentiment of Melancholia', FE 28, p. 309.

For him, an action stopped too soon results in melancholy; an action carried through to the end results in joy. Emotion, therefore, depends upon tendencies and their conflict or harmony.

This is the view of Whately Smith. He differentiates between two uses of the term emotion. The first use is in the specific sense as the 'emotions' of fear, desire, etc. The second, he calls 'affective tone' and is identical with 'emotion' in the generic sense. This emotion is either positive or negative depending upon whether there is harmony or conflict in the relations of instinctual (wish) tendencies.[2] Incompatibility of these physiological mechanisms involved in these tendencies gives rise to negative emotion; positive emotion, on the other hand, takes rise in their 'harmony and reinforcement'.

Drever's view is of the same kind:

> Emotion, as we have said, is 'feeling-tension', and 'feeling-tension',

---

[1] 'Les phénomènes de l'émotion se produisent quand un être vivant et conscient est exposé brusquement à une modification du milieu physique et surtout du milieu social dans lequel il est plongé, quand il n'est pas préparé par une éducation antérieure a s'y adapter automatiquement et quand il n'a pas soit la force vitale nécessaire, soit le temps suffisant pour s'y adapter lui-même au moment présent. Il y a alors une dépense nerveuse incoordonnée, inutile, qui a tous les caractères de l'épuisement . . . L'émotion ne se distingue de ces autres faits que par la brusquerie du phénomène et par les circonstances extérieures qui le déterminent,'—Janet, *L'Etat mental des hystériques*, 3rd edn., Paris, 1931, pp. 93–4.

[2] Smith, W. Whately, *The Measurement of Emotion*, London, 1922, pp. 151–2.

Differentiation

we maintain, arises when the appropriate action does not follow immediately upon the impulse or stimulus.—J. Drever, *Instinct in Man*, Cambridge, 1917, p. 267.

As with Bull, the concept of delay is important. We found the same notion in Crile (Chapter XIII). Emotion is something which occurs instead of direct action. Drever differs from Whately Smith and Janet in one major way. They use the co-concepts of positive and negative, conflict and harmony, while Drever refers *all* emotion—like Angier—to the single concept of conflict.[1]

The view of Frink combines these notions with the psychoanalytic view:

> An emotion, one might say, is an undischarged action, a deed yet retained within the organism. Thus anger is unfought combat; fear unfled flight. Perhaps it would be more accurate to say that an emotion is *a state of preparedness* for action, which however in many ways is almost action itself.—H. W. Frink, *Morbid Fears and Compulsions*, London, 1921, p. 153.

The reason why the deed is retained within the organism is because of a damming (again the hydraulic model) of the libido. In his analysis of anxiety he makes the conflict theory more specific. The opposing forces are wish-energy *versus* repression which blocks, dams, inhibits.

> The essential cause of morbid anxiety or fear is a damming up of the libido. The fear is an overflow phenomenon, the result of pent-up energy forcing a way of escape despite opposition or repression. The dammed up wish-energy which the repression withheld from action now breaks out as feeling. The effect of the repression has been to transform this energy into fear. Morbid fear, in other words, is really desire—in the broad sense, sexual desire—which various inhibitions have diverted from more natural channels of expression.—*Ibid.*, p. 153.[2]

Paulhan, finally, sums it up concisely:

> Whatever affective phenomenon we take, we can observe the same fact: the arrest of a tendency. From the most ordinary emotions to the highest and most complex feelings, we can always verify this law.—F. Paulhan, *The Laws of Feeling* (transl. from the French by C. K. Ogden), London, 1930, p. 16.
> ... by an arrested tendency I understand a more or less complicated reflex action which cannot terminate as it would if the organization of the phenomena were complete, if there were a full harmony between the organism or its parts and their conditions of existence, if the system formed in the first place by man, and afterwards by man and the external situation, were perfect.—*Ibid.*, p. 17.

[1] Drever, *op. cit.*, Appendix III, 'The "Joy" Emotions', pp. 266–9.
[2] See also Chapter XIII, pp. 160–3, on the relation of anxiety and sexual desire.

This view that emotion either signifies or is the result of something imperfect or disordered we shall come to in detail in the next chapter where we shall refer to Paulhan again. But first let us draw the conclusions up to this point.

These views make a questionable implication about the nature of man. If we assume that where there is emotion there is conflict (inhibition, blocking, arrest) and also assume alongside that where there is conflict there is a 'lowering', an imperfection, then we take a view of man which hardly allows him emotion. It becomes semi-pathological (Janet), destructive (Luria), substitutive (Tuttle),[1] inappropriate (Drever), disharmony (Paulhan). As a sign of human frailty it is best got rid of. The metaphysical model is a monism in which no incompatibilities exist. Or the model is that of a well-oiled machine which never clogs, heats up or misfires. It implies—and the biological analogies in these theories further reveal the attitude—that the right state for man is an animal state without problems and conflicts, and where, if there is any emotion at all, it must only represent harmony and appear as joy. Drever's negative notion of tension—like that of Bousfield in Chapter VI—also brings this out.

A conflict is a clash of opposites. It is how we stand to this clash that governs how we see emotion. If, like Herakleitos we say, 'War is the father of all and the king of all . . .',[2] or like Jesus, 'I came not to send peace but a sword',[3] or as Pope puts it: 'But all subsists by elemental strife/And passions are the elements of life',[4] then a conflict theory does not have to lead to a view of emotion as a malady as in the theories of the next section. We can separate the two assumptions, accepting only the first: where there is emotion there is conflict. It appears in connection with a fundamental phenomenon of life—the clash of opposites.

However, even this notion can be questioned; for example, there can be conflict without emotion and emotion without conflict,[5] and although emotion is not necessarily the result or even accompaniment of conflict, it might be the source of conflict. The alteration of the train of ideas and the parallel change in the conventional ego, the usual habitus, at the appearance of emotion might be so difficult that conflict (intrapsychic or between man and world) might well ensue. Or as Hartmann says: 'Security does not come from the

---

[1] Tuttle, H. S., 'Emotion as Substitute Response', *J. General Psychol.*, 1940, pp. 87–104. A conflict theory in that Tuttle says: '. . . *thwarting* is the most significant factor in explaining the nature of typical emotional states' (p. 99).

[2] Fragment 44 (Bywater's arrangement), EGP, p. 136.

[3] Matthew X. 34.

[4] Pope, A., *An Essay on Man*, Epistle I, line 169.

[5] See P. T. Young, *Emotion in Man and Animal*, N.Y., 1943, pp. 322–3.

affects, nor does harmony . . . the character of affect is tyrannical; each has the tendency to suppress the others. . . . [1] This fits in with the nature of emotion as brought out in Chapter VIII: each emotion is a *total* event. As a manifestation of the general or total person, it subordinates all special and partial aspects. Emotion overwhelms. The special and partial aspects of the psyche tend to resist this overwhelming.

In this way we can take conflict not as the cause of emotion, but as the *result* of the appearance of emotion on the scene—but only when the emotion is resisted, inhibited, blocked, opposed. As such, conflict does not necessarily have to be an essential condition of emotion at all. It so often is, however, because the conventional habitus is usually an unemotional habitus and thus opposes emotion. It does not usually start from Herakleitos' premise: 'It is the opposite which is good for us.' [2] And so, where there is emotion there is usually conflict.

For the *purpose* of this conflict, the clash of opposites, we can turn to Jung:

> The stirring up of conflict is a Luciferian virtue in the true sense of the word. Conflict engenders fire, the fire of affects and emotions, and like every other fire it has two aspects, that of combustion and that of creating light. On the one hand, emotion is the alchemical fire whose warmth brings everything into existence and whose heat burns all superfluities to ashes (*omnes superfluitates comburit*). But on the other hand, emotion is the moment when steel meets flint and a spark is struck forth, *for emotion is the chief source of consciousness.* There is no change from darkness to light or from inertia to movement without emotion.—C. G. Jung, 'Psychological Aspects of the Mother Archetype' (1938), *Coll. Works*, IX, 1, p. 96 (italics mine).

This destructive-creative paradox of emotion, its 'Luciferian virtue', leads into the last chapters of our amplification.

[1] Hartmann, N., *Ethik*, 3rd edn., Berlin, 1949, p. 437.
[2] Fragment 46, *loc. cit. sup.*

XVII

EMOTION AS DISORDER

UNTIL NOW this recurrent theme has been only an implication; here it comes to full statement as the dominant hypothesis. We have already seen emotion viewed as an energy disorder (Chapter VI), as a disorder of the *milieu intérieur* (X B), as the disorder of conflict (XVI). In Chapter X C, emotion was presented in terms of 'explosions', 'delays', 'disintegrations', and it was connected to a second kind of willing which interferes with the rational ordered kind. Then we have seen such notions as 'bouleversement' (Burloud) and 'Erschütterung' (Stern)—and even Lewin's 'Umschichtung' can be taken as disorder. The idea of disorder given in Chapter VII differs from what we shall encounter here because there the disorder was due to quantitative excess. Emotion was simply excess, and as the excess of anything can be disordering, so emotion was disorder. Here, however, emotion is disorder because of its irrational or unordered essence. Disorder also entered into Chapter XIII where some genetic theories proposed a common, simple root for all emotion, calling it—in one way or another—desire. Desire was then linked with the Fall, the separation from the natural state and perfect order, and with evil. Also, in Chapter XII, where emotion was explained by the subject-object gap, this void was taken as an imperfection, giving us again an 'unnatural' view of emotion.

The scores of *prima facie* disorder theories are abundant in the literature. They are reviewed by Leeper[1] and again by McGill.[2] The following serve only as examples:

> Emotion is a kind of malady which by its inner pressure produces in man agitation and irresolution. It is the want of direction and certainty and the conflict between inner tension and adequate expression which makes strong emotions resemble madness.—C. Wolff, *The Psychology of Gesture*, London, 1945, p. 36.

[1] Leeper, R., 'A Motivational Theory of Emotion to replace "Emotion as a Disorganized Response" ', *Psychol. Rev.*, 1948.
[2] McGill, V. J., *Emotions and Reason*, Springfield, Ill., 1954.

. . . in the emotional behavior segment there occurs a total disruption of the person, because a reaction system to some overwhelming stimulus fails to operate. Lacking the appropriate or customary reaction the resulting disturbance of the individual is followed or accompanied by the operation of many reflex responses of a visceral sort. But let us note that these reflex responses are replacement actions. . . . they do not serve as appropriate responses to definitely correlated stimuli. These . . . reactions we must look upon as really biological processes. The person's psychological personality is for a moment, at least, in abeyance.—J. R. Kantor, *Principles of Psychology*, N.Y., 1924, p. 349.

The following definition presents the criteria for identifying emotion: *An emotion is an acute disturbance or upset of the individual which is revealed in behavior and in conscious experience, as well as through widespread changes in the functioning of viscera (smooth muscles, glands, heart, and lungs), and which is initiated by forces within a psychological situation.'*
—P. T. Young, *Emotion in Man and Animal*, N.Y., 1943, p. 405.

Howard and Carr also find disorder to be the criterion of emotion, and they add that this disorder makes emotion meaningless.

I wish now to advance the thesis that in the emotional state, in its true form, what is experienced is an enlargement and irradiation of the original blur. Introspectively, as well as objectively, emotion is a state of disruption. All the sensational, imaginal, and affective elements of the experience are exploded out of their natural patterns, are confused and mixed and meaningless. Some theorists maintain organic sensations are the characteristic elements in the emotions: others emphasize the feelings. Introspection upon genuine emotional states will . . . show that none of the sensational or affective elements are definitely in the focus of experience, but that, on the contrary, experience is without focus or margin, a confused and scattered state of consciousness.

I have always been interested in that question, as to the value of emotional states, and the conclusion to which I come is that they have absolutely no value at all, but represent a defect in human nature.—D. T. Howard, 'A Functional Theory of the Emotions', FE 28, pp. 146–7.

What is the differentia of an emotion? Why do we term the somatic reaction an emotion when we flee from danger, but do not call it an emotion when we run just as energetically to win a race?

The distinction proposed is that of the orderly and co-ordinated character of the non-emotional adjustments as opposed to the relatively unco-ordinated and somewhat chaotic course of events in the emotional reactions. H. Carr, 'The Differentia of an Emotion', FE 28, p. 233.

The biological utility of the emotions . . . has been somewhat overemphasized. . . . In order to promote survival, Nature would have been wiser to have endowed organisms with less emotion and more cunning and intelligence.—*Ibid.*, p. 231.

The problem which Howard and Carr leave us with goes well

beyond theory of emotion, and yet it is fundamental to all theory of emotion. The question is raised: what place has emotional upset in human life? This question leads to a second and wider one: what place has disorder—and with it suffering and evil—in the general scheme of things? It is well to be clear that the judgment against emotion—it has questionable biological utility (Carr), it represents a defect in human nature (Howard), it resembles madness (Wolff), etc.—is not made on objective data alone, since the same data can be interpreted very differently, e.g. Chapter XVIII. Rather, this judgment betrays a subjective attitude which depends upon a model of viewing things dear to philosophers with an over-rational and idealistic turn of mind.

In sum, the disorder view of emotion uses a moral and ontological model the foundations of which lie deep in antiquity. The *Phaedrus* myth of the disorderly and irrational horse is a classic formulation. Already there, order, goodness, reason and the upper regions of the body belonged together—the liver being associated with the lower emotions of the irrational, dark horse. Another contribution to this model—the notion of stability and the denial of motion—came from the Eleatics. From the Stoics[1] the concept of Nature was added to order, goodness, reason and stable impassivity. The Church Fathers perfected the model by identifying it with God, Whose perfection could not allow the attributes of disorder, change, corporeality, evil and the irrational. Important here is the *identification of the irrational with evil*. Tertullian writes:

> It is the rational element [of the soul] which we must believe to be its natural condition, impressed upon it from its very first creation by its Author, who is Himself essentially rational. . . . The irrational element, however, we must understand to have accrued later, as having proceeded from the instigation of the serpent. . . . Now from the devil proceeds the incentive to sin. All sin, however, is irrational: therefore the irrational proceeds from the devil, from whom sin proceeds; and it is extraneous to God, to whom also the irrational is an alien principle.—Tertullian, *De Anima*, 16, ANCL, XV, pp. 442–3.

And when in the fourth century, Nemesius, in interpreting Aristotle's *orexis*, writes '. . . yearning starts movement',[2] it is to be

---

[1] As Hartmann (*Ethik*, 3rd edn. Berlin, 1949, p. 342) points out, the Stoic concept of Nature is not a 'natural' Nature which would welcome affects and passions as part of 'natural' man. It is a concept of Nature referring to an ideal metaphysical rational order; thus, affects are 'unnatural'. Hartmann's analysis of the war against emotion in terms of the identification of the 'natural' with evil, does not go quite far enough. It is not just the 'natural' but also the 'irrational' and the 'dynamic'—in short any principle which does not fit in with the stable pleromatic view of the rationalist's God that leads to the war against emotion.

[2] Nemesius of Emesa, 'De Natura Hominis', 16 (Library of Christian Classics IV, p. 348), London, 1955.

seen on this model. God cannot have this faculty of *orexis* because, as most perfect of the perfect, he lacks nothing and therefore needs nothing. Yearning means a defect, a lack, a deprivation of some good (*Privatio boni*) which is the very definition of evil given by Augustine. Thus is developed a moral position against the desires and motions of the soul which are evidence of human imperfection and the Fall away from the divine order. Man, were he perfect, would need nothing, would desire nothing, and would have no emotion.

This moral stand against needs and wants, although bound up with the identification of the irrational, the unnatural and motion with evil, arises, as we see it, due to a concretistic vision of perfection as a pleroma (e.g. Parmenides and Plotinus) in which any imperfection is conceived as an *emptiness*. This spatial image we have already encountered in such ideas as that of the Fall, the subject-object split, and in the Eleatic arguments—all of which we have touched upon in previous chapters in connection with negative attitudes toward emotion. Other examples appear in those theories of art which demand all space be filled, or in the physicist's old dictum, 'Nature abhors a vacuum'. A break in perfection is a break in order, reason and nature. This gap is evil. *The root metaphor of the disorder view is a kind of ontological agoraphobia, which identifies irrational emptiness with evil.*

A clear example of theory of emotion built on this model is put by Descuret in the middle of the last century. For him, emotion (passion) arises out of desire, which arises from 'need', which in turn signifies emptiness. ('Un besoin est l'expression d'un manque ou d'un vide', and he calls this need 'une sorte de voix intérieure réclamant une satisfaction'.)[1] Or, as Nemesius put it, '. . . yearning starts movement'.[2]

The notion of the need as the voice of emptiness demanding satisfaction is with us in many ways still today. It appears in depth psychology where instincts and complexes demand fulfilment, in concepts of homeostasis and cybernetics, in Gestalt psychology where incomplete 'Gestalten' demand completion, and in the psychology of motivation. For example Masserman states: 'Behavior is basically actuated by the physiological needs of the organism and is directed towards satisfaction of those needs.'[3] Again and still the

---

[1] Descuret, J. B. F., *La Médecine des Passions* (3rd edn.), Paris, 1860, p. 19.

[2] Such an ontological agoraphobia is perhaps a particularly Western and concretistic notion, since in Buddhism the Void is not a break in perfection nor an empty negation. The Void is a positive absolute, such as the void which gives form to the Chinese jar and which must exist for the jar to exist. It demands nothing, and thus it originates no motion. (Cf. *Dictionnaire encyclopédique du Bouddhisme*, entry 'Byo' = 'pot'.)

[3] Masserman, J., *Principles of Dynamic Psychiatry*, Philadelphia, 1946, p. 102. Others for whom the concept of needs is central are K. Horney and H. A. Murray.

model is that a need equals a disbalance.[1] It means something is not in order, something is lacking. It arises from an emptiness as Descuret says. And this hollow is evil.[2]

As background this model which unites disorder and evil does not become explicit because modern views no longer risk statements about evil. For Galen, the moral and the 'scientific', i.e. physiological behaviour, were not split apart. Not only was disorder an evil, but sin itself was disorder. *Hamartema* (sin) referred to all those things which were not performed correctly, and so functional disorders, whether sufferings of the flesh or sufferings (*pathos*) of the soul were pathological and sinful conditions. As Entralgo says: 'There can be no doubt that for Galen the entire moral life falls within the province of the physician, and sin is a disorder of the human soul which can be referred to the formula by which he defines disease: *diathesis para physin*, "a preternatural condition" of the "nature" of man.'[3] The passions belonged among these unnatural conditions because of this same model which joins reason, order, nature and goodness. Passion, by defying the bounds of reason, becomes at once an unnatural and evil disorder.

Today the science of emotion tries to keep a clean cut away from the morality of emotion—and not without good reason, since centuries of moralizing had obfuscated the facts. Nevertheless, the moralizing continues to colour the facts because of the continuity of the conceptual model. Theories of emotion which depend on such key concepts as 'abreaction', 'social adaptation', 'well-adjusted', 'autonomic balance', 'homeostasis', 'compensatory feedback' imply

[1] The German psychologists, Herbart, Waitz, Schilling, Volkmann and Nahlowsky, (KB, pp. 127–40) each discuss emotion in terms of the concept of balance. For them emotion is always a disturbance of inner balance so that 'emotion' and 'balance' become contraries. The more Romantic C. G. Carus (*Vorlesungen über Psychologie*, Leipzig, 1831, pp. 376–7) on the other hand, sees emotion as a 'middle condition of the soul between health and illness', a condition which has a balance or pattern of its own. He elaborates a 'compass of emotion' of twenty-four different emotional directions, the centre of which is a 'pure and vitally vigorous peace of soul'.

[2] Theory of emotion based on 'needs' has always to confront the difficulty that there are two models for accounting for needs. The first is this ancient model of disbalance and disorder. The second goes back to Aristotle and is presented today clearly by A. Maslow ('The Instinctoid Nature of Basic Needs', *J. of Personality*, 1953–4, p. 327); '... recent developments have shown the theoretical necessity for the postulation of some sort of positive growth or self-actualization tendency within the organism which is different from its conserving, equilibrating, or homeostatic tendency.... This kind of tendency to growth or self-actualization ... has been postulated by thinkers as diverse as Aristotle and Bergson.... it has been found necessary by Goldstein, Rank, Jung, Horney, Fromm, Rogers, May, and Maslow.' On this second view, as Maslow says, what man wants is 'what he needs (what is good for him)'; but what is good for him is not restricted to the maintenance of homeostasis. Emotion might then be based on the needs of new growth and the emergent possibilities of creativity. See further, Chapter XVIII.

[3] Entralgo, P. L., *Mind and Body* (transl. from Span. by A. Espinosa), London, 1955, p. 66. I am indebted to this work for the substance of this paragraph.

211

an ideal condition of harmonious order and are only understandable on the moral model of perfection. There are always some bright standards of order, perfection, balance and reason against which are held in defective comparison disorder, disbalance and the irrational. Stability is the essence of this model; dynamic processes are only servants of needs arising from breakdowns and gaps in stability. Statistical methods only further this static kind of thinking by providing laws and norms against which deviations are charted. For one example of this model in recent literature there is the attempt of Bindra to solve the 'Leeper-Young controversy' as to whether emotion is ordered or disordered behaviour. Bindra finds it can be both, the division between order and disorder made according to a criterion of stability. For him, what is ordered is rational and stable. 'Behaviour is organized to its highest degree when it is stable (hence predictable) with respect to both its sequence of responses and its outcome or goal. Behaviour's lowest degree of organization exists when it shows neither a stable sequence ... nor a stable outcome...'.[1] No mention is made of evil, but no mention need be made since the concept of disorder (at the *lowest* end of the scale) nowadays includes it and implies it. Today as for the ancients, disorder is something negative, sinful and sick.

There are three varieties of the disorder view of emotion. The first one is extreme, unconditionally declaring all emotion is disorder. This is the view of Young, Howard, Carr, and others too many to mention. The second variety finds only part of emotion to be disorder. This is the view of Bindra who draws a line between organized and unorganized emotional behaviour according to the criterion of stability. Descuret draws his line between good and evil passion according to a rational line of moral duty.[2] This attempt to find a place within reason for a part of emotion again uses the model going back to Plato's division between the rational and irrational horse. Nemesius makes the same division: 'The irrational in us is partly not susceptible to reason, and partly obedient to reason' (*loc. cit. sup.*). The Church Fathers, too, did not relegate all passions to the Devil; they were not all disorders and sins. Tertullian held, on the model of God's divine anger and divine desire, that:

> In our own cases, accordingly, the irascible and the concupiscible elements of our soul must not invariably be put to the account of the irrational (nature), since we are sure that in our Lord these elements operated in entire accordance with reason. God will be angry, with

---

[1] Bindra, D., 'Organization in Emotional and Motivated Behaviour', *Canad. J. Psychol.*, 1955, p. 161.

[2] Descuret, *op. cit.*, p. 28.

perfect reason . . . and with reason, too, will God desire. . . .—Tertullian, *De Anima*, 16, ANCL, XV.

Nemesius even went further by saying: '. . . these passions are necessary components of a living creature, for life could not endure without them'.[1] This second variety of theory only condemns as disorder the lowest end of the scale which is outside the confines of reason. But, of course, it is just this aspect which is problematic.

The third variety is similar to the theories of Chapter XV about reason and emotion and Chapter X C about the two kinds of willing. Emotion is not reason and not order, yet there is an order and reason in emotion.[2] There are, in fact, two kinds of reason and order, and the idea of disorder only enters in when one kind of order is judged from the viewpoint of the other. This is how Bergson attacks the problem of disorder:

> Now, suppose there are two species of order, and that these two orders are two contraries within one and the same genus. Suppose also that the idea of disorder arises in our mind whenever, seeking one of the two kinds of order, we find the other. The idea of disorder . . . would not admit a theoretical use. . . . It denotes the absence of a certain order, but *to the profit of another*. . . .—H. Bergson, *Creative Evolution*, London, 1928, p. 234.

Bergson's solution simply denies disorder; it is but another kind of order. This is not wholly satisfactory. The problem might better be formulated to admit order and disorder as complementary coordinates which are necessary to define each other. There is no order without disorder and *vice versa*. This is borne out by experience in the world of the psyche and in the world of nature (physical sciences). Every extension of the realm of order brings with it an extension in the realm of disorder, and it is just this challenging increase in the latter which gives the material and impetus to extend the realm of order. In fact, it makes the realm of order possible. Witness to this is given by theoretical developments in physics, where the advance of the realm of order continually opens out new disordered and

---

[1] One is reminded of the Rabbinic tale in which all the passions of the world were finally brought under control and locked up, assuring mankind at last of peace and order; but then the people came to the Rabbi to complain: there were no more eggs.

[2] According to F. H. George, 'Machines and the Brain', *Science*, 127 (1958), p. 1274, recent thinking about emotion in the field of brain models seems to be abandoning the disorder view of emotion (misfire or backfire). As was put in Chapter XV, emotional behaviour is also a kind of rational, meaningful behaviour. George says: 'Work on electrical stimulation of the hypothalamus of cats has shown what is called "sham rage", but recent demonstrations of the cortical representation of the autonomic system, coupled with the apparent meaninglessness of sham rage (hence its name), have convinced most people that the hypothalamus is only a relay centre for the "emotional" system. Ultimately emotional behavior can best be understood in the light of reasonable behavior. . . .'

irrational aspects, new unknowns to order. For theory of emotion this view of disorder means that *every extension of consciousness yields the by-product of new emotions.* The wider the consciousness the more susceptible it is to new encounters with irrational, unconscious and disordered emotions. These do not cease as consciousness develops, as the rational and idealistic upward-striving man might hope.[1] Rather they are the necessary complement to the extension of order. In fact, they make that extension of order possible in the same way that the problems set by the irrational and disordered aspects of nature make possible the extension of order in the physical sciences.

To return to the third variety of disorder theory, we find it accepts emotion as disorder; but it gives a positive and meaningful interpretation to this disorder mainly by saying, as Bergson, that disorder is not only disorder, but is profitable and useful. Thus Kant, who held in accordance with the great tradition of rational philosophy that the emotions and passions are 'abnormal events' and 'diseases' of the mind because they are irrational, and who endorsed the Stoic doctrine of apathy, still could find some use in them.[2] Forti proceeds in this manner, finding positive value in the disorder:

> The theory which we have just sketched allows one to eliminate the difficulties summed up by the famous 'paradox' of emotion. The odd thing with emotion is that it seems to be an exorbitant and disturbing phenomenon, the role and persistence of which one cannot explain.
> But if one takes it at its origins, its positive aspect becomes more apparent. With all his being an individual defends himself, not without having some notion of aim and of the steps to lead him there: such is the instinctive reaction. Understandably this reaction presents a disordered and excessive aspect since it proceeds from a kind of sudden mobilization of all forces. However, in spite of its confused and tumultuous character, the event maintains on the whole, a real efficacy.'—E. Forti, *L'Emotion, la volonté et le courage*, Paris, 1952, p. 10, my translation.

His concept of emotion as 'une réaction instinctive' (p. 7), solves the paradox. It is a disorder, but as an instinctive reaction it has a real use.

The theory of Strasser,[3] as extreme as the first variety of disorder views, nevertheless tries to find some reason for and meaning in the disorder. For him emotion is out and out disorder. Its ground is a 'disorganization of levels' (p. 184). It has all the characteristics of pre-intentional behaviour, such as: the coming to the fore of automatic, vegetative and reflex levels; the fascination with an over-

[1] L. J. Saul's *Emotional Maturity* (Philadelphia, 1947) gives a good picture of such an idealized condition; maturity for him seems to exclude emotionality, especially in its more irrational or 'irresponsible' aspects.

[2] Kant, *Anthropologie*, 73 and ff.

[3] Strasser, S., *Das Gemüt*, Utrecht/Antwerpen/Freiburg, 1956.

powering Good or Evil; simplified, primitive, 'absolute' reactions;
the impossibility to act meaningfully (pp. 183–4). Like Stern, he calls
emotions 'Erschütterungen des Menschen' (p. 187). And further,
'In den Emotionen entschwindet die personale Würde des Menschen.
Er überlässt sich Urgewalten, die nun ohne Geleise, ohne Ordnung,
ohne Form, ohne Ziel verpuffen' (p. 185). And Strasser agrees with
Plessner[1] that an emotional attack is not behaviour; it is the end of
behaviour. It might well belong to the behaviour of animals and therefore be useful (and not disorder) for them, as a kind of instinctive
reaction as Forti proposes. But for humans, an emotional breakdown
is an end to meaningful behaviour (p. 187).

We can compare Strasser's statement, 'The personal dignity of the
human being disappears in the emotions', with Whitehead's statement,
'My importance is my emotional worth now . . .' (Chapter XV).
Strasser's whole position runs counter to the views of that chapter
because of his split of emotion from reason. Thus he speaks of
emotion as a 'breakdown' which has a pathological implication. And
thus he writes: 'Being endangered through emotional breakdown is
precisely the price man must pay for his Reason' (p. 187).

Although Strasser splits emotion radically from reason and spirit,
he finds it yet has a signification and intention. This is a 'last intention', the intention of letting go of all intentions, like a monarch
who abdicates (pp. 185–6). Therefore, emotion is not altogether
irrational and unspiritual because the *conditions which it requires* are
rational, spiritual, intentional. Reason and order and spirit must
first be there before they can abdicate or be overthrown. Thus he
concludes that although emotion itself is arational, it is nevertheless
conditioned by reason.[2]

This strained, peculiar attempt of Strasser to find for emotion
some reason, some intention, does not mitigate the extremity of his
'disorder' theory. He leaves us with the hopeless psychology of the
rational academic tradition, now wearing the fancy plumes of 'philosophical anthropology'. Reason must hold off emotion at all costs
until, helpless, it abdicates to the dark violations of passions. As we
pointed out in Chapter XV, pp. 188–9, reason becomes impotent and
emotion meaningless when they are sundered. It is not their separation, but their union which is therapeutic, or as was said in Chapter
XIV: reason must become impassioned in order to deal with emotion.
Strasser's 'abdication' hardly fulfils this condition. His image of
reason (intentionality) looks more like compulsion, like a system of
paranoid defence of an old crumbling (*abbröckeln*) king. One wonders

---

[1] Plessner, H., *Lachen and Weinen* (2nd edn.), Bern, 1950.
[2] Strasser, *op. cit.*, p. 188. "In diesem Sinne ist der emotionale Ausbruch als ein
ungeistiges, aber durchaus geistbedingtes Phänomen zu bezeichnen."

about the so-called reason and dignity of a personality, forever endangered by emotional breakdown. Strasser's book—a phenomenological analysis of emotional life—wilfully ignores the unconscious aspects of the problem, as well as all evidence from psychopathology about split-personality and repression. Only in the light of this ignorance can we understand his position.

Wolff and Paulhan, quoted earlier—like Nemesius, Forti and Kant—after taking emotion as disorder, complete their views by finding some signification for this disorder.

> An affective phenomenon is the sign of a disturbance which may sometimes accompany an extension of systematization about to be effected in the organism, but it is always the sign of an imperfection and disorder of activity.—F. Paulhan, *The Laws of Feeling*, London, 1931, p. 144.
>
> The emotional stage is a transitional period between the instinctive and objective phase. Emotion has thus a definite role: it opens out a path for thought by enlarging consciousness. Every functional development follows a utilitarian design imposed by nature and in irrational emotional whims can be discerned the acquirement of knowledge of the self and of the world. . . .
>
> To acquire knowledge of the self and of the world is a tremendous task. It is in fact the final goal of wisdom.—C. Wolff, *op. cit.*, p. 37.

This last provides both a conclusion to this chapter and an introduction to the next. We have been told that emotion is a thoroughgoing breakdown of one's behaviour, consciousness and worth. The personality is shaken, in abeyance, blurred and even disappears. This malady resembles madness and is the dark price we must pay for the light of reason. Yet, emotion has 'une réelle efficacité'. It has to do with the extension of order and perhaps with that higher systematization called wisdom. Therefore, there is a place for this disorder within the scheme of things because it is the necessary co-ordinate of all order. It can also be taken as serving a larger concept of order, either (1) by compensation (re-dressing a lost balance), or (2) by being in itself a new kind of order *in statu nascendi*, or (3) by being the dissolution of a non-serviceable order and so making possible a new systematization. In the last instance, Oscar Wilde's statement is neatly apt: 'The advantage of the emotions is that they lead us astray.' [1]

[1] Wilde, O., *The Picture of Dorian Gray* (Chap. 3), London, 1891. Compare 'astray' with Dejean's 'déroute' (Chap. XV, above).

XVIII

EMOTION AS CREATIVE
ORGANIZATION

WE SHALL ENCOUNTER in these views the same kind of
expositions which we came across in the first two chapters where the
arguments turned on the *reality* of emotion. Here the argument
concerns the *value* of emotion, and again we find polemics mixed with
theory.

As we have just seen even the disorder views of emotion can lead
to a positive evaluation of emotion. Some other positive evaluations
have been where emotion was presented as energy (Prince, McKinney)
as the innermost core of the personality (Chapter IX), as an emergency reaction to maintain homeostasis (Cannon), as motives and
drives (Chapter II), as giving rise to representations (Chapter XIV),
and also where it was taken as a still useful, phylogenetic reaction-
pattern. Many other *special* significations for emotion were given in
Chapter XV. Here, however, these views hold for one *general*
signification: *emotion furthers the development of personality.*

Leeper presents this view after first coming down hard on the
disorder views found in most textbooks. He attributes the cultural
origins of the disorganization theory of emotion to (1) the age of
rationalism, which came to life again in (2) Freud and psycho-
analysis, and in (3) modern rational technology with its social milieu.
In the last section, we tried to expose a fundamental model of
disorder which lies even further behind these 'cultural origins' which
Leeper mentions.

Leeper's own view is a blend of polemic and theory, being as much
argument against as declaration for:

> Such disorganization theorists, however, have not defined their key
> terms, have not written consistently, and have not related their gener-
> alizations to a wide range of factual knowledge. Disorganization pro-
> perly means that subordinating activities are operating at cross purposes
> rather than in ways congruous with some main tendency or function. In

terms of such a definition ... emotions produce *organization* rather than disorganization—viscerally, behaviorally, and in conscious experience. They disrupt preceding and incongruous activities, but all integrating activities do the same. Disorganization seen in intense emotion does not give the clue to the general influence of emotion because, as in physiology, extremes cannot be taken as evidence of normal effects. Especially awkward have been the attempts to force the positive emotions to fit the characterization of emotions as disorganizing.

Some of these writers have recognized that emotion often accompanies marked integration of behavior, but have insisted that emotion, 'being always disruptive', has nothing to do with this organization seen in 'emotional behavior'. However, if we use the same logic in thinking about emotion as we use in thinking about physical motives, we are led to the conclusion that emotional processes of all sorts (except perhaps in rarely intense forms) are organizing in their influence and should be studied as an aspect of the motivation of higher animals.—R. W. Leeper, 'A Motivational Theory of Emotion to Replace "Emotion as Disorganized Response" ', *Psychol. Rev.*, 1948, pp. 20–1.

McKellar[1] agrees wholeheartedly with Leeper. McGinnies states: 'Emotion appears to represent a highly organized and directed state of the organism'.[2] And Stratton, writing on sthenic emotions, find they 'increase our adequacy' and 'supplement our routine modes of response'.[3]

If we turn again to the idea of Wundt and Lehmann, restated in our terms, that the main characteristic of emotion is its alteration of the conventional habitus, then the theories in the last section saw this change as disorganizing, while here it is taken to be organizing. Here, the view favours the emergent forms of behaviour which disrupt and replace the older ones which are 'incongruous' (Leeper) and 'inadequate' (Stratton). The disorder is not emotion, but due to a conflict ('subordinating activities ... operating at cross purposes') between the old and the new, or to the breakdown of the non-serviceable old form. Thus emotion comes out of this position quite clean and orderly. It is 'highly organized' (McGinnies), 'increases our adequacy' (Stratton), and 'produces *organization*' (Leeper).

What Leeper (and each who enters the controversy on his side) misses is that he stands upon the same philosophical background of rationalism which he attacks. Since he must justify the positive value of emotion in terms of order, he too denies that emotion—except when it is extreme—can be disorder. By challenging the view that emotion must always be disorder, he grasps the other horn of the rationalist dilemma by holding that emotion must always be order.

[1] McKellar, P., *A Textbook of Human Psychology*, London, 1952.
[2] McGinnies, E., 'Emotionality and Perceptual Defense', *Psychol. Rev.*, 1949.
[3] Stratton, G. M., 'The Function of Emotion as shown particularly in Excitement', *Psychol. Rev.*, 1928, p. 363.

The same exclusion of irrational disorder appears in both views.[1] Just as it was not necessary in the last chapter to condemn emotion as useless because it is disorder, so it is not necessary to justify emotion in this section as order because it is useful. Only a paradox answers this problem: emotion is disorder and useful. It can be both chaotic and creative.

An aspect of the organizing function of emotion appears in its relation to *learning*. There is evidence for the view that emotion negatively affects the learning process.[2] On the other hand, Beck[3] makes out a case, based on his view of emotion as a molar event (Chapter VIII), for emotion as a necessary element in knowing. Zilboorg[4] presents the same view concerning the effectiveness of insight in psychotherapy. Prescott[5] stresses the importance of emotion in education: 'Undoubtedly, emotions are the most potent and frequent factors in the change of attitudes.' And Wiener hints:

> ... that the sort of phenomenon which is recorded subjectively as emotion may not be merely a useless epiphenomenon of nervous action, but may control some essential stage in learning, and in other similar processes.—N. Wiener, *The Human Use of Human Beings*, 2nd edn., N.Y., 1954, p. 72.

One way in which emotion might control learning is suggested by Heiss's theory which conceives emotion as an accompaniment of drive, such as we saw in the hypotheses of Chapter III. But on Heiss's view, emotion is not an impotent epiphenomenon. It is the original carrier of experience ('ursprüngliche Erlebnisträger'— *op. cit.*, p. 253), and above all, emotion is a mediator between outer stimuli and inner drive mechanisms.[6] The special function of emotion is to direct and control the more mechanical, instinctual and physiological aspects of behaviour which emotion accompanies. Therefore, the more developed is the emotional faculty, the more are the drive

---

[1] Compare Bergson and Bindra above, Chap. XVII.

[2] See Allport (Chapter XI, p. 138) for this view. Also P. T. Young, *Emotion in Man and Animal*, N.Y., 1943, pp. 29–30.

[3] Beck, S. J., 'Emotional Experience as a Necessary Constituent in Knowing', FE 50, pp. 95–107. (See also Chapter VIII for more of Beck's view.)

[4] Zilboorg, G., 'The Emotional Problem and the Therapeutic Role of Insight', *Yearbook of Psychoanalysis*, 9, N.Y., 1953, pp. 199–219.

[5] Prescott, D. A. (ed.), *Emotion and the Educative Process*, Washington, 1938, p. 86. (See also Chapter XI above.)

[6] 'Demzufolge hat der Affekt und das affektive Geschehen eine *doppelte* Funktion. Einmal ist der affektive Bereich ... durch die inneren angeborenen Funktionen bedingt. Das meint der Satz, dass jeder Trieb affektbesetzt ist. ... Zum andern aber ist das affektive Geschehen in einem stärkeren Masse als der triebhafte Mechanismus nach aussen geöffnet. Ueber den Affekt hinweg gewinnt der Aussenreiz einen Zugang zum Triebmechanismus, der um so mächtiger wird, je mehr das affektive Vermögen entwickelt ist.

'Dies gibt dem Affekt seine eigentümliche Funktion innerhalb der psychischen

aspects of behaviour open to direction through emotion. Again the model is like a continuum (Chapter XIV) in which the upper (here 'outer') end can direct and determine the lower or inner. On the model of levels (Chapter IX) this view says that through emotion the innermost personality becomes accessible to cultural influences. Thus emotion serves learning.

Does emotion help or harm learning? The usual resolutions of this discussion depend either upon the theory of emotion (e.g. disorder views find emotion harmful, etc.) or upon the kind of emotion and its degree (e.g. extreme anxiety and hatred being assumed harmful, etc.). However, the real issue here more likely depends upon the view one takes of learning. If learning is a partial activity of the will and intellect, and these functions are educated apart from emotion according to the traditional split of reason from emotion (such as we saw in Chapter XV and in the 'two kinds of willing' in Chapter X C), then it becomes well probable that emotion harms learning. If, on the other hand, there is another kind of learning which involves the whole man and which aims at experience rather than, or as the basis of, knowledge, then emotion might be necessary to learning.

Briefly, this view of learning takes *knowing as an emotional experience*. A plain example are initiation ceremonies in which knowledge is imparted along with pain and terror. The Zen master kicks, beats and slaps his pupils in the process of awakening a new consciousness. 'Concrete experiences are valued more than mere conceptualization.' [1] Other examples are religious rites and mysteries in which revelation of dogma is an emotional event. Plato's views on education emphasize music and its effect on the whole man.[2] The general notion is that experience with the mind is not enough; the whole man, including the 'inner' man and the flesh must also be changed. Etymologically, this is brought out in the Hebrew *l'da'at* = to know, meaning to experience with the flesh, a connotation found in our meaning of knowing as being familiar and intimate with. The word 'philosophy', now so pure and dry, itself means *love* of wisdom, while 'inform' means also to inspire and animate. Another witness to the view that learning is, or arises from, emotional events is the ordinary notions of 'experience' and 'maturity'. These terms,

Dynamik. In seiner Abhängigkeit von äusseren Geschehen wird der affektive Apparat aus einer Begleitfunktion des Triebgeschehens zu einer Instanz, die das Triebgeschehen und die triebhaften Mechanismen determinieren kann.

'So müssen wir bei den höher entwickelten Lebewesen von einer affektiven Steuerung der Triebmechanismen sprechen, die offenbar um so bedeutsamer und wichtiger ist, je mehr der Bereich der Affektivität entwickelt und entwickelbar ist.'— R. Heiss, *Allgemeine Tiefenpsychologie*, Bern and Stuttgart, 1956, pp. 261–2.

[1] Suzuki, D. T., 'The Awakening of a New Consciousness in Zen', *Eranos Jahrbuch* XXIII, Zurich, 1955, pp. 275; 293–4.

[2] Compare H. Read, *Education through Art*, London, 1943, and F. Schiller, *On the Aesthetic Education of Man*, London, 1954.

unless specified within a certain context, tend more and more to refer in the mouth of the general to an impalpable psychological residue of a rich emotional life beyond intelligence measurements and academic learning. Knowing is a process of the soul and flesh, not only of the mind.

Learning so conceived is favoured by emotion; in fact, it cannot take place without emotion which, as has been stated variously and often, changes the whole man, consists of bodily events, and is a movement of the soul. The importance of the *body* in this kind of learning is brought out in the preceding paragraph. This would fit in with Malebranche's view that the essential principle of all the emotions is that they incline us 'to love our own body and what is useful for its preservation'.[1] Or as Landauer said, affects, associated with different organ zones, make us aware of ourselves as a whole. 'Thus affects tend towards integration . . . they are sought after, even when consciously experienced as unpleasurable' (Chapter XIII, p. 158). And Goldstein (whose view we shall come to a few pages farther on), agrees: '. . . the individual can and does bring himself into these emotional conditions because they make for better self-realization'.[2] '. . . even though experienced as disturbance, emotion may not really be a state of disorganization, but rather one of reorganization with special significance within the totality of behavior.'[3] In sum, emotion furthers the development of personality and in that sense serves, and is an essential aspect of, the learning process.

Emotion, which makes one aware of and love one's body, which furthers learning, adaptation and integration into a whole, is still not necessarily creative. Organization and re-organization are not the same as a new, creative organization. However, there are views which link emotion to *creation*.

Affective activity therefore seems to impregnate every manifestation of our thought. It might even be said that, using the pure imaginative memories stored in our sensory-mnemonic accumulations as its intellectual material, it is then the sole architect which creates every edifice of reason, from the humblest construction of the lowest animal to the most elaborate triumph of the man of genius.—E. Rignano, *The Psychology of Reasoning*, London, 1923, p. 389.[4]

[1] 'Les passions de l'âme sont des impressions de l'Auteur de la nature, lesquelles nous inclinent à aimer nôtre corps, et toutes les choses qui peuvent être utiles à sa conservation.'—N. Malebranche, *De la Recherche de la Vérité*, Vol. II, Bk. 5, Chapter I, 1674.

[2] Goldstein, K., 'On Emotions: Considerations from the Organismic Point of View', *J. Psychol.*, 1951, p. 47. [3] *Ibid.*, p. 38.

[4] See also Chapter XIV, p. 168, for further reference to Rignano's view of emotion based on biological memory.

In the sphere of the motility of expression of internal states, man converts the energy of his visceration into catabolable energy which does no work and so his behavior in this sphere of movement is a 'spendthrift' behavior; discharged, i.e. expressed, for its own sake it uses energy reserves and tends to 'spend' man as, for example, in states of intense emotional excitement without outlet for action. However, converted into changes in the world of matter through the motility of effectuation, this 'emotional' energy is the matrix and source of all human achievement through which man frees energy from matter and so not only pays the operational cost of maintenance of life as a process of visceral being but of living as a process of productive, 'creative' becoming.—P. I. Yakovlev, 'Motility, Behavior and the Brain: Stereodynamic Organization and Neural Coordinates of Behavior', *J. Nerv. Ment. Dis.*, 1948, p. 333.

For the emotional factor yields in importance to no other; it is the ferment without which no creation is possible.—Th. Ribot, *Essay on the Creative Imagination* (transl. by A. H. N. Baron), London, 1906, p. 31. (See also Chapter IV, p. 49, for fuller view from Ribot.)

Our individual tensions are simply the new thing growing through us into the life of mankind. When we can see them steadily in this universal setting, then and then only will our private difficulties become really significant. We shall recognize them as the travail of a new birth for humanity; as the beginning of a new knowledge of ourselves and of God. —J. MacMurray, *Reason and Emotion*, London, 1935, p. 18. (See also Chapter XV, p. 191, for fuller view from MacMurray.)

It is a revealing fact that every artist, when asked how his vocation came to him, invariably traces it back to the emotion experienced at his contact with some specific work of art.—A. Malraux, *The Creative Act* (transl. by S. Gilbert), N.Y., 1949, p. 121.[1]

These statements, different as they are, take emotion as a kind of energetic matrix (Yakovlev), ferment (Ribot), tension (MacMurray) such as we saw in the energy views of Chapter VI. For Rignano and MacMurray, this energy is purposive, while for Yakovlev the energy is more a quantity. The essential point in all is that emotion is the ground of creation; it makes creation possible.

Just how emotion works in the creative process is a mysterious and stupendous issue, involving such questions as the nature of inspiration, prophecy, and the creative act.[2] Wordsworth describes the

[1] 'Il est révélateur que pas une mémoire d'artiste ne retienne une vocation née d'autre chose que de l'émotion ressentie devant une oeuvre. . . . Dès que les documents nous permettent de remonter à l'origine de l'oeuvre d'un peintre, d'un sculpteur—de tout artiste—nous rencontrons, non un rêve ou un cri plus tard ordonnés, mes les rêves, les cris ou la sérénité d'un autre artiste.'—A. Malraux, *La Création artistique* (Skira), 1948, p. 117.

[2] Housman, A. E. (*The Name and Nature of Poetry*, Cambridge, 1933) gives a short description of the creative process, illustrating its link with emotion, and in particular with the flesh:

'. . . I would go out for a walk of two or three hours. As I went along, thinking of nothing in particular, only looking at things around me and following the progress of the seasons, there would flow into my mind, with sudden and unaccountable emotion,

222

process as follows:

> I have said that Poetry is the spontaneous overflow of powerful feel-
> ings; it takes its origin from emotion recollected in tranquillity: the
> emotion is contemplated till by a species of reaction the tranquillity
> gradually disappears, and an emotion similar to that which was before
> the subject of contemplation, is gradually produced, and does itself
> actually exist in the mind.—W. Wordsworth, *Lyrical Ballads with Other
> Poems*, Vol. I, 2nd edn., London, 1800.

Malraux's statements would deny that the origin of art lies in
emotion as such, as Wordsworth seems to hold. It is not just emotion,
but rather the emotion spreading and igniting from one artist to
another via a work of art. In other words, art takes rise in a specific
emotion, the emotion of artists as expressed in a work of art. This
compares with the traditional notion of the 'aesthetic' or 'creative'
emotion as described in the older textbooks (Bain, Ribot, Lehmann),
and in Clive Bell.[1] But this kind of solution is no solution. It posits
different kinds of emotions: religious, moral, aesthetic, etc., and then
attributes religious, moral and aesthetic activities to these emotions.
It simply says creativity is due to the creative emotion.

Another theory for explaining the role of emotion in art is given
by Langfeld. He denies the views presented so far. He would refuse
Wordsworth's more Romantic position that art arises from emotion
per se. He also criticizes the idea that emotion is purposive (Rignano's
metaphor of emotion as architect) and the idea that emotion is a
quantitative energy source. He bases art on a *conflict* theory of
emotion:

> It can therefore be said that emotions are at the root of aesthetic
> creation, but not as some mysterious driving force that guides the artist
> in his endeavors, or supplies the energy for his effort. Nor can it be said
> that a man is emotional because he is an artist, but rather he is an artist
> for the reason that he is emotional, or more explicitly, because his life
> is full of conflicts, which he is best able to overcome in artistic expression.
> —H. S. Langfeld, 'The Role of Feeling and Emotion in Aesthetics',
> FE 28, p. 348.

sometimes a line or two of verse . . . there would usually be a lull of an hour or so, then
perhaps the spring would bubble up again. I say bubble up, because, . . . the source of
suggestion thus proffered to the brain was an abyss . . . the pit of the stomach'
(pp. 49–50).
   'Poetry indeed seems to me more physical than intellectual. . . . Experience has
taught me, when I am shaving of a morning, to keep watch over my thoughts, because
if a line of poetry strays into my memory, my skin bristles so that the razor ceases to
act. This . . . is accompanied by a shiver down the spine . . . constriction of the throat
and a precipitation of water to the eyes. . . . (pp. 46–7).
   'And I think that to transfuse emotion—not to transmit thought but to set up in the
reader's sense a vibration corresponding to what was felt by the writer—is the peculiar
function of poetry' (p. 12).
   [1] Bell, C., *Art*, London, 1914, pp. 6 ff.

Langfeld gives the thesis again more recently.[1] Conflict is 'at the root of emotional states' and these states are expressed in art—'All art expresses emotion'. And so art becomes a way of solving problems and is a kind of 'escape' or flight into unreality. This widespread and pernicious view of art as a kind of neurotic phenomenon ('In statistical studies of personality inventories we find indications that artistic activity is related to disorders of personality'—Langfeld) comes about wholly because of the conflict and disorder models of thinking about emotion.

It would seem Read endorses this conflict view:

> The emotional conflict creates a tension which is relieved by the act of poetic utterance, in some way, or to some degree, the poetic quality of the utterance is related to the intensity of the conflict . . . whenever we uncover the springs of modern poetry—post-Renaissance subjective type of poetry—there we soon detect a conflict of this nature. *Hamlet* and *King Lear* are the prototypes of such psychic conflicts, resolved in poetry.—H. Read, 'Poetic Consciousness and Creative Experience', *Eranos Jahrbuch* XXV, Zurich, 1957, p. 379.[2]

But the difference between him and Langfeld (and Kris whom we come to below) is significant. Both Langfeld and Kris are not free from Freudian notions of sublimation and from a psychoanalytic view of emotion as something which must be released. Read, in sympathy with Jung, takes both conflict and art as *sui generis* authentic aspects of the healthy psyche.

Continuing on, we find again and again the thesis that emotion is required for creativity. Harding[3] gives a splendid collection of auto-biographical passages from creative artists showing that the creative state is a condition of emotional excitement. Bowra says: 'For Tasso the key was a rich melancholy, for Wordsworth an awe akin to fear, for Dante love, for Coleridge joy, for Rilke anguish.'[4] In accordance with psychoanalytic theory, Kris finds that creative art is a release of unconscious passion 'under the protection of the aesthetic illusion'.[5] But important as emotion is in the process of creation,

---

[1] Langfeld, H. S., 'Feeling and Emotion in Art', FE 50, p. 517.

[2] Read quotes Maud Bodkin's hypothesis as to the archetypal pattern of tragic poetry: 'The pattern consists of emotional tendencies of opposite character which are liable to be excited by the same object or situation, and, thus conflicting, produce an inner tension that seeks relief in the activity either of fantasy, or of poetic imagination, either originally or receptively creative.'—*Archetypal Patterns in Poetry* (Vintage edn.), N.Y., 1958, p. 21.

[3] Harding, R. E., *An Anatomy of Inspiration and an Essay on the Creative Mood* (3rd edn.), Cambridge, 1948.

[4] Bowra, C. M., *Inspiration and Poetry*, London, 1955, p. 4.

[5] Kris, E., *Psychoanalytic Explorations in Art*, New York, 1952, p. 63. See also R. Arnheim, 'Emotion and Feeling in Psychology and Art', *Confin. psychiat.*, 1958, pp. 69–88, for more argument against the importance of emotion in art. A. M. Hocart ('Ritual and Emotion'), *The Life-Giving Myth*, London, 1952) writes in the same vein

Kris and Bowra, and Gordon too, emphasize that the emotionally inspired state is not enough. 'Mere emotion does not produce works of art, nor anything else. Emotion may be essential as the occasion for creative work, it may be the theme of creative work, but it is never sufficient for its achievement.' [1] The achievement depends upon 'effort' (Gordon), the role of the 'ego' (Kris), 'technique', 'intelligence', 'discipline' (Bowra). This means that emotion is not an equivalent of art since art requires certain specialized functions for the elaboration of the emotion; nevertheless, emotion is the fount and matrix on all these views of such elaborations called poems, paintings and songs.

Again we come to the kind of problem already familiar: the way in which emotion is related to creative activities will be explained according to typical models for dealing with emotion. On one view, creativity is the result of emotional *conflict*; on another, it has to do with the *unconscious*; on a third, emotion is seen as *energy*; on a fourth, creativity is the result of emotional *purposive forces*. Elsewhere we can find it said that creativity arises from the *objective values* revealed through emotion (Reid, Chapter XV); and also the thesis that in the creative man, emotion *cognizes* and *signifies* new important problems to work out, which the ordinary unemotional man misses. [2]

Bergson links emotion and the creative process through *representations*.[3] He defines emotion as 'an affective stirring of the soul' (*op. cit. inf.*, p. 43), and then distinguishes between two kinds of emotion:

> In the first case the emotion is the consequence of an idea, or of a mental picture; the 'feeling' is indeed the result of an intellectual state.
> . . . It is the stirring of sensibility by a representation, as it were, dropped

against the view that 'ritual is essentially emotional, is in fact the child of emotion'. For him, as for Kris and Arnheim, emotion is conceived negatively, as a sort of disordering intensity and so its effects are seen as harmful.

[1] Gordon, K., 'Imagination and Emotion', *J. Psychol.*, 1937, p. 134.

[2] Neumann, E., 'Der schöpferische Mensch und die "Grosse Erfahrung" ', *Eranos Jahrbuch*, XXV, Zurich, 1957, pp. 19–20: 'Im Gegensatz dazu gehört die verstärkte emotionale Reaktion zu den betonten Merkmalen des schöpferischen Menschen. Denn auch ein im Naturwissenschaftlichen schöpferischer Mensch, der eindeutig und sogar einseitig nur der einen Ding-Welt-Seite der Wirklichkeit zugewandt ist, wird von ihr tiefer erregt, beunruhigt und beeindruckt als der sogennante normale Mensch. Nur diese wache Erregtheit lässt ihn überhaupt bemerken, was Tausende vor ihm nicht bemerkt haben, und führt dazu, etwas als Problem, das heisst aber als etwas Neues, Unbekanntes und noch nicht eindeutig Eingereihtes, zu entdecken.'

[3] Compare Chapter XIV above on the relation of emotion and representations. Emotion was said there to be the basis of imagination. Or one can put it in the language of Knapp—so similar to the thesis of Cuvier, Jung, etc., in Chapter XIV—who says emotion is 'fused with fantasy', 'inextricably interwoven with fantasy' (P. H. Knapp, 'Conscious and Unconscious Affects . . .', *Psychiatric Research Reports* 8, 1957, pp. 60; 65). Thus, the way to creative imagery would lie in the fantasy images of one's own emotions. Psychological techniques for unweaving the images from the emotion are discussed above in Chapter XIV, artistic techniques are not our province.

into it. But the other kind of emotion is not produced by a representation which it follows and from which it remains distinct. Rather is it, in relation to the intellectual states which are to supervene, a cause and not an effect; it is pregnant with representations, not one of which is actually formed, but which it draws or might draw from its own substance by an organic development . . . the second kind of emotion can alone be productive of ideas.—H. Bergson, *The Two Sources of Morality and Religion* (transl. by R. A. Audra and C. Brereton), 1956 (reprint of 1935 edn.), N.Y., pp. 43–4.

These two ways in which emotion and representations are linked we have already noted in Chapter XIV as 'emotion arises from representations' and 'representations arise from emotion'. Bergson connects only the second kind of emotion to invention and creativity, and for him it is the basis of everything new. 'That a new emotion is the source of the great creations of art, of science and of civilization in general seems to be no doubt' (p. 43). 'Creation signifies, above all, emotion . . .' (p. 45).

These new emotions are manifestations of the *élan vital* as it creatively surges forward through the 'ashes' of extinct emotions. Works of art and the ideas, images and attitudes of morality and religion, are worked out expressions or representations of a new emotion. The emotion comes first; after it the formulations.

To the same effect Collingwood writes: 'What an artist is trying to do is to express a given emotion. . . . A bad work of art is the unsuccessful attempt to become conscious of a given emotion; it is what Spinoza calls an inadequate idea of an affection.' [1]

Again, as with Bergson, the emotion is prior to the work of art; while art is the conversion or transformation of emotion from the psychophysical level to the level of imaginative formulation. And since 'the artist finds expression for an emotion hitherto unexpressed' (p. 238), out of emotion the artist shapes the new.

Out of emotion the new arises. This main idea found in Leeper, in Bergson and Collingwood, is central to Goldstein's theory. We have already seen above his views on the order-disorder controversy in terms of self-realization, i.e.:

> . . . order and disorder are not simply different forms of functional organization; they can be defined only in terms of their relationship to the basic trend of the organism, that of self-realization. Whether there is order or disorder can be judged only from the positive or negative value which the condition holds for the organism's self-realization.— K. Goldstein, 'On emotions: Considerations from the organismic point of view', *J. Psychol.*, 1951, pp. 37–8.

[1] Collingwood, R. G., *The Principles of Art*, Oxford, 1938, p. 282; also pp. 273–4 for the 'skeleton' of his theory.

And so man can and does bring himself into conditions of emotion and insecurity when such states help self-realization (p. 47). Self-realization is not the way of security ('. . . *an essential characteristic of man, his not being primarily concerned with security. The search for security is neither the only nor the highest form of self-realization of man*', p. 49). 'Security' behaviour, like all behaviour, is based on emotion. But as Bergson might have said, it has become extinct; it is no longer vital. It is characterized by relative rigidity and emotionlessness and is similar to Goldstein's concept of pleasure. 'Pleasure . . . is a phenomenon of "stand-still"', *it is akin to death.*' 'Pleasure is equilibrium, elimination of danger, quietness' (pp. 48-9).

Opposed to this kind of behaviour is emotional behaviour, characterized by colour, variety, vitality, freedom—and insecurity. Therefore, emotions (as Landauer said) may well be experienced as unpleasant, yet be sought out because they lead to self-realization.[1] And so we come to the similarity between Bergson and Goldstein: both use the model of the *old versus the new*, and both link emotion to the new and to the highest. By connecting emotion to the *élan vital* and to self-realization (the summum bonum in each system), emotion becomes at once a creatively organizing activity.[2]

The curative effects of emotion—and not just love, hope and joy, but also the so-called negative emotions—reported in the older literature (e.g. Scheidemantel,[3] Tuke and Féré) and in the case reports of depth analysis become explicable in a new way. Hitherto, the release of emotion had a therapeutic effect when emotion was seen as conflict, as energy, or to do with the unconscious; that is, when

---

[1] On this thesis *all* emotions can lead to self-realization. There is no division between beneficent and maleficent emotions. Nietzsche writes (*Der Wille zur Macht*, 931): 'The emotions are altogether useful, some direct, others indirect: In respect to their usefulness, it is utterly impossible to set up any value schema. . . . At the most one could say that the most powerful are the most valuable, in that there are no greater sources of energy.' In one of the last papers written before his recent death, N. Kemp Smith ('Fear: Its Nature and Diverse Uses', *Philos.*, 1957, pp. 3–20) presents a beautiful brief for the positive values and cultivation of the emotion of fear, and describes how it can serve self-realization.

[2] Goldstein's short paper is studded with hypotheses of types we have seen. Like Chapter IX, he treats emotion in terms of the centre of the personality and in terms of tonal qualities. Like Chapter II, he finds emotion to be a driving force. He separates anxiety from other emotions (Chapter XIII). He finds experiences always accompanied by emotions (Chapter III), and implies, as in Chapters I, IV, X B, that it is going on all the time. He also uses a quantitative criterion of disturbance (Chapter VII). As in Chapters XI and XV, he views emotion as a way of adapting to particular situations. Emotion can indicate a lack (Chapters XVI, XVII). However, the fundamental hypothesis around which the others are clustered is that emotional behaviour, as opposed to security behaviour, leads to self-realization.

[3] Scheidemantel, F. C. G., *Die Leidenschaften als Heilmittel betrachtet*, Leipzig, 1787; also L. H. C. Niemeyer, *Commentatio de Commerico inter animi pathemata*, Göttingen, 1795; S. A. Tissot, *Traité des nerfs et de leurs maladies*, Lausanne, 1789.

emotion was seen as bad it was curative to release it. Now emotion is curative because it is creatively organizing. It creates, produces, re-orders, integrates, breaks down the old and static, furthers self-realization. Therapy *realizes*, not just *releases*, emotion.

This gives a clue about the method of therapy to be derived from this view of emotion. We might suppose that emotion could be prescribed to create the new man. Féré discusses this:

> Aristotle thought that the passions might be powerful arms in the hands of those who could make them serve them: but, as Seneca remarked, they are unfaithful arms, for one cannot take them up and lay them down at will, 'habent et non habentur'.
>
> The profound emotions can act, it may be well, it may be ill, and no human sagacity is capable of foreseeing the result. They are 'moral crises' which can have sometimes a happy, sometimes a deplorable effect. One cannot 'dose' the emotion one seeks to provoke; one can only in general restrain oneself to timid attempts.—C. Féré, *The Pathology of Emotions* (transl. by R. Park), London, 1899, p. 285.[1, 2]

How can emotion be dosed? One way is the seeking out of emotional events and situations in the Romantic manner: war and adventure, travel and sports, gambling and love affairs, solitude, crime, etc. The aim is to stimulate the emotions, to set fire to new emotions, which give rise to new integrations and new representations out of which grow human culture and self-realization. This can, of course, become morbid sentimentalism or cheap sensationalism with its cult of experience and its code of 'live dangerously'.

Less radical dosage is occupational therapy. This does not actively provoke emotion, but it encourages it to fulfil the creative function described for it by the views of this chapter. This means, in particular, activities of the imagination: the creative arts, intimate relationships, the life of religion.

But there is another way of dosing emotion which is also 'occupational therapy' in the broad sense. Here, there is nothing to seek out nor any particular way in which to express and create. This prescription is the simplest and the most difficult, for it consists solely in following the emotions in daily occupation, allowing them to transform life just as it comes, into a creative process of self-realization.

In looking back over this and the last chapter we find the main difference between them—and the main issue of the order-disorder

---

[1] The last phrase is my translation of '. . . on ne peut donc en général que se borner à des essais timides', which seems preferable to Park's '. . . one can in general, therefore, bear them in timid attempts.'

[2] Most recent discussion of the fatal effects of emotion can be found in *Psychosom. Med.*, 1957, pp. 182–98. (C. P. Richter, 'On the Phenomenon of Sudden Death in Animals and Man', W. B. Cannon, ' "Voodoo" Death'.)

controversy—to consist in the kind of question which each answers. The question for the views of Chapter XVII is primarily: what is the *nature* of emotion? They answer: it is disorder, just as Chapter II answered, it is a distinct entity, and Chapter VI said, it is energy. The views in this chapter conceive the question to be: what is the *meaning* of emotion? They approach the problem in terms of signification as in Chapter XV. The facts noted by Young in the last chapter are no different from those noted here. For example, he admits many ordered and useful aspects: Emotion may result in a useful and creative aftermath. Emotion may have segments of highly organized physiological reactions. Emotion may also provide a useful outlet for extra energy as in laughing and crying. But for him, because he is concerned with what emotion *is*, these aspects are only ingredients of emotional behaviour. They are not emotion itself, which *is* only and always disorder—whatever it might lead to or mean. Chapter XVII starts and ends with the bare fact, the sense data of blur and disorder, and declares this is the phenomenon called emotion. What it means develops out of what it is. Chapter XVIII takes the fact of disorder only as starting point, only as a ground for its *meaning*. It says: we can only really tell what a phenomenon is after we have seen what it becomes. Therefore, its being is ultimately what it becomes. The model of the problem is the ancient one of *being versus becoming*.[1] Our suggested solution we have given already: emotion is the disorder which means creation.

Because of this approach in terms of signification, and because, as we saw in Chapter XV, signification is an approach via the final cause, we are given little in these theories about the origins of emotion. (Bergson, for instance, speaks of a 'new' emotion, but does not say much of its origin.) Also neglected is the material or energetic aspect and the problems of physiological location. And when an attempt is made to account for the creativity of emotion, the theory turns on one of the views (energy, conflict, representations, etc.) we have already seen. In other words, these theories are not complete; only the final cause of creative organization is adequately treated.

Emotion as creative organization can be understood upon two different models. The first considers emotion to serve the general homeostatic balance of the organism; it appears when there are problems, conflicts, inadequacies, emergencies in order to restore and conserve natural equilibrium. It organizes and motivates behaviour into a new pattern of response and adaptation compensatory to the

---

[1] This controversy between being and becoming can also be accounted for on the basis of Jung's functional types of sensation and intuition (*Psychological Types*, London, 1923). The former perceives facts; the latter possibilities. Possibilities distort facts, while facts constrict possibilities. They are mutually exclusive.

old. Creative works of art, morality and religion would not occur if the natural organism were in balance.

The second way considers emotion as creatively dynamic, spontaneous, going beyond the system of equilibrium by producing the totally new, in what Kierkegaard might call a 'qualitative leap'. The need to which it refers, as mentioned in connection with Maslow's statements (p. 211 above), is not homeostatic but self-actualizing. Man, on the former view, is a creature of Nature within whose wisdom emotion finds a place. On the latter view, man is a creator who finds in emotion the place of the Spirit.

XIX

ADDENDA ON EMOTION
AND SPIRIT

THERE ARE no theories as such which strictly account for emotion as spirit; there are only suggestive passages which bring the two concepts into significant relation so that an exploratory chapter—even if only of notes and hints—becomes required for the full amplification of our theme. The dominant thesis here, mentioned at the close of the last chapter, is: *emotion is the place of the spirit*. Let us hear another view of William James on emotion, a view so widely ignored that it might perhaps be worth some attention:

> Conceive yourself, if possible, suddenly stripped of all the emotion with which your world now inspires you, and try to imagine it *as it exists*, purely by itself, without your favorable or unfavorable, hopeful or apprehensive comment. It will be almost impossible for you to realize such a condition of negativity and deadness. No one portion of the universe would then have importance beyond another; and the whole collection of its things and series of its events would be without significance, character, expression, or perspective. Whatever of value, interest, or meaning our respective worlds may appear indued with are thus pure gifts of the spectator's mind. The passion of love is the most familiar and extreme example of this fact. If it comes, it comes; if it does not come, no process of reasoning can force it. Yet it transforms the value of the creature loved as utterly as the sunrise transforms Mont Blanc. . . . So with fear, with indignation, jealousy, ambition, worship. If they are there, life changes. And whether they shall be there or not depends almost always upon non-logical, often on organic conditions. And as the excited interest which these passions put into the world is our gift to the world, just so are the passions themselves *gifts*.—Gifts to us, from sources sometimes low and sometimes high; but almost always non-logical and beyond our control. . . . Gifts, either of the flesh or of the spirit; and the spirit bloweth where it listeth; and the world's materials lend their surface passively to all the gifts alike. . . .—W. James, *The Varieties of Religious Experience*, London, 1906, pp. 150–1.

Whether or not emotions are 'our gift to the world' we have already taken up in relation to the innermost theories and empathy (Chapter IX), and in relation to emotions as qualities of the objective situation (Chapter XI). Of interest here, in this view of James is what could be meant by the idea that emotions are gifts of the spirit.

Notions of 'spirit' are familiar from theories in other chapters. For example, Strasser (Chapter XVII) said emotion was a 'spirit-conditioned' phenomenon, but his notion of spirit differs deeply from the one we shall encounter here. 'Geist' for him is identified with the first system of intellect, reason and order and not with that spirit which alters this order. In Chapter VI, we came upon the term as ground of emotion both in the principle of an immaterial, universal energy and in the ancient doctrine of the 'animal spirits'. Also, if we follow the first dictionary meaning and take 'spirit' as the 'animating or vital principle in man (and animals)' (OED), Chapter II, which presents emotion as an activating force, and Chapter IX, which presents emotion as the inner essence of life, could both be taken as examples of the view that emotion is the place of the spirit. Again there is the statement from Jung (Chapter V) that the primitive mind experiences autonomous affects as 'spirits' which come from without and move him.

There would seem to be a sort of primal identity of emotion and spirit, or at least a persistent confusion in describing emotional and spiritual experiences. Even the term 'Geist', psychologically understood, is bound up with emotion, 'since it goes back to the Indo-Iranian *gheizd* whose root means "to move powerfully". Thus its original meaning is "motive force". In early usage, Geist simply designates "vital force" . . .' [1] Onians gives the word a definite emotional connotation; it is akin to the Old Norse *geisa*, 'to rage', and the Anglo-Saxon *gaestan* (terror).[2] The Semitic term for spirit (*ruâh*) has a distinct emotional meaning. Ruâh is a synonym for anger and 'is used to cover such emotions as sadness, trouble, bitterness, and longing, which are regarded as "located in the ruâh" '.[3]

We can look elsewhere for this indistinction between emotion and spirit. A passage attributed to Pascal puts it like this: 'The more spirit one has, the greater the passions . . .' [4] We have already seen how this works in theories of creative states where inspiration and emotion blend (Chapter XVIII). For example, the 'internal commotions' of Mohammed which Massignon says are the beginning of the experience of inspiration in Islam could also be defined simply as

---

[1] Wili, W., 'The History of the Spirit in Antiquity', *Spirit and Nature*, Papers from the Eranos Yearbooks, N.Y. and London, 1954, p. 77.
[2] OET, p. 150, fn. 3.
[3] ERE, Vol. 11, p. 785a.
[4] Ducas, A., *Discours sur les passions de l'amour de Pascal*, Algiers, 1953, p. 56.

emotional experiences.[1] In other words it appears as if inspiration begins in emotion, or that the spirit depends on emotion. Sherrington says plainly: 'The spirit whether of brute or man is impotent of accomplishment unless it have emotion. Without emotion could a bird build its nest?' [2] The same idea can be found in the eighteenth century: 'As sails are to a ship, so are the passions to the spirit.' [3] In plain speech we still can refer to the inspired or spirited man as the passionate man—even if today's spirituality is anything but passionate! Plato recognized that 'the lunatic, the lover and the poet' find their common denominator in emotion. He describes four kinds of *mania* or frenzy: prophetic, initiatory or Dionysian, poetic and erotic.[4] According to Onians this is true too for the Arabs for whom spirits or *ginn* are responsible for love, madness and prophecy.[5] The spiritual and emotional would seem to overlap in these states. For Plato, the passionate—even ambitious—aspect of the soul was spirited, an idea which is most likely a historical source for another dictionary meaning of 'spirit' = 'the emotional part of man as the seat of hostile or angry feeling' (OED). The spirit of prophecy, frenzy and desire has its locus for the Greeks and Hebrews in the bowels and belly,[6] giving us a 'visceral' view of spirit comparable to the location of emotion as discussed in Chapter X B. A thalamic location of the spirit is to be found in a recent book by the distinguished biologist, Sinnott:

> In the thalamus, so to speak, the whole body comes to focus. It is the seat of the emotions, the place where motives and desires are born. If the cerebral cortex is the dwelling of man's rational part, those qualities in him that we call spiritual may be said to center in the thalamus.—E. W. Sinnott, *The Biology of the Spirit*, London, 1956, p. 128.

To go to the bottom of the matter, the basis for the hypothesis that emotion is the place of the spirit is the testimony of experience: the descent or upwelling of the spirit is experienced first of all as emotions. Here we can look to religious texts and to the witness of saints, mystics and prophets, to the literature of epics and myths, or to the reports of anthropologists or psychopathologists upon possessions divine or diseased. The experience of spirit is sudden, uncontrollable, unaccountable, molar and total, suffusing flesh, senses and mind. The chief marks of emotion brought out in preceding chapters— gross physiological changes, facial expressions, alteration of the flow of energy, quantitative excess, movements of the innermost

---

[1] Massignon, L., 'L'Idée de l'Esprit dans l'Islam', *Eranos Jahrbuch*, XIII, Zurich, 1946, p. 277.

[2] Sherrington, Sir C., *Man on His Nature*, 2nd edn., N.Y., 1953, p. 296.

[3] Nathan Bailey's *Dictionary* (1736). [4] Plato, *Phaedrus*, 265.

[5] OET, p. 487. [6] OET, pp. 488-9.

personality, the experience of importance and signification, the symbolization of representations and the production of spontaneous representations,[1] disorder of the conventional posture and habitus, the emergence of something new, etc.—are also the chief characteristics of such experiences and such behaviour. Both share the common denominator of *passio*, of *being moved*.

Being moved by what? For the ancients, the invisible, involuntary source of emotion was in a force of the same nature: *pneuma*. Duprat reviews the ancient doctrines of the passions and concludes that this 'breath', the *pneuma*, is presented either as 'the cause pure and simple, or as the indispensable agent for the production of the passions'.[2] And, just as we have had images for the source of emotion of water (the fluid model), of fire or heat, and of matter or earth (the deep strata of the psychological person, or the concrete body), we come now upon the fourth element: *air*. The words for spirit (*spiritus, ruâh, animus, pneuma*) all express a central notion of air, which varies from a violent blowing or blast to simply breathing. Even those words so dear to the tough-minded schools of psychology —'animal' and 'organism'—refer originally to a creature suffused with the airy spirit which moves (or motivates) animals and organisms and which they serve as instruments (OED). And this 'air' penetrated the deepest parts of the person, for even that inmost dark source of strong emotion, the liver, was held by the Greeks to be restored by breathing.[3] Today, this connection of spirit also with the supposedly less 'spiritual' aspects of flesh is to be found in one of the meanings of the word 'gut' = 'spirit; force of character' (OED), or 'guts' as courage.[4] That air was in some way the source of the emotions continues as a hypothesis until the Enlightenment, as for instance in the subtle vapours of the animal spirits, and in the Romantic medicine of Stahl's combustible phlogiston which was only finally overthrown by the discovery of oxygen.[5]

Today, modern experimentalists bring this 'air theory' up to date.

[1] 'The hallmarks of spirit are, firstly, the principle of spontaneous movement and activity; secondly, the spontaneous capacity to produce images independently of sense perception; and thirdly, the autonomous and sovereign manipulation of these images.' C. G. Jung, 'The Phenomenology of the Spirit in Fairy Tales', in *Spirit and Nature*, Papers from the Eranos Yearbooks, N.Y. and London, 1954, p. 8.

[2] Duprat, G. L., 'La Psycho-Physiologie des passions dans la philosophie ancienne', *Arch. f.d. Gesch. der Phil.* XI, 1905, p. 411.

[3] OET, p. 87.

[4] In this light we might understand the ancient practice of haruspicy, the performance of divination by inspection of entrails or the liver. If emotions are taken as being located there, and if the emotions are conceived as the specific forces and motives which determine behaviour (Chapter II) or conceived as reflections of the objective psychic situation (Chapter XI), then it is reasonable to expect that an examination of these dark and bloody regions should lead to accurate predictions. Today, less concretely, we explore another dark region, the unconscious, in attempting to puzzle out a man's fate.

[5] SS, p. 176.

Addenda on Emotion and Spirit

Doust and Schneider have revised Jung's association test, correlating capillary blood-oxygen saturation with emotions produced not only through word stimuli (as with the original association experiments) but also through colour and smell,[1] and other sensory stimuli at

[1] That stimuli to the sense of smell are among the most powerful evokers of emotion has long been known in literature, in the amatory arts, in those curious books on cosmetics of the High Renaissance, and in modern animal experiments. As Cobb points out (ECM, p. 35), modern theories of brain localization following Papez (Chapter X A) began with investigations of the rhinencephalon, nose brain, or what MacLean (RDPM, p. 109) calls the 'smell brain', said to be, from the point of view of phylogeny, one of the oldest parts of the human system. With some exceptions, brain researchers since Papez have usurped this area for emotion, tending to neglect the relation of emotion and smell. (There is a definite etymological relation between emotion, spirit and smell in the word *ruâh*. This term, besides referring to emotion and spirit as we saw above, is also cognate to the Semitic words for scent, odour and smell (ERE, XI, p. 784b). The Arabic *rûh*, is that breath by means of which one smells odours and 'discerns spiritual qualities' (Massignon, *loc. cit. sup.*).) Several hypotheses have been offered to account for the strength of scent-aroused emotion. According to MacCurdy, 'our culture taboos the indulgence of smelling as a branch of aesthetics' (*The Psychology of Emotion*, London, 1925, p. 558). This collective cultural repression makes smells particularly emotional because they arouse unconscious images (MacCurdy, Chapter XIV above). According to Cobb (ECM), smells stir emotions because of their common organic substrate, the rhinencephalon. Rosenzweig ('The Affect System: Foresight and Fantasy', *J. Nerv. Ment. Dis.*, 127, 1958, p. 114 f.) agrees, finding odours arouse the 'affect system' (MacLean's 'visceral brain') because 'in primitive vertebrates attempts to relieve the stresses of the internal environment were governed by affective responses mainly to various olfactory messages'. An odour is 'a coded signal, representative of a particular quality . . . of the perceived object'.

But on the general view of emotion given in this chapter, emotion stirred by scent is particularly powerful because scent is the privileged manifestation of spirit. Scent caused emotions would be direct encounters with the spirit, or qualifying essence, of an object. The pneumatic source of emotion would be physically inhaled. This says that each object has its own 'air', its own 'smell', or affective quality which is its spirit. Such speculations are in line with Hartshorne's thesis of an 'affective continuum' (an objective realm of sensory and feeling qualities) which is the realm of the spirit (Chapter XV). Cannot *Gestalten* in the field be patterned for the nose as well as for the eye or ear? We might hazard it a little farther by saying that emotion, as the vision of the psyche which perceives an objective world of value facts (Chapter XV), discerns spiritual qualities by means of a subliminal sense of smell. Might not intuition have actually a sensory basis? An experiment on the cat, for instance, reveals an increase in electrical activity in the olfactory bulb corresponding to increased alertness. The olfactory bulb in this animal seems to behave like an Aristotelian 'common' sense organ: 'It must be emphasized that the observed increase of activity in the olfactory bulb was elicited not only by odours but also by visual, acoustic, somatic, or gustatory stimulation' (A. Lavin, *et al.*, 'Centrifugal Arousal in the Olfactory Bulb', *Science*, 129, (1959), pp. 332–3). It is as if the cat's sense of smell were the psychic sense par excellence for evaluating the environment. Because our olfaction is underdeveloped, it may work in an unconscious and instinctive manner; it may arouse interest and give information below the threshold of awareness. The 'spirit' of a place or object might actually be sniffed out and breathed in, just as the early Greeks and Arabic physicians conceived it. (Vision for Homer involved lungs or breath, qualities were breathed in (OET, p. 73); and thus the importance of 'airs', 'waters' and 'places' in the formation of temperament and the treatment of emotion for Hippocrates (*The Medical Works*, ed. by Chadwick and Mann, Oxford, 1950, Chapter: 'Airs, waters, places').)

The epiphany of spirit to the sense of smell, as scent-qualities stimulating intense emotion, connects spirit again to the body, from which throbbing home it has been torn in order that it be enshrined in the cool blue empyrean for transcendental worship by delicate men of Christian intellect and culture. In all this we must remember that

235

regulated intervals, ordinary conversation, hypnotic dreams, suggestion, etc. They state:

> Common to each of these emotions, however produced, is an oximetric change, the direction and extent of which seem to be consequent both upon the intensity of the affective charge and also upon its hedonic quality, for pleasure is euoxaemic and its absence connotes anoxaemia.[1]
>
> The intimate relationship between emotions, awareness, anoxaemia, and E.E.G. activity is well seen in the interdependence of all these variables, since to change one is to produce change in all the others. . . . Our present findings indicate that deliberate induction of anoxaemia by critical choice of suitable stimulation frequencies in any convenient modality of sensation evokes differential changes both in affect and awareness.[2]

A pneumatic view of emotion, just as the views of other chapters, has bearing on modern emotional problems and gives indications for therapy. Perhaps, the emotional state sought for by those who turn to alcoholic spirits is *au fond* a spiritual state access to which is not available otherwise. This is not to pretend that the problem of neurotic *alcoholism* can be dealt with this simply, but it could be profitable to entertain this meaning of drinking spirits. It would imply that the therapy of neurotic alcoholism ought not to consist only of physiological and disciplinary measures, but would have to include an alternative access to that spirit found in drink. If Dionysian *mania* is akin to prophetic, poetic and erotic frenzy, then the craving for ecstasy and inspiration, i.e. for another perspective of conventional reality, for unwilled and irrational behaviour, for the autonomous appearance of images, must be satisfied if the craving for drink is to be healed in depth.

The alteration of emotional conditions through *breathing exercises*, a method so fundamental in the East, would, on this pneumatic view of emotion, take on a privileged position. This, too, goes beyond the physiological and disciplinary measures of correct breathing, but means as well the *qualitative awareness* of the way in which the world is inhaled and exhaled, taken in and given out, introjected and projected. Every mouthful of food, word spoken, item purchased and

the phenomenology of odour is largely unexplored. It is useful for our purposes to note how the ranges of emotional and olfactory behaviour run parallel from the simplest mechanistic reactions of lower animals which we can be said to share through the rhinencephalon to those odours cultivated by aesthetes or exuded by mystics (M. Summers, *The Physical Phenomena of Mysticism*, London; 1950, p. 62) at the highest reaches of human emotion.

[1] Doust, J. W. L., and Schneider, R. A., 'Studies in the Physiology of Awareness: An Oximetrically Monitored Controlled Stress Test', *Canad. J. Psychol.*, 1955, p. 77.

[2] Doust and Schneider, 'Studies in the Physiology of Awareness: The Effect of Rhythmic Sensory Bombardment on Emotions, Blood Oxygen Saturation and the Levels of Consciousness', *J. Ment. Sci.*, 1952, p. 652.

deed performed would be part of the fundamental cure of disordered emotion. This is the refinement of 'breath', of the spirit as the source of emotion. It is a therapy of the whole—body, psyche and world.[1] Thus, too, particular importance must be paid to the cultivation of the sense of smell as in the classic works of the East, where the arts of fragrances, spices and teas are so carefully dwelt over—noble task indeed in a world of deodorants, air-conditioners, tobacco and smog.

Let us call a halt here and draw together some conclusions from these notes. The muddles arising from mixing 'emotion' and 'spirit' could be sorted out in several ways. We might make one dependent upon the other, for example, taking emotion as primary. Then it is the prime stuff out of which spirit emerges and without which spirit is impotent. Or we can say spirit is first and its manifestations in human life are experienced as emotions. Again, we might clear things up by saying the two categories only partly overlap; so that where it might be true 'that the more spirit one has, the greater the passions', it might not be true that the more passion one has, the greater the spirit. Inspiration might be but a special kind of emotion. This raises the question whether all emotion is 'airy', has a spiritual source, or only some. (The hypotheses presented here definitely state all emotion has this essential airy component, whether the air be taken as oxygen (Doust and Schneider) or as 'pneuma' (Duprat).)

More easy is to deny the notion of spirit altogether by reducing it to a certain sort of emotional behaviour: those emotions in which affections of voice, dilated nostrils, alterations of breathing and blood oxygen, hyperventilation, heightened metabolism are paramount.

But if we try to come to grips more earnestly with the statement that emotion is the place of the spirit none of these solutions will do. They will not do because we run the risk of repressing what this view of emotion has to tell us. If we admit that there might be spirit in emotion—in any emotion, even those dark ones of the liver which do not mean spirit in the academic and polite sense of that word— then any rejection of emotion is a refusal of the spirit. As long as we can identify spirit with intellect and reason (the contemporary meaning of the German word *Geist* is a perfect example) and deny spirit a place in emotion, we can carry on with these prejudices that emotion is only flesh and only body. In these prejudices against emotional states, in calling them violators of the real human spirit (e.g. Strasser) we contribute to the drying up of inspiration, prophecy, poetry, spiritual love and spiritual drunkenness. For these things we

---

[1] An excellent discussion of the medical philosophy of 'breath' can be found in O. C. Gruner, *The Canon of Medicine of Avicenna*, London, 1930, pp. 125 ff.

live in a dark age. The explanation for this darkness, on the view here, is the denial of emotion—or rather the affirmation that emotion is 'material', reason 'spiritual', whereas the pairings might be better reversed, since today's conscious mind is only too often the rational instrument of materialism in all sorts of forms while the emotions demonstrate spirit. Thus the spiritual problems of the age are reflected in emotional disturbances.[1] As MacMurray said (p. 222 above):

> Our individual tensions are simply the new thing growing through us into the life of mankind. When we can see them steadily in this universal setting, then and then only will our private difficulties become really significant. We shall recognise them as the travail of a new birth for humanity; as the beginning of a new knowledge of ourselves and of God.

Spirit cannot be willed; it comes in through the back door. It is a gift which bloweth where it listeth, and might very well be found in just the place we are not looking. Therefore, it is particularly to be found in emotion whenever emotion is neglected and repressed. Modern man in search of spirit might turn to his emotions and his psychosomatic symptoms to see what spirit might be distilled from them.

Through a phenomenology of spirit we would surely encounter criteria for distinguishing it from emotion, but for the purposes of a chapter concerned with emotion the distinctions are less relevant than is the exposition of a primal identity. On the views given here, this identity consists mainly in the experience of being moved. This is the 'passivity' of the ego which Kris considers the hallmark of inspiration.[2] We might attempt to account for this 'mover', this *pneuma*, in the light of things already said about emotion in earlier chapters. From the point of view of the phenomenology of the psyche, the ego is passive only to dominants greater than it, in particular to the psyche as a whole. If emotion is a massive, total event setting the whole individual in action (Chapter VIII), then it is to this wholeness that the ego is passive during inspiration. We need not go beyond the human psyche in locating spirit, theologically or metaphysically. Spirit could be conceived as the dynamis of the whole person; the quality and intensity of it depending upon the complexity and differentiation of this wholeness. Thus Bowra writes: 'Inspiration, according to many poets, creates a state in which they see *as a whole* what normally they see only in fragments as parts of a temporal process, and are able to grasp from outside in the *full pattern* of its

---

[1] See report by World Health Organization Study Group on the Mental Health Aspects of the Peaceful Uses of Atomic Energy which emphasizes the 'emotional' aspects of the 'second industrial revolution'. Also, P. Entralgo, *Mind and Body*, London, 1955, p. 144, on the objective spirit of the times as a cause of disorder of emotion.
[2] Kris, E., 'On Inspiration', *Psychoanalytic Explorations in Art*, N.Y., 1952.

movement what normally they know from inside in separate and limited stages of development. It is not surprising that in such circumstances they feel that they have passed into eternity[1].' This experience of transcendence, eternity, power, truth, beauty and light which Bowra says mark inspiration, belong also to those moments which Jung calls experiences of the Self, of psychic totality. We are led to conclude that it is through emotion, the most convenient way to suffer the helplessness of the ego, that the individual can encounter his wholeness and thereby have access to the grace and might of spirit.

[1] Bowra C. M., *Inspiration and Poetry*, London, 1955, p. 10.—Italics mine.

PART III

Integration

'Felix, qui potuit rerum cognoscere causas.'—Vergil.

'Instead of explanatory hypotheses being treated with the *maximum* scepticism when they are *new*, and the *minimum* when they are *old*, a reversal of this policy might be profitable.'—Prof. J. H. Woodger, *Physics, Psychology and Medicine*, Cambridge, 1956, p. 37.

'Damn the torpedoes—full steam ahead!'—Adm. D. Farragut, *Battle of Mobile Bay*.

A. PRELIMINARY

LOOKING BACK on the last chapter we can conclude with the absurd intelligence of *Alice in Wonderland*: 'Everybody has won and all shall have prizes.' Everybody has won because, to quote Cobb[1] again, 'no person with only one point of view can explain the whole phenomenon of emotion'. Or as English and English[2] declare: 'Emotion is virtually impossible to define . . . except in terms of conflicting theories. . . .' The great variety of hypotheses has been necessary to shed light on the phenomenon from many sides. They do not annul or disprove each other. As Wikler says:

> From a monistic standpoint the terms 'psychic', 'organic', 'physiologic', 'biochemical', etc., only denote different frames of reference which may be used to describe the organism in its environment. One is no more fundamental than any other, and phenomena described in one frame of reference do not cause the phenomena described in any other. Conclusions derived from data in one frame of reference cannot be proved or disproved by comparison with data derived in another frame of reference. . . .[3]

In other words we have been dealing, as we said in the Introduction, with a complex phenomenon which requires a complex system of explanation. A demonstration of this by means of the testimony of theories is a main result of the second part. The conclusion that emotion is a complex phenomenon is nothing new, since emotion has been defined as such by writers as diverse as Stout,[4] Ribot,[5] Lehmann,[6] Laignel-Lavastine,[7] Jaspers,[8] Young,[9] Woodworth and Marquis,[10] McKellar[11]—to name but a few. Even such exact attempts

---

[1] ECM, p. 110.

[2] English, H. B., and English, A. C., *A Comprehensive Dictionary of Psychological and Psychoanalytical Terms*, N.Y./London/Toronto, 1958.

[3] Wikler, A., 'A Critical Analysis of Some Current Concepts in Psychiatry', *Psychosom. Med.* 1952, pp. 16–17.

[4] Stout, G. F., *A Manual of Psychology*, 5th edn., London, 1938, p. 369.

[5] Ribot, Th., *The Psychology of the Emotions*, London, 1897, p. 12 (*La Psychologie des sentiments*, 3rd edn., Paris, 1899, p. 12).

[6] Lehmann, A., *Die Hauptgesetze des menschlichen Gefühlslebens*, 2nd edn., Leipzig, 1914, pp. 312, 420.

[7] Laignel-Lavastine, M., *The Concentric Method in the Diagnosis of Psychoneurotics*, London, 1931, p. 15.

[8] Jaspers, K., *Allgemeine Psychopathologie*, 4th edn., Berlin/Heidelberg, 1946, p. 91.

[9] Young, P. T., *Emotion in Man and Animal*, N.Y. and London, 1943, p. 405.

[10] Woodworth and Marquis, *Psychology* (20th edn.) London, 1949, p. 366.

[11] McKellar, P., *A Textbook of Human Psychology*, London, 1952, p. 82.

at the precision of emotion as in the operationalist construct theories presented by Beebe-Center come to the conclusion:

> Feeling and emotion are truly all-pervasive. Almost any dependent variable taken as an index of feeling or emotion will be found to be correlated in some degree with a tremendous number of other dependent variables.[1]

More important, some even view this *complexity as the essential characteristic of emotion*, thereby making it the dominant hypothesis for a theory. For example Landis writes:

> It seems that emotion can best be characterized as a relationship existing between many diverse elements of experience and reaction.[2]

And Lindsley, whose theory we saw in Chapter X A, says:

> Emotion is one of the most complex phenomena known to psychology. It is complex because it involves so much of the organism at so many levels of neural and chemical integration. Both subjectively and objectively its ramifications are diffuse and intermingled with other processes. Perhaps therein lies the uniqueness, and possibly the major significance, of emotion.[3]

Cason writes:

> The theory which we wish to propose is that feelings and emotions are organic patterns of interacting activities which simultaneously involve many different kinds of processes, although the different processes may not be involved to the same degree. In addition to conscious experiences and associated language habits, the affectivities always simultaneously involve processes that are physical, chemical, neurological, endocrinological, visceral, sensory, muscular, conscious, unconscious, etc.; and the causal factors operate in both directions between each activity and practically all of the other activities involved in the total organic pattern. ... and the total interacting pattern is more complicated than is generally assumed. .... The emotion does not depend upon the bodily processes; it is the organic pattern of interacting activities.[4]

In the interacting-pattern theory which has been described above, the causal factors seem to operate in practically all directions between almost all of the different kinds of organic activities involved in the total pattern. The claim that all factors operate in all directions would be nearer the truth than the claim that only one kind of function is, or is the cause or condition of an affectivity.[5]

[1] Beebe-Center, J. G., 'Feeling and Emotion', in *Theoretical Foundations of Psychology*, ed. by H. Helsen, N.Y., 1951, p. 306.
[2] Landis, C., 'Emotion', Chapter XVI in *Psychology* by Boring, Langfeld and Weld, N.Y., 1935, p. 398.
[3] Lindsley, D. B., 'Emotion', in *Handbook of Experimental Psychology*, ed. by S. S. Stevens, N.Y. and London, 1951, p. 473.
[4] Cason, H., 'An Interacting-Pattern Theory of the Affectivities', *Psychol. Rev.*, 1933, pp. 287-8.
[5] *Ibid.*, p. 291.

Where Cason's view that emotion 'is the organic pattern of interacting activities' is a forthright definition of emotion in terms of
its complexity—and thus comes closest to what we are trying to
achieve—it falls short in systematizing this complexity. Complexity
alone does not provide explanation. The variables, processes, levels,
relations, patterns must be combined into a systematic explanation.
Lindsley attempts this in his theory (Chapter X A), but it is in terms
of neuro-chemical levels only. What is missing is a model for grasping
the whole complex, or 'relationship' as Landis calls it.

Reid, who says '. . . the word "emotion" has a very complex,
multidimensional referent . . .',[1] sums up the problem, with which
we are left at the end of Part II, as follows:

> An emotion is not a private mental state, nor a set of static qualities
> abstracted from such a state, nor a hypothalamic response with intense
> autonomic discharge, nor a pattern of behavior viewed in purely objec-
> tive terms, nor a particular stimulus-situation. . . . An emotion is not
> any one of these distinguishable things, nor is it the entire set of them
> viewed as constituting a merely additive whole. . . .
>
> . . . different investigators or theorists or practitioners with special
> vested interests will be disposed to select and emphasize different com-
> ponents in this total referent. An introspectionist psychologist may talk
> mostly of sensations, images, and feelings; a psychoanalyst will stress
> the role of unconscious processes . . . a physiologist . . . will probably
> be trying to locate neural 'centers' . . . behaviorists are inclined to ignore
> on methodological grounds, all of these several kinds of 'intervening
> variables'; whereas, finally specialists in interpersonal dynamics, with
> their field theories, tend to think of emotion as a 'social category.' . . .
>
> Now *some* combination of these points of view is probably what is
> required for an adequate over-all theory of emotion.[2]

The problem before us is just the one Reid presents: a combination
of these points of view. This is the aim of the work as set out in
Part I. In order to achieve, or at least approximate, this integration
we cannot use any of the methods which we refused in Part I, nor
can we use the methods of integration which we refused in the second
part. The method there was essentially reductive, i.e. a systematization
of data according to a single dominant hypothesis. This ultimately
results in one-sidedness. Emotion, in each group of theories, emerged
as a physiological function, as an aspect of a genetic root, as an
energetic phenomenon, as disorder, as conflict, etc. The light brought
by these dominant hypotheses illumined certain aspects of emotion
(hence we called them 'views') but it left in shadow other aspects
equally relevant which were in turn illumined by other models of
theory. In order to encompass the problem from all sides, we cannot

---

[1] Reid, J. R., 'Introduction' to ECM, p. 31.   [2] *Ibid.*, p. 30-1.

use this kind of simplification. Our method, on the other hand, must be complex if it is to succeed. It must combine the points of view without starting from any single one of them, without a 'special vested interest', which is the fundamental mistake in all of the methods used in the last chapter. We can recall Broad on this point:

> ... each of these great men will have seen some important aspect of the subject, and the mistake of each will have been to emphasize this aspect to the exclusion of others which are equally relevant.[1]

But *combination* alone is not enough. As Reid says: 'An emotion is not any one of these distinguishable things, nor is it the entire set of them viewed as constituting a merely additive whole.' The method must do more than combine; it must *integrate*.

Where we find the preceding models inadequate for dealing with the problem of emotion, it does not mean we discard all models. As Gilbert[2] writes: 'Every psychologist, whether he knows it or not, follows a model. He has a simile (a "root metaphor") in mind.' Our model—that of the fourfold root given in Part One—is an assumption like all the other models. It differs from the others in that it is complex, rather than monistic or dualistic, and thus suits the problem. Besides, though complex, this model is economically *elegant*; it is not a mere enumeration of a stunning array of variables. Our argument for the choice of this model as exemplified in the Aristotelian types of causes was also given in Part One.

Here, we must add that our choice does not rest on the authority of Aristotle and his statement that only these four causes exist. Such logical arguments are not enough to demonstrate or convince. Schopenhauer, who also uses the model of the fourfold root in answer to the question 'why', points out the principle, or model of explanation, is an assumption which cannot be proved[3]. Aristotle says:

> These people demand that a reason shall be given for everything; for they seek a starting-point, and they seek to get this by demonstration, ... But their mistake is what we have stated it to be; they seek a reason for things for which no reason can be given; for the starting-point of demonstration is not demonstration.[4]

According to Aristotle, the model of explanation is given and undemonstrable. Schopenhauer agrees, interpreting it in terms of Kant's

[1] Broad, C. D., *Five Types of Ethical Theory*, London, 1930, p. 1.
[2] Gilbert, A. R., 'Recent German Theories of Stratification of Personality', *J. of Psychol.*, 1951, p. 3.
[3] Schopenhauer, A., *Ueber die vierfache Wurzel des Satzes vom zureichenden Grunde* (*On the Fourfold Root of the Principle of Sufficient Reason*, London, 1889). Chapter II, 14.
[4] Aristotle, *Metaphysica*, 1011a (*Collected Works*, ed. by W. D. Ross, Oxford).

categories of the cognitive faculty. Ultimately, they present a *philosophical a priori* as ground of their four principles. We offer another kind of basis to the four causes of Aristotle, suggesting for them a *psychological a priori*.

A system of a fourfold root principle leads both Aristotle and Schopenhauer to abandon demonstration because it yields a sense of satisfaction, of completion, of totality, so that there is the experience of both necessity and sufficiency which is what is demanded of explanation. When Aristotle says that these four causes exhaust the way in which the 'why' can be understood[1] and that he cannot name any others or more fundamental than these,[2] one might be convinced by the philosophy (logic and evidency) of his statement. But one can also be convinced by the psychology of his statement. It is an expression of his satisfaction that these four causes answer the question 'why'—that 'why?' which Schopenhauer calls 'the Mother of all Sciences'.[3] The 'psychological desire'[4] which wonders, which inquires, which seeks for demonstration and raises the question 'why' is fulfilled. The questing mind of the great Aristotle (and of Schopenhauer) is suddenly stilled. The question on this level is answered. Logical or not, rationally demonstrable or not, this is a *psychological* fact of first importance.

This leads one to ask if there is not a psychological ground to these four causes, a fourfold root principle of which Aristotle's causes are one example. Here we can point to parallel phenomena, i.e. a model of a fourfold root has provided some remarkably long lasting, eminently satisfying and perpetually recurring explanations. For example, there are the four humours of Hippocrates—a fundamental and influential system of explaining human nature lasting two millennia. Schopenhauer's fourfold root of the principle of sufficient reason has already been mentioned. There are also the great natural systems of 'explanation' (which strike the mind as so necessary and sufficient, so evident, that they are never questioned): the four directions, phases of the moon, elements, seasons. Whenever a fourfold root is used to circumscribe phenomena it seems to be self-evident and to include its own demonstration. Or, to push the point further, this model is used to account for the undemonstrable.

The ultimate undemonstrable as *causa sui* is, of course, the province of theology and it is just here that we meet again with this model, e.g. the holy *tetraktys* of the Pythagoreans (EGP), the fourfold

---

[1] Aristotle, *Physica* II, 198a.
[2] Aristotle, *Metaphysica*, 993a.
[3] *Op. cit.*, Chapter I, 4.
[4] See Part I, p. 16, for discussion of Reichenbach's statement: 'The satisfaction of psychological desires, however, is not explanation.'

theological ontology of Eriugena,[1] the 'quattuor coaequaevae' of Augustine's theology, the fourfold religious mandalas, the four-legged mythological beast on which the world rests, and the four letters used ubiquitously for the name of God.[2]

In other words, the four causes of Aristotle provide explanation as the minimum requirements for total comprehension, because they are a form of the symbol of the fourfold root. This is a symbol of completion and fulfilment, the undemonstrable ground of being itself. As such it is what Jung[3] calls a symbol of the Self. It represents a psyche which no longer asks 'why'. The question, as for Aristotle, is answered—or rather, has disappeared.

In addition to making clear our model, we must also make clear our method for this chapter. The empirical method: collection of theories, classification, analysis and critical exposition is behind us. Also behind us is the amplification of the phenomenon, emotion, through all the statements made about it. This means that we can be spared going through the theories again in detail. The method we have used up to now no longer serves, because we do not need to derive categories empirically out of the material at hand. We already have our categories of organization given by the model. Therefore, we need only apply our model directly to the material and organize it accordingly.

It might look finer and neater if the four general categories appeared to emerge out of the twenty random categories which in turn emerged out of the material itself. But, as pointed out in the Introduction, the categories of Part II have nothing to do with the problem of integration. They are in no way connected to the system based upon the fourfold root metaphor. To try to fit them in would falsify what has been our intention all along: to make it very clear that data are always organized according to certain fundamental models. Since we accept the necessity of a model, we do not need to camouflage it behind a pseudo-empiricism. We do not need to force one set of categories into the other. Our categories, to say it again, are not extracted from the theories themselves; they are taken over from our model. But they are taken over consciously from antiquity in the light of modern depth psychology, and so they are not modern substitutes or disguises for some half-conscious and ancient model of

[1] Eriugena (Johannes Scotus), *De divisione naturae.* See W. Pauli's short discussion in C. G. Jung and W. Pauli, *The Interpretation of Nature and the Psyche*, Appendix III, London, 1955 (*Naturerklärung und Psyche*, Zürich, 1952, pp. 192–4).

[2] Allendy, R., *Le Symbolisme des nombres*, Paris, 1948, p. 92.

[3] Jung's researches into this symbolism have influenced us greatly here and a more careful exposition and amplification of this model can be found in his works, *Psychologie und Alchemie* (1944), *Symbolik des Geistes* (1948), *Gestaltungen des Unbewussten* (1950), *Aion* (1951), *Von den Wurzeln des Bewusstseins* (1954), Zürich. (Engl. transl., see *Collected Works*, Vols. IX, XI, XII, XIII.)

thinking such as we encountered in many of the other systems of operations in Part II.

With the end of differentiation and analysis of the material comes also an end to the detailed way of discussion. The integration in this chapter will be attempted in as broad and general strokes as possible. But this integration—in the form of a structural outline—does not stand altogether on its own, since it presupposes having gone through the experience of the previous chapter. Without that confrontation with the pandemonium of theory, the freely presented, generalized and *a priori* approach would seem high-handed. It would be hard to see the inter-relation of the material and the categories; whereas after going through all the hypotheses it becomes clear how well-suited our method is to the material. The reader who skips the bulk of the book in order to get to the conclusion will have missed far more than he gains.

The limitation of the method to the broad and general does not limit the scope. It remains the same as in Part II. We shall expect the general theory to cover the whole ground covered by all the different theories in the preceding chapter.

B. THE CONCEPT OF '*CAUSE*'

Any dictionary, encyclopedia or philosophical handbook reviews this concept. From its supposed first appearance in a statement by Leukippos, through its great differentiation in the logic books of the seventeenth century where at least forty different kinds of causes could be listed,[1] to the present scientific scepticism which avoids the term (and with it avoids explanations), the concept has gone through much amplification. Even the particular Aristotelian use has been expanded by commentators, especially Arabic and Scholastic. The history of the concept 'cause' coincides with a good tract of the history of Western thought. Fortunately, this problem is not our problem, because we use the term as given by Aristotle (Part I, p. 19 f. above). 'Cause' gives the answer to the question 'why'. It provides explanation. This, the broadest use of the term, is analogous to *aitia*, *ratio*, *Grund*, or 'reason'. It is generic and goes beyond the specific problems of causality as cause-and-effect. These problems do not belong to the concept 'cause' as such, but to one of its specifications, the *causa efficiens*. (The position we take up is clearly opposite to that of Ryle, who, in his chapter on emotion,[2] definitely limits the concept of 'cause' to *causa efficiens*, as part of his argument for getting rid of emotions as states of mind.) The efficient cause is only one of

[1] Wolf, A., *Spinoza's Short Treatise*, London, 1910, pp. 190–5.
[2] Ryle, G., *The Concept of Mind*, London, 1949, pp. 86–8; 113–14.

the four basic answers to the question 'why'. It is but one mode of explaining an event. Let us begin with this notion.

C. *CAUSA EFFICIENS*

We shall not be led away from Aristotle's clear presentation of the efficient cause ('What initiated a motion') by any of these variations and reductions: (1) Reduction of it to the formal cause in the manner of Platonists, so that the form or pattern of an emotion is said to be the power, force or agency that sets the emotion going. (2) Reduction of it to the final cause in the manner of Leibniz, which would mean that the final outcome or purpose of an emotion initiates the emotion. (3) Reduction of it to the material cause in the manner of Marxists, which would endow the material stuff of emotion with the power of self-activation. (4) Nor do we accept that the efficient cause is really extrinsic or secondary (Occasionalism), a mere instrument in some hidden plan of a prime mover, because the problem of efficient causality, or 'what initiated a motion', remains. (5) Neither do we admit the scepticism of Hume who finds that efficient causality cannot be demonstrated. We have already dealt with the issue of demonstration above. Because Hume's position led to the corollary position (Kant) that causality must—because it is undemonstrable—be an *a priori* category of the mind, modern science finds the concept too subjective, too anthropomorphic. It prefers to state the problems of cause-and-effect in terms of laws or functions, or what are called 'if-then' statements. Whether or not efficient causality is demonstrable, whether or not it is restated in conditional language or in the form of probability curves, it remains one fundamental answer to the question 'why'.

Further, (6) we cannot admit the classical limitation of efficient cause to the cause-and-effect relation only. Traditionally, the efficient cause must exist prior in time (succession) to that of which it is said to be the cause. Now, priority in time cannot be established for certain classes of events which bear on emotion—the realm of depth psychology and the realm of physics. Traditionally, the efficient cause must exist distinct in space (contiguity) to that of which it is said to be the cause. But as we said in the Introduction, all four causes are to be taken as aspects of an event, not as a bundle of discrete phenomena. The causes are merely ways of dividing up a complex for comprehension. The efficient cause is not separate, neither in time nor in space, from the event of which it is an aspect. We do not take cause-and-effect as two distinct events, but as related aspects of the same event. This qualification is important. Without it, that is if we stick within the traditional cause-and-effect limitations of efficient cause, we are led to a mechanical and isolated view of the human person. In theory of emotion, the human person becomes an effect, a *patiens* stimulated by an *agens*. Man would be cut off from his environment because the efficient cause is spatially outside of and distinct from man. Man would be overwhelmingly dependent upon his past through a chain of succession because the efficient cause ('what initiated a motion') lies in the past temporally distinct from the present event. Where this mechanical view of man may be justified in the realm of certain abstracted physiological systems, it is not so for the whole person. We must keep particularly in mind our refusal of this sixth or last limitation of the efficient cause, because most discussions of the stimuli of emotion still retain this mechanistic view of man, dividing into discrete events subject and object, cause-and-effect, action and reaction.

Starting, then, from Aristotle's 'What initiated a motion', or to use the language of today, 'what was the stimulus', let us draw together to form one type of theory and one aspect of our theory those hypotheses which answer the question 'why' in terms of stimuli. This aspect comes to the fore particularly in Chapter XI (situation), Chapter XII (subject-object relation), Chapter XIV (representations) and Chapter XVI (conflict). In general, the idea that these theories express is: Emotion can best be explained by hypotheses about the stimulus. These hypotheses can be classified as follows:

I. The efficient cause can be described psychologically, as:

   A. Representations arouse emotion (Chapter XIV):
      1. Either conscious representations (ideas, sensations, perceptions, images).
      2. Or unconscious representations.
      3. Or a combination of both, i.e. symbols.
   B. Conflicts arouse emotion (Chapter XVI):
      1. Conflicts between physiological systems, e.g. cerebral, motoric, damming of sexual discharge, etc.
      2. Conflicts between psychological systems. These can be further divided into:
         a. conflicts conceived dualistically (ego *vs.* non-ego or primary system *vs.* secondary system). Between the two systems there is a threshold, repression, a structural barrier, etc.,
         b. conflicts conceived pluralistically, between various levels, drives, motives, needs, tendencies, instincts, traits, etc.
      3. Conflicts between the individual and his environment. These are described as frustrations, perceptual conflicts, motor delays, timing disorders, etc.

251

C. Situations arouse emotion (Chapter XI) and these situations can be described in terms of:
1. The meaning of the momentary objective psychic constellation of which emotion is a reflection.
2. The presence of emotion in the present situation as:
    a. in a work of art (Chapter XVIII),
    b. in one's own or another's gestures, speech, expression (Chapter XV),
    c. in emotional qualities objectively given by the environment.
3. Social, economic and/or historical factors in the situation, which arouse emotion because of learning or conditioning.
4. Quantities, intensities, or some measurable property of the situation, produces emotional response (Chapter XII).

II. The efficient cause can also be described physiologically on the level of:
A. Specific processes of arousal:
1. In the brain (Chapter X A).
    a. due to self-activation of the cortex, or as perceptions taken as physical stimuli,
    b. due to removal or cessation of cortical inhibition,
    c. due to activation of the diencephalon.
2. In the blood, glands and gut and their connections to the autonomic nervous system (Chapter X B).
3. In the postural set of the muscles, tendons and joints (Chapter X C).
B. Instinctual 'forces' or activities which initiate emotion as an accompaniment (Chapter III, in particular).
C. Constitution or genetic endowment, when conceived physiologically as unconditioned affective response, startle, stress, sexuality, etc.
D. Physical energy as electrical, chemical or nervous energy, certain amounts of which or certain (downward) directions of which start emotion (Chapter VI and VII).

III. Emotion is also said to exist without an efficient cause:
A. Emotion is a genuinely spontaneous event without a stimulus.
B. Emotion has no stimulus because it is never 'initiated'. It is going on all the time. This continuous activity can be described as:
1. Isomorphic with other events (Chapter IV).
2. A dynamic background of a physiological kind (Chapter X B).
3. A qualitative accompaniment of the innermost regions of the person (Chapter IX).

4. A repercussion or rebound of values and qualities in the situation (Chapter XI and XV).

C. Emotion only appears to be spontaneous, but it is actually initiated by:

   1. The spirit (Chapter XIX).
   2. The unconscious (Chapter V).
      a. we are unconscious of the stimuli,
      b. or the stimuli lie in a region outside of awareness called the unconscious.
   3. Genetic endowment, which releases emotions when built-in processes come into action within a specific time-cycle of maturation (Chapter XIII).
   4. Events which properly belong under formal, material or final causes.

In keeping with all that has gone before in Part II concerning the analysis of these hypotheses, let us now paraphrase this outline developing a unified hypothesis about the efficient cause of emotion. We shall make this integration in terms of *the symbol as efficient cause*, conceiving the symbol in the specific way of Chapter XIV. We saw in Chapters XI, XII and XIV that it is not the outer object or situation as such which gives rise to emotion, but the representation of the object or situation. We saw too that these representations were not in themselves enough to evoke emotion: first, because emotion could arise independent of conscious representations and, second, for representations to be effective in arousing emotion, they must be connected to an instinctual image. It was this concatenation of inner and outer, of conscious and unconscious representation, which we called a symbol.

This means that *situations* arouse emotion when they are apprehended symbolically. All the various situation hypotheses—the forms of art, the patterns of gesture and expression, the environmental qualities (in landscape or restaurant), the 'Gestalten' and meanings—only arouse emotion in so far as they are symbolic. Further, this means that the objective psychic situation, said to be (Chapter XI) the realm of which emotion is a subjective repercussion, is constituted of symbols. These reveal themselves through emotion as was said in Chapter XV. Emotion is thus the symbolic apprehension of the objective psyche and emotional behaviour is adapted to this exceptional world (Chapter XV). To put it another way round, the field of symbols external to the subject is emotional. The symbol is not something 'outside' which arouses emotion 'inside'. Outside in the world, emotions are apprehended as symbolic qualities; inside in the person, symbols are lived out in emotions. As we saw in

Chapter IX, the realm of emotion cannot be limited to the 'within'. In Chapter XI we saw that the objective psyche is both 'within' and 'without'. For situations to be symbolic they must be apprehended by or evoke not only the primary system of ego-consciousness, but also the secondary system variously called magical, unconscious, instinct, unconditioned genetic endowment, biological memory, etc. Again, however, there is the paradox that the secondary system is not only 'innermost', but is in immediate rapport with the 'outside'. It is experienced as innermost because it is experienced as value, as importance. It is urgent that the concept of emotions as located only in the inmost and subjective realm be abandoned. *Emotional behaviour corresponds with the symbolic aspect of objective reality.*

It is just this symbolic apprehension of reality that gives rise to *conflict*. Conflict, as we said in Chapter XVI, is not primary or necessary to emotion. It can be the result of emotion. The various conflicts between structures, systems, tendencies, etc., are due to the activation of both systems, of the whole person, by the symbol. The conflict which ensues is due to the appearance of emotion on the scene. Normal reality (the conscious sign aspect of reality) and symbolic reality are experienced at the same instant. At one and the same moment there is the habitual way of behaving and apprehending and an emotional one. Because usually the habitual behaviour is too rigid to admit a second aspect, there is conflict and disorder. We are in conflict with the environment because society generally refuses the symbol, favouring the conventional habitus. We are in conflict with ourselves because the emotion is resisted. If, however, the emotion is experienced—not necessarily lived out concretely but witnessed attentively—there is no conflict. Rather than a conflict between levels because of insistence upon a partial, habitual attitude, there is a unified participation of all levels. This is a moment of truth, a moment of transcendence in which inner and outer, conscious and unconscious, are linked by the symbol and lived as conscious emotion. This kind of experience is known not only to mystics and artists, but to every child, and to every adult too, who has once allowed himself emotion. The achievement of it in therapy is described in terms of symbolic realization (Chapter XIV), in terms of emotional reason (Chapter XV), and in terms of living imagination and emotion in daily life (Chapter XVIII). The simplest example of such liberating moments where the symbolic and conventional are joined is humour and laughter. Other examples with the same type of effect are fairy tales, parables and the riddles of spiritual masters.

In another sense, conflict can give rise to emotion because any conflict as a clash of incompatibilities can become symbolized as a pair of contending opposites, the archetypal image of duality. But

254

again it is not the conflict situation as such, but the conflict as symbol, which produces the emotion.

The hypotheses concerning *genetic endowment* and those concerning *conditioning* can also be harmonized with the thesis that the symbol is the efficient cause. Emotion depends on learning in so far as its arousal is always within a concrete context—even if not always by a concrete image. The context is social, historical and economic. It is a learned context; and in this sense, emotion is learned behaviour because one aspect of the symbol which arouses emotion has been learned. This aspect (which we have called in Chapter XIV the conscious representations) is subject to conditioning and is in fact a product of learning. Therefore, emotions can be manipulated by the control of conscious representations. This is well-known to be the case wherever man has lost connection to the life of instinctual nature. Then his emotions fall prey to the conditioning of the professional manipulators of jargon and image.

However, the other aspect of the symbol—i.e. instinctual behaviour pattern and its image, or whatever one chooses to call the unconscious, non-represented meaning which makes the conscious representation 'click' and live—is part of genetic endowment. Given with constitution, it is archetypal, perpetually repeating with only slight variations the same theme. Fortunately it is iconoclastic, breaking shabby products of conditioning, attempting to view the world *sub specie aeternitatis*. It is what the writers in Chapter XIII call the unconditioned basis of the affective response. It is this second aspect of the symbol that gives learning its limits and is the ground of its possibilities. In fact, it conditions conditioning.

It has not been established that specific images are constitutionally given. What is given is the capacity to behave and to apprehend representations symbolically. Like instinct and traits and our physical constitution, this capacity is not given all at once at birth. From one point of view it comes to natural fruition through maturing; from another, the capacity changes in qualitative leaps as gifts of the spirit. As the capacity grows and decays, the symbolic representations evoking emotion change. They are part of the unfolding motion of alteration, growth and decay, as discussed at the end of Chapter XII. There are emotions appropriate to what tradition calls the stages of life, in so far as there are different symbols effective at different moments in life. What we laughed at once is no longer funny; while symbols not yet ripe evoke no emotion. The child knows little of pity, of mercy, or of a father's holy rage. Therapeutically this means, as we said in Chapter XIV, that the education of emotions is changing their symbolic fixations. Not hate, nor desire, nor fear are to be changed, but the inappropriate symbols (of Mother or Father, say) which evoke these emotions. They are inappropriate because they are personal and on the level of conscious representations, while the emotion actually is initiated by the symbol of 'Mother' or 'Father', that combination of personal and objective psychic levels. Also, as said in Chapter XIV, alteration of the symbols alters the emotion. This is so because each of the causes, in this case the symbol as efficient cause, is the emotion itself in one aspect.

The efficient cause as symbol depends thus both on learning and on the genetic endowment as a built-in symbolic capacity (or as spiritual gifts) come into action within a limited time-cycle. The capacity can be taken as an accompaniment of instinct, as one set of hypotheses holds. But it can also be independent of instinct. A broader formulation would be that the capacity to apprehend and behave symbolically accompanies (is an aspect of) all traits whether narrowly instinctual or not. As such, emotion can be admitted to accompany any action or idea, providing the action or idea is experienced symbolically, through having been given an unconscious meaning. It is of value for therapy to note the specificity of the time-cycle. Failure to live in accordance with the growth and change of symbols in the stages of life (not at all rigidly the same in each individual) yields distorted emotion. Poverty of emotion is also due to the failure to recognize the pattern of genetic unfolding. Symbols of archetypal stages, say—puberty, young adulthood, the middle of life, the approach of death—become neglected, lapsing into the burden of unlived life.

From what has just gone before, little need be said about how the hypotheses concerning the *spiritual*, *spontaneous* and *unconscious* origin of emotion fit in. The symbol as efficient cause is credited with spirit because it appears irrational, autonomous (unconditioned) and creative. These were three attributes of spirit mentioned in Chapter XIX. The spontaneity of emotion is therefore only relative. Emotion is spontaneous viewed from the primary system of the conventional habitus with its world of conscious representations, because its arousal can be independent of this system. It depends rather upon the unconditioned level which symbolizes the representations of the primary system. This level is not spontaneous (wild) in that it does have patterns of organization, regularities of repetition, definite meanings, and probabilities, as for example shown by clinical predictions (or also by the formal similarities of emotional behaviour patterns and emotional images the world over, which both the study of emotional expression and the study of universal religious and art symbols shows). As said in Chapter XI, it can be ordered according to the fields of Gestalt psychology, the essential meanings of existential phenomenology, or typical forms of Jung's analytical psychology.

Furthermore, true spontaneity would demand 'uncaused' emotion, while an examination of each emotion will always reveal a definite symbol as its efficient cause. In so far as this unconditioned aspect of the symbol is not presented to consciousness, the origin of emotion can be said to be unconscious, indicate unconsciousness, or lie in the unconscious depending upon how we use the concept.[1]

We are left then with the problem of integrating that group of hypotheses which describe the efficient cause *physiologically*. Here we must beware of merging two orders of events. We prefer to keep clear the distinctions between *physis* and *psyche*, though they may well be to a large extent isomorphic (Chapter IX) or pass into each other at a vanishing point along the same continuum (Chapter XIV). Therefore, we shall not try to locate or represent the capacity for apprehending and behaving symbolically in the diencephalon, cortex, or any partial system. In so far as the symbol is a coordinated achievement of all levels, parts or systems, its corresponding physiological representation would be the whole body. This is not to deny that partial physiological systems can initiate emotion. Drugs, quanta of electricity, intensities of sound and light, etc., can and do evoke affects. The question is whether or not these affects are complete, or only emotions on the physiological level. According to the statement we quoted from Wikler (p. 243 above), events in one system of operations do not cause events in another. In our view, emotions produced by drugs, shocks and excessive physical stimuli can only be considered complete (not 'sham' or 'cold') emotion when the physical events are apprehended symbolically by the psyche, that is, when physical events are represented by a symbolized image and receive a meaning beyond that of a conscious sign. It is not known what in fact goes on when physical methods are used in altering emotional conditions, but it is our hypothesis that their effectiveness depends upon their being apprehended symbolically. Otherwise, according to our view, the events are merely affects on the physiological level, that is, instinct or drive processes due to endocrine and/or thalamic-autonomic events. On this level it is only fortuitous whether they have a therapeutic effect, because the symbolic meaning might or might not appear. Physical therapy of emotion has another effect when combined with psychotherapy. This, we can hypothesize, is not only—as is usually thought—because one must approach the human person from 'two sides', physical and psychological, but because physical therapy might only be effective in altering the whole emotional state when it is at the same time apprehended in terms of a

[1] Detailing the relation of these concepts—unconscious, spirit, objective psyche—goes beyond the scope of this work. In respect to emotion, they are terms standing for orders of events which in places coincide, while in other contexts they represent valid distinctions. The similarity and distinctness of these notions in respect to emotion can be noted in Chapters V (unconscious), XIX (spirit) and XI (situation).

meaningful symbol. In respect to emotion therapy, the physical side would depend upon the psychological side which would have for its goal the elaboration of these physical events into symbols. An attempt would be made to relate the physical event (drug or shock, say) to the patient's own actual symbols of his healing process (a healing herb of life, or food from the mother, or shocks of initiation, say). To put it simply: the pill works when it has a symbolic meaning for the patient.

Emotion evoked by *intensities* or *quantities*, whether in the physiological or psychological sector, is due to the breaking down of the primary system of the conventional habitus. There is an 'abaissement du niveau' which allows the levels of symbolic functioning to come to the fore, interpreting these intensities symbolically. Moreover, symbols are intensities; they are felt subjectively as such, and they mobilize quantities of energy not usually at the disposal of the conventional habitus. Under the influence of a symbol (during emotional behaviour), there is an alteration of intensity in both psychological and physical spheres. This holds true also for the asthenic emotions (depression and boredom) which appear to be the very contrary of intensity. Depression is a severe intensity, but of a negative sort; while boredom is caused by the accumulation of energy in new symbols, the old ones having lost their intensity. Again, for therapy, it is a question of turning to the symbol which is the image of the boredom or depression.

Let us conclude the first answer to the question: *why is there emotion? There is emotion because the world is being apprehended and lived through a symbol.* This is the radical shift in perception and behaviour spoken of by psychologists. The symbol is the efficient cause of emotion; it is its stimulus. Where there is emotion there is a symbol. Or, as the cause is an aspect of the event itself, *the symbol is thus the emotion itself in the aspect of an exciting image.*

D. *CAUSA MATERIALIS*

The hypotheses of efficient causality were statements answering the question 'why' taken to mean, 'What is the stimulus-cause of emotion?' Hypotheses of material causality are statements answering the 'why' in another sense: 'What is the nature, the stuff of emotion?' The material cause, by dictionary definition (OED) is 'that of which something consists or out of which it is developed'. In order to group the hypotheses of this class of cause we must first get at the various criteria of matter that have been offered through the ages. A foremost distinction must be made at the outset: the concept of matter, like that of the material cause, is *relative*. It is not an absolute, either as a meaningless fiction of unreality as the idealists would have it, or as the one and only principle of reality as the materialists maintain. We avoid both extremes by following the central line of tradition begun with Aristotle, using the concept of matter as co-ordinate with the concept of form and the material cause as relative to the other causes.

In spite of the contributions to the notion of matter given from every side, there are six essential groups of criteria. They are all inter-related and we divide them into these groups for the sake of more easily grasping this complex idea. Let us review them, discovering at the same time the explanations of emotion *via* the material cause governed by these fundamental ideas of matter.

(1) Matter is an *abstract principle*. As the universal substrate of all things it exists only in abstraction; in and for itself it is unknowable. It is therefore invisible and incorporeal (Eriugena). The universal abstract substrate, *materia prima*, is unknowable; *materia secunda* is knowable as formed things come into being. As substrate of all existents, it is the potential of all existents. It is of course without quality, but can be apprehended quantitatively. (This accords with one meaning of its supposed root, *matrum* (Sanskrit)—measure.) This is the notion of matter derived from Aristotle and the Scholastics. This notion gives the view that emotion is energy, that invisible, universal substrate of all things, such as we saw in Chapter VI. Further, this idea of matter supports the quantitative approach of Chapter VII.

(2) Matter is *chaos*. It is the mother of all things, the feminine principle; so, it is the passive and suffering principle. Without qualities, without forms, it is even without being. In this sense it is the deprivation or absence of being. It is impure, dark, evil and dead. This view derives from Plato, Philo and Plotinus. When emotion is approached through the material cause, and matter is given these meanings, emotion is found to be a feminine weakness, unconsciousness, yet also the source and mother of everything new. This view of matter also gives the ground to the views of emotion found mainly in Chapter XVII: emotion is a formless blur, a chaotic disorder, the dark price paid for the light of reason, where the person is deprived of all human worth. We also find here the views of Chapter XIII, which reduced emotion to this notion of matter, as primordial non-being, a negative, evil (and sexual, as the darkly feminine) first principle.

(3) Matter is *res extensa*. Body and matter are the same thing, for matter is an extended, physical substance. It is visible. It is distinct from the invisible mind and external to it. Matter is solid and impenetrable, but infinitely divisible into infinite parts or atoms. When emotion is taken from this notion of the material cause, we have the

259

hypotheses which explain emotion through the body. The physiological processes external to the mind said to explain it are represented in space as visible areas, zones, centres and organs. This view supports the conclusions that emotion cannot be completely accounted for nor accurately located since *res extensa* is infinitely divisible.

(4) Matter is *building stuff*. It is *hyle*, wood, timber. (This accords with one meaning of another supposed root, **dmā*, **dom*, **dem* = the timber of a house (*domus*).) Interpreted by Kant, matter as building stuff is the sense content of consciousness. The material cause with this notion of matter dominant yields the hypotheses of Chapter XIV: emotion consists of representations (sensations, ideas, images, perceptions). These are the building stuff, the contents of emotion.

(5) Matter is *inertia*. As the passive principle deprived of active form, it can be imaged as an inert solid resisting change. 'Mass . . . is the essential characteristic of matter . . . what we think of first in connection with mass is the inertia with which a body resists being set in motion by forces.' (Schrödinger[1]). Thus we only know matter as inertia is overcome, is changed, and work is done. This notion of the material cause comes to the fore in the hypotheses which explain emotion as a conflict: the conventional habitus resisting change. Emotion is then manifest in muscular tensions (Chapter X C). Emotion is known only at the moment when there is this overcoming of resistance, at the moment when the ego is in process of alteration.

(6) Matter is *a field of force*. The solid, impenetrable *res extensa* is in fact a field of particles, waves, quanta of motion. These are invisible, but objectively valid constructs known through behaviour. Here we have the view that the material stuff of emotion is the play of invisible forces. These forces can be 'within' as physiological constructs (hormones, nerve cells, centres) or as psychological constructs (complexes, instincts, traits). Or they can be 'without' as constellations of the objective psyche. Emotion is ultimately reducible to nuclear dynamic units.

Apparently we are given at least six different hypotheses about the material of emotion. But an integrated answer can be given to the question of the *material cause* if we take it as *energy*. This energy is, first of all, an abstract principle said to be unknowable in itself, but which is posited as the universal substrate of all existents. In this sense energy is not a 'real thing' and emotion consisting of energy is also not 'real', as was said in Chapter I. It can be reduced to quantitative formulae of direction and intensity like other descriptions of

---

[1] Schrödinger, E., 'The Spirit of Science', in *Spirit and Nature*, Papers from the Eranos Yearbooks, N.Y. and London, 1954, p. 332. ('Der Geist der Naturwissenschaft', *Eranos Jahrbuch*, 1946, Zürich, p. 507.)

energy. Quantitative approaches are, in fact, the inevitable way of describing emotion and the inevitable method of therapy as long as emotion is explained only through the material cause. This we saw in Chapters VI and VII.

Also in Chapter VI it was said that emotion is the conscious or psychic form of universal energy. When this *materia prima* is experienced from within it is both the matrix and source of all creativity (Chapter XVIII) but also it is a chaos, a disorder and a blur (Chapter XVII). Emotion is the way energy appears to consciousness, but in and for itself it is said to be ungraspable. However, we can hypothesize on this view, that those two basic descriptions of energy —negative and positive—correspond to *the two fundamental emotions*: anxiety and love (Chapter XIII). Anxiety is the negative experience from within of prime energy, without content, without quality, without personal form. Love, also said to be the fundamental emotion, is the experience of the same energy, without form, without qualification or personal content of any kind, but now in the positive aspect.[1]

But energy is rarely so perceived, since such experiences require the end of all forms and the union of the individual with the prime substrate, for better or for worse, in love or in dread. Usually energy is perceived as *materia secunda*, that is, as it is formed, or 'comes into being' to use Aristotle's language (or as 'work is done' in modern language). Here we have the different general specifications of energy —nervous, thermal, chemical, psychic, etc.—mentioned in Chapter VI. Just as chemical energy or nervous energy is known through certain specific chemical and nervous processes, so emotional energy is known through specific emotional processes. These are the specific gross demonstrations of the body and the specific representations in consciousness; without these palpable contents, there is no emotion. From the point of view of material causality alone these *demonstrations and representations* (Chapters II, X B and XIV) *are the emotion*. The James-Lange theory would have to be extended: if from one sad, the tears and sobs, *and also* the depressed thoughts, feelings and images are removed, where is the emotion? The demonstrations alone are not the emotion; the demonstrations and representations together are the stuff and material of emotion; without which emotion can be said to exist only in the abstract, *in potentia*, as *materia prima*.

Concrete and visible emotional energy (*materia secunda*) is the *res extensa* of the human body. But this *res extensa* is not just limited to the enclosure of our skins; rather the human body is a situation,

---

[1] Pleasure and pain are not primary *emotions*, but *sensations* (see Bousfield, Chapter VI). As such, pain and pleasure might be the corresponding experiences of positive and negative energy within the realm of sensation.

an interacting field of energy. This energy is polarized or located in discrete nuclei. These are posited as complexes, motives, needs, drives, traits; as genes; as organs, zones, hormones, nerve centres. They are never completely accounted for nor accurately located because they are ultimately only explicable (from the material point of view) in terms of abstract energetic nuclei known through spatial behaviour, whether the search for them is carried on through physiological dissection (general organ, tissue, cell, nuclear electro-chemical charge) or psychological analysis (general attitude, complex, factor, nuclear drive). Different levels of description provide different terms. These terms however do not refer to the same thing in different aspects (isomorphism), which would mean identifying complexes with organs, drives with hormones, or using 'vital energy' as a psychophysical alloy. Complexes and organs (in the sense of Freud's erogenous zones), drives and hormones (Chapter X B), brain waves and emotions (Chapter VII) may be to a certain extent isomorphic, but all correlations are not identities. There is no one-to-one correlation between these different systems of operations. The important thing here is to see that the idea in all the systems of description is the same: emotion is based upon dynamic nuclei of energy. They can be self-activating or reflexive, conditioned or not, continuously active or working in bursts as quanta, inhibited or released or constellated, etc. But always explanations through the material cause depend upon hypotheses of a network of energetic units, i.e. matter as a field of force. The many specific descriptions can only be integrated by a high-level hypothesis, such as the general concept of energy taken as the relatively closed (non-intradermal) field of the human body situation, polarized in interacting nuclei.

Just as invisible, abstract nuclei of energy are known as chemical energy through behaviour of substances and processes in the chemical field of matter, so the same quanta are known as emotional energy through behaviour in the human field of matter, the body. The field of the body is the stuff of emotion, and so emotion is an aspect of the field of the body. This means *emotion is the body*, concrete and visible, here and now. The body-situation is the locus of emotion; it is the *res extensa*, the spatial demonstration of emotion. (Thus we come to the idea expressed so often: the more body in an event the more the emotion.) Its internal processes and organic substances are emotional and its interaction with the environment is emotional. Everything the body is and does is emotional, in so far as the body is the material cause of emotion. This means that all life, physiological and social, is emotional—or as was said in Chapter IX, where emotion is there is life. This accounts for the facts of the clinic. Disturbances called psychosomatic or interpersonal are often due to the failure of the patient to take into account the emotional aspect of his physiological and social life. He neglects the emotional aspect of his body and that the energetic processes which occur in this field are primarily emotional, only secondarily chemical or electrical. For example, he neglects that his feeding and sleeping habits, his sexual and his digestive and excretory functions are emotional—not just physiological mechanisms—all of which is part of the great contribution of the Freudian school towards understanding these events. Thus, preoccupation with emotions is the *via regia* to get at these disturbed processes; it is the immediate way that consciousness can know from within the body as a field of energy (Chapter VI).

The energy of this field is ordered. Again the description of this order can be made in many ways, from chemical enzymes to animal spirits. But again, on the level of an integrated and general hypothesis, the order of this *energy is the homeostatic balance of the whole person in his situation.* And it is just this homeostasis which is the material cause in the sense of the fifth meaning of matter above—that which is acted upon and altered. The field of the body persists in a homeostatic convention. It is ordered into specific attitudes, organic and postural sets, and it is lived as the first system in daily life. This is the inert 'mass' carried by its own momentum, resisting change. This inertia is the stuff of emotion; emotion as potential energy. It is due to this resistance that emotion can be disorder, an 'Umschichtung' of the field releasing potential energy. This potential as it is converted takes the forms of, say, tears and sobs, depressed thoughts and feelings, when the set is altered. As the clinician knows, the more set this matter, the more dynamic the emotion. The greater the mass, the greater the force to set it in motion. But since mass and energy are convertible ($m = e$), the more massively rigid and solid the person in his situation, the more the potential energy.[1] This means that there are not two separate energy systems, first and second, but from the energetic point of view the second system is the potential energy of the first system. It becomes actualized as kinetic energy, emotional behaviour, when the conventional set of the system is altered by a symbol.

Always we must keep clear the distinction between abstract prime energy with its descriptions of abstract invisibles (quanta, nuclei, genes, archetypes, traits, etc.) and energy as *materia secunda*, i.e. the concrete organization of energy in chemical, neural, emotional, etc., forms, the human body situation being the concrete organization of

---

[1] The conversion of this potential energy can occur in many forms, each of which is a kind of emotion. The two main categories, classically, are sthenic and asthenic, that is, the potential energy can 'explode' outwards or dissipate inwards in the emotions we call exhaustion, misery and despair.

emotional energy. In the first instance, emotion as the psychological aspect of the universal substrate can be said to be going on all the time, just as energy is always 'going on'. This continuous activity is wider than its specific forms within the personal sphere of gross demonstrations and conscious representations. It is wider even than the human body situation. The activity can be going on 'without', going on 'in the field'. as the theories of Chapter XI held. *Because emotion is the psychological aspect of general energy, emotion is 'going on' all the time everywhere.* It is a potential aspect of all things. This high-level hypothesis can be useful in thinking about the role of emotion in parapsychology (Chapter V).[1] It can be useful to the hypotheses of the kinds we saw in Chapters XI and XV where emotion was related to the objective psyche or to an affective continuum as the realm of the spirit. The ontologically real world apprehended through emotion is not some 'other', occult or transcendent world; it is the same world consisting of the same energy as the physical one, but grasped in its emotional aspect. Or, to put it simply, individual things are fields of energy the psychological aspect of which is emotion. This aspect is immediately given through emotion, primarily as 'importance', 'value', 'significance', 'meaning'—Chapter XV. Furthermore, as things affect the psyche through emotion, *the psyche affects things through emotion*. The facts of parapsychology point to this; so too we might interpret the psychosomatic category of 'accident proneness', in which physical objects are 'staged' or 'arranged' in accordance with the emotion of the victim, turning events into symbols. Also, art and holy objects, the material things of vogue and mode, the fetishes of children, primitives and the insane

[1] For example, we can speculate that the magical behaviour of objects and fields (e.g. haunted houses) described by psychic research workers and anthropologists can be accounted for by the view that emotion is energy. Objects and places 'saturated' (Chapter V, pp. 62–3) by emotion—through curses, *crimes passionnels*, taboos, unresolved sins and emotional tensions, etc.—suffer a transformation of energy from physical into psychological. Due to emotion the field changes from one which is predominantly physical to one predominantly psychological, so that the field no longer obeys the laws of physical energy only. The emotional aspect of energy comes to the fore, whereas before it had only been potential or 'occult'. The conversion is due to a saturation of the object by an excess of emotion (Chapter V, p. 62, Albertus Magnus). This psychological intensity transforms objects into symbols. (This does not necessarily involve an 'emergence' theory of energy, from physical to psychological, such as we saw in the view of Prince, Chapter VI; only the hypothesis that emotion is transformation, such as we shall discuss under final cause below.) Therefore, mediums, shamans and witch-doctors are 'energy transformers'. Either by gift or training their emotional life is particularly non-subjective. They are thus open, without personal involvement, to the emotional aspect of the field which is occult to 'normals'. Through them energy is converted from physical to psychological, or vice versa, always through the emotions, requiring great emotional discipline and yielding great emotional exhaustion. Hence, too, periods of major emotional crises in the life of the individual—puberty, childbirth, approach of death—and in the life of primitive society—change of seasons, change of rulers—are the times *par excellence* when such events occur. These are the critical times of energy transformation, the moments when archetypes constellate.

are all just things, but things which have been affected radically by the psyche through emotion. Emotion is a bridge, a two-way bridge, uniting subject and object—Chapter XII.

If emotion is this two-way bridge, then the world of nature has an emotional aspect given along with its physical, chemical and electrical aspects and, also, our own emotions—whether we know it or not— are continually interacting with the world of nature. Every 'cut' between subject and object is arbitrary. Man and world are fundamentally inseparable because the same basic energy constitutes man and world. This is evident on the physical level, i.e. we are composed of the same elements as the world about us. But on the psychological level we experience the cut because we neglect our emotions and thus miss the emotional aspect of things. We have such little and such primitive emotional awareness that the world about us is either dead and without value or falsely overcharged due to the coarseness of our emotions. We have left undeveloped the faculty of apprehending the world as emotional. Therefore, occupation with one's own emotions in an attempt to restore and refine one's own emotional life is at the same time a restoration and refinement of the relation between oneself and world. Psychotherapeutic practice attests to this: the more the individual admits his capacity to lust, weep and rage, develops his emotional awareness, begins to recognize his emotions as affecting the world around him, the more he begins to find himself a part of an emotionally meaningful world.

But not only for psychotherapy is this view of emotion useful; it has bearing on the problems of science and the problems of ethics and aesthetics. If the world of nature has an emotional aspect, then science can no longer cut out a field of truth without emotion. Emotion is a potential aspect of every energetic event, even the most abstract and 'objective'. Furthermore, scientists can no longer neglect their own emotions since they are continually affecting the world of nature by these emotions, whether they know it or not. The romantic reaction against science on the part of moralists and aesthetically inclined intellectuals as well as the curious self-occupation of scientists with the morality of contemporary science reflect this concern over the emotional aspect of science. By ignoring the emotional aspect of objects, the scientist feels justified in separating his own emotion from reason in order to be more 'objective', more in accord with the field of 'truth' he investigates. He distrusts his own emotional consciousness because it is often an uncouth instrument owing to neglect. Thus forms a vicious circle; and the neglected emotional life of the scientist affects his field, perverting and distorting his aims into ugly and destructive events. The mushroom cloud representing the incredible achievement of science in our times is also our times' symbol of the ugly and the evil. A realm of truth without its emotional aspect is no longer truth of any value.

Philosophy has long said that truth cannot be separated from goodness and beauty, This is not an idealist's shibboleth; it has a natural ground. If emotion is the psychological aspect of universal energy, the realms of ethics and aesthetics are on firm footing. They are not subjective, not projected on to a dead physical world whose truth science has pre-empted. Rather, the emotional qualities of goodness and beauty are objectively given by the world of nature as part of its truth. That we are blind to the emotional aspects of things does not mean that they are not there. Moral and aesthetic education, education of the emotions, goes hand in hand with the development of science and reason if reality is to be experienced as it really is and not as a cut out, partial system of operations. Moralists and educators have long cried for this but always on the basis of some moralistic ought; while here we try to expose the rational ground of this ought in the very material substrate of all things.

To conclude with the material cause of emotion we return to the statement that the concept of matter, like that of material cause, is relative. It is not in itself sufficient to account for emotion. So we can appreciate why those groups of theories which try to account for emotion through denying its reality (Chapter I), quantification (Chapter VII), physical location (Chapter X), a negative single root (Chapter XIII) disorder (Chapter XVII) are not sufficient. They have seized upon one aspect of the phenomenon, the material aspect, and sought their explanations only in material causality. Thus they are led into the paradoxes of the concept of matter: its unreality, its negativity, its invisibility, its chaos. Only a high-level hypothesis that the material cause of emotion is energy, the same prime energy of the universe, goes beyond these entanglements. Such an hypothesis says everything and nothing; therefore the energy must be qualified as *materia secunda*. This is the human body situation. This is the potential energy of the conventional set which is converted during emotional behaviour and known by work done as the demonstrations of the body and the representations of the mind,

E. *CAUSA FORMALIS*

Matter and form are correlates. For Aristotle, form is 'prior to matter and more real'—(*Metaphys.* Z3, 1029a). ('For the form, or the thing as having form, should be said to be the thing, but the material element by itself must never be said to be so'—*Metaphys.* Z10, 1035a.) That the material element by itself is not sufficient to account for the thing is evident from the discussion just behind us. On the other

266

hand, we need not assume with Aristotle the priority of form or that the statement of the essence of a thing is the thing. Neither matter nor form is prior or enough in itself to explain. Both are necessary; neither is sufficient. From the point of view of the fourfold root there is no priority of one cause over another. The form or essence is only one aspect of the explanation.

Just as there have been explanations of emotion through the initiating cause and others through the material stuff, there are explanations of emotion which turn mainly on essence. These explanations answer the question 'why', neither in terms of stimulus cause nor substantial basis, but rather in terms of the *essential quality which defines emotion*, differentiating it from all other events. The search is for that which makes a thing what it is and not some other thing. This essence is '. . . something besides the concrete thing, viz. the shape or form'—*Metaphys.* B4, 999b).[1]

The answers to this sense of 'why' as given by the theories fall into two main kinds. The first identify the essence of emotion with a specific *pattern*. This is the classic approach to emotion through studies of expression. The second identify the essence with a specific *quality*. This is the classic approach through qualitative analysis of inner states and the naming of these states, as fear, hope, joy, etc. It is this pattern or quality which is held to be the distinguishing characteristic of emotion, that shape or quality differentiating and defining it from all other events. Let us outline these patterns and qualities.

[1] We can easily stumble over the Aristotelian construction of form because it is so different from our notion of form today. It unifies in one concept the notions of essence, active power, substance, shape, reality or actuality, idea, and definition. With the history of philosophy behind us, these are now all distinct concepts. We no longer identify the shape of a thing with its essence; under the impact of idealism essence and appearance have been driven wide apart. Nor do we identify the definition or name of something with its essence; due to nominalism and modern linguistic analysis names and things have no inner or necessary relation. Ideas taken as passive impressions made upon the mind are radically different from reality and from active power. Substance to us today is just the contrary of essence and form. It connotes solidity; essence some vague and ghostly spirit. We presume matter for the reality and actuality of things, not form which is just an accidental shape of matter. For us matter tends to be prior and to be power. Form is only 'the visible aspect of a thing, now usually shape or configuration' (OED). In short, the meanings implied by 'form' have gone over to the concept 'matter'. The older view of form is also brought out by the roots of its modern synonyms: pattern, figure, shape, type. Pattern is a doublet of Patron. The two words were not distinguished until about 1700. The root of pattern is thus via the French *patron* to the Latin *patronus, pater*, implying the creative active father principle. Figure, from (ME) *feinen, feignen*, (OF) *feindre*, (Lat.) *fingere*, connotes action through the meanings 'invent' and 'forge'. Shape, from the Old English *gesceap*, Teutonic **skap*, also means 'create', 'make'. Type, from the Greek, even more strongly implies action, meaning 'strike', 'beat', 'impress'. Form itself still has the colloquial usage of liveliness, conversational powers, high-spirited good functioning bringing out the old meaning of *actus*. So, whereas now it is necessary to relativize the concept of matter and to labour the importance of form and the formal cause, it once was *the primary cause* to which the final purpose of a process and its initiation could ultimately be reduced.

267

Integration

I. Emotion is a pattern.

A. The pattern is inherited as an ancestral, instinctual reaction (Chapter XIII).

B. It is molar; a generalized whole pattern (Chapter VIII).

C. It is a physiological pattern, either as:
1. External facial expression (Chapter XV),
2. Internal and external gross demonstrations (Chapter X B and C).
3. Internal patterns of activation (Chapter X A).

D. The pattern is a motion of the subject-object relation (Chapter XII).

II. Emotion is a quality.

A. There is one primary quality of all emotion:
1. The quality is conflict (Chapter XVI).
2. The quality is unconsciousness (Chapter V).
3. The quality is inwardness (Chapter IX).

B. Each individual emotion is a blend of qualities:
1. These qualities are given by representations (Chapter XIV).
2. These qualities are given by proprioceptive visceral sensations (Chapter X B).
3. The unique qualitative difference of each emotion is the product of a limited number—said to be 2, 3, 4, 5, 6, 11 or 14 —distinct and fundamental emotional elements alone or in combination (Chapter II).

III. Emotion is neither pattern nor quality.

A. It is a formless blur and disorder (Chapter XVII).

B. It can be only quantitatively distinguished (Chapter VII).

C. It cannot be distinguished from other events (Chapter I).

Of the three parts of the outline, the third can be dealt with handily. The denial of formal quiddity is the result of explaining emotion through material causality only. Thus emotion is not real (Chapter I) or is chaos (Chapter XVII) or is only a quantitative event (Chapter VII) such as we saw in our discussion of the material cause. Emotion is always only blur and chaos and it never differs from other behaviour, except quantitatively, if one neglects the formal cause, that qualitative essence which differentiates it from other behaviour as was pointed out in Chapter I.

In order to integrate the other two parts of the outline—pattern and quality—a general hypothesis is again needed which can join not only the different descriptions of emotion as a pattern, but which can unite this pattern of behaviour with the qualitative essence of

268

emotion. A hint about the formal cause has already been given in the last section where it was said that emotion is the psychological form of energy. This means that we take *the formal cause of emotion to be the soul*. What we mean by this will become clearer as we go along. (The terms 'soul' and 'psyche' will be used interchangeably, although there tends to be a difference in the literature. 'Psyche' is more the biological concept, a kind of natural concomitant to physis and perhaps reducible to it. 'Soul' has metaphysical implications which some psychologists consider inappropriate to psychology as a science. As was said in the conclusion to Chapter VI, the concept of soul is ambiguous; it is traditionally connected with morality, immortality and God.)

Looking again at the outline we find that what differentiates the psychological patterns which are emotion from other psychological patterns such as feeling, sensation, will, etc., are several particular criteria. The pattern is inherited, overtly physiological, molar and part of the subject-object relation. (Emotion is, of course, further differentiated from other psychological activities by its final, material and efficient causes. Sensation, feeling, will, etc., are also 'soul', but they are not also symbolic and energetic in the same way as these concepts were described in the foregoing sections.) Here, however, we have to do with criteria within the formal cause alone which distinguish emotion from other activities of the soul. These criteria can all be integrated by the concept *total*. *Emotion is a total pattern of the soul*. It is the soul behaving as a whole, or as was said in Chapter VIII, emotion generalizes a reaction. It does this because emotion is the soul as a complex whole, involving constitution, gross physiology, facial expression in its social context as well as actions aimed at the environment. Emotion is the soul in its ancestral and learned past, physiological present and social aims. In the moment of living emotion, fear say, I am living as a result of my evolutionary inheritance and personal experience, in terms of my body here and now, and as a part of the world upon which I have intentions. It is this totality which differentiates emotion from partial psychological events such as feeling,[1] sensation, will, etc. Thus its essence is complex as was said

---

[1] The difference between emotion and feeling might be formulated as follows: It is simply a distinction between whole and part. Feeling is a particular psychological function disposable to consciousness (see Jung, *Psychological Types*, Definitions). Emotion is an activity of the psyche as a whole. Feeling it is possible to have in one's hands; emotion is always partly beyond ego control. In individuals where feeling is relatively undeveloped, i.e. unconscious in the sense of unadapted, it will be emotional since it will tend to be under the influence of the unconscious, thus becoming symbolic. In our culture where the function of feeling and its products is given rather short shrift, feeling has indeed become emotional so that the confusion between these concepts in the literature (particularly Freudian) does reflect the real state of affairs. In that feeling is a partial function, emotion as a whole activity always comprises elements of feeling (evaluations on the good-bad or pain-pleasure scales), just as emotion includes

in the preliminary to this chapter and thus the method for explaining it must be complex as was maintained all along.

Just as the pattern hypotheses of our outline can be integrated by the concept total, so the quality hypotheses can be integrated by the concept of *central*. Just as inheritance, physiology, facial expression, etc., give partial descriptions of the total pattern, so too are conflict, unconsciousness and inwardness partial descriptions of the central quality.

The *conflict quality* of emotion occurs in two ways. First, there can be specific 'conflict' emotions, just as there are specific emotions of 'joy', 'hope' or 'fear'. Conflict is a type of emotion; it is not identical with the generic concept emotion any more than is 'joy', 'hope' or 'fear'. All emotion does not have the quality of conflict, but all emotion takes on the quality of conflict the more the central quality is not acknowledged. This is the second way in which the conflict quality occurs: partial and peripheral systems assert themselves against the centre, e.g. emotion is resisted as has been discussed in Chapters X C, XVI and again under *Causa Efficiens*. Thus we have situations or events becoming symbols for the problem of opposites.

One basic psychological experience of this problem is the opposition between the first and second systems, whether conceived as only intrapsychic or as reflected in the outer world. Therefore, conflict qualifies so much emotion because, as has been said, emotion activates both systems and because one tends to resist the whole event in favour of a part. The conflict quality is due to a failure to recognize the central quality of emotion and to yield to it. In fact, emotion is the psyche's answer to the conflict of opposites for it is an activity of the whole.

The *unconscious quality* of emotion can be similarly accounted for. It is not due simply to a fall into unconsciousness, into an unadapted, magical, primitive, physiological world. Emotion is not unconsciousness; rather it is only unconsciousness in so far as it relativizes consciousness. In emotion both systems are behaving at once; we are partly conscious and partly unconscious. The whole psyche is behaving as a whole. So, in emotion we live the truth of ourselves just as we are, partly adapted and partly not. We expose ourselves as a whole and reveal our personality from its middle point. Thus the essence of character is said to come out in the trials of love and battle, or '*in vino veritas*'. Thus, too, we resist emotion, especially in public. But the more refined our emotions are the less unconscious-

---

sensations (perceptions and proprioceptions—X B and X C), thoughts (cognitive elements—XV), and intuitions (inner images—XIV, creative novelties—XVIII, inspirations—XIX, and the reflection of a situation as a whole—XI). See above, Part II, p. 60, footnote.

ness—in a negative sense—they carry with them. Then the unconscious quality of emotion is a compensation in the positive sense of supplement to conscious behaviour. This is so whether we take emotion as the necessary disorder which is corollary to every extension of consciousness (Chapter XVII) or as the new and creative (Chapter XVIII). This implies that conscious behaviour requires emotion for completion, so that emotions are welcomed as necessary to wholeness by psychologically developed people.

The quality of inwardness occurs when the subject identifies himself with the central quality of emotion. That which is central in the senses of leading, important, vital, essential—although it marks the subjective experience with significance—is not the subject itself. The inward feeling is the subjective side of any central event. It says: 'This event means *me*!' An emotion has this central quality of making life 'mean me'. An emotion tells me: 'This is my experience.' But experience is given me as well as is mine: I am as much lived by life as I live it. Just as the conflict quality results from the way the subject *resists* emotion as a central process, so the inward quality results from the subject's attempt to *identify* himself with this central process. One presumes emotion to be not just 'me', but '*mine*'. Thus one sets out to locate it within. But as has been repeatedly said, the psyche is not only within and such old-fashioned spatial models fail to give the proper image. And so the centre does not have to be pin-pointed in the heart, liver or endothymic ground (Chapter IX) or in the diencephalon, etc. (Chapter X A). As was said at the end of Chapter X A, it might be more fruitful to theory of emotion to examine the concept of centre than to look for concrete centres. The central quality of emotional experience does not mean, 'I am living from this one point', but rather, 'I am living out of my centre'. When I fear, crave, beg for mercy I do so out of the midst of myself, out of myself as a whole. The centre is ultimately both the midmost darkness (Chapter IX) and the person in his circumference. It is the psyche as all and as one. Inwardness is the quality of the soul-complex from within; but a complex is not to be modelled after spatial solids. A complex is a functional process which has no spatial inside. Even its centre is the process in its entirety.

We must keep in mind here that central and total, inner and outer, quality and pattern are ways of talking about one single complex, the psyche. By tradition the psyche is one, even if divisible into many factors. By upholding the unity in diversity of the soul we do not mean isomorphism (Chapter IV). We do not posit a necessary identity between the diversities such as inner and outer, quality and pattern, etc. These pairs become dualities bridged through the concept of isomorphic unity. Our view makes such bridges unnecessary.

The split between these different dualities is not fundamental; it is due to the disappearance of the soul from psychology and the split can be healed by restoration of this concept to its proper use. As was touched upon in the discussion of animal spirits (Chapter VI), the soul, from the seventeenth century onward, either became identified with mind or matter, or it dropped from psychology altogether. A host of substitute concepts have since been put forward—from Descartes' functions of the pineal gland to contemporary 'isomorphism'—to bridge a gap caused by its loss. There is no need for substitutes because the classic notion of the soul as a unity in diversity, or as that complex functional relation of body, mind, world and spirit omits need for such bridges. The bridge is there in every action of life. We simply do not realize that we stand upon it, that the primacy of the soul is the first reality. It was said in Chapter XV: my reality is my psychic reality, my emotional worth here and now. Or as the Existentialists put it: the here and now, both within and without, both body and mind is united in an emotion.[1] Instead of this unity, contemporary psychologists too often see the partial functions of the soul as separate islands linked with elaborate constructions. But the soul itself is the union of mental functions, social relations and physiological processes. It joins body, facial expression and pattern of inheritance. It is the relation of subject and environment (Chapter XII), the relation of cortex and thalamus (Chapter X A), the relation of instinct and imagination (Chapter XIV), the relation of conventional and spontaneous will (Chapter X C). In the various chapters these partial functions were said to be related to each other during emotion. This is because emotion is the total pattern of the psyche which includes all; the central quality which connects all. As one author says, emotion 'puts together elements of experience'.[2] Therefore all the relations between all the partial functions of man's life depend upon emotion. And emotion cannot be correlated directly and only with any one set of functions, either physiochemical (Chapter X B), specific test results,[3] outer stimuli perceptions, body patterns, or facial expressions. As systems of operations cut out by the observer for study, each partial function is incommensurable with every other. The laws of one system do not apply to another. Explanations in terms of one system cannot account for the others. Isomorphic correlations or the notion that the functions are different 'languages' state that these functions are ultimately equal, even identical. But the 'languages' cannot be translated into each other directly; there are no point-to-point equalities between the different systems. The psyche

---

[1] Bollnow, O. F., *Das Wesen der Stimmungen*, Frankfurt a/M, 1941, pp. 20-2 (M. Heidegger, *Sein und Zeit*, p. 136 f.).
[2] Knapp, P. H., *op. cit. sup.*, p. 60.   [3] Landis, C., Part I, pp. 12–13, above.

as a whole—and in each person slightly different—is the original text through which all translations and correlations must be referred. The similarity in form between the different orders of events, the very ground of the isomorphic thesis, is the one form itself, the soul.

Therefore whether we speak of emotion as the total pattern of the psyche or as the central quality of the psyche we refer to the same model: emotion as the soul in its wholeness. The formal cause is the psyche observable in 'objective' behaviour and 'subjective' experience. The psychic aspect of emotion is given to introspection as those unique qualitative feelings, specific vegetative and muscular proprioceptions, and patterns of representations of each emotion. But further, the psychic aspect of emotion is the formal cause in the fundamental sense of cause: as ground of possibility. The psyche is the faculty, the very facility by which behaviour and experience are possible. Without psyche there is neither experience nor behaviour. Energy or matter alone is an abstraction. It cannot be said to experience. Nor can it be said to behave except in some particular form as chemical, electrical or emotional. It is the psyche which organizes energy in the form of emotion. It is the psyche which is the formal ground of human experience and behaviour. And emotion, as the energetic stuff of the psyche as a whole before it is differentiated into partial functions, is the primary state or activity of the soul. As Chapter IX held, emotion is the essence of life; where emotion is, life is; it is the heat which distinguishes the living from the dead.

A psychology of emotion without psyche is also without logos. It fails to understand or explain. The soul is necessary for explanation, and where it is barred it comes in under disguise. Isomorphism is not the only example of this. As we saw in Chapter VI, the energetic concepts (psychonic, bio-, vital energy) were such substitutes. Chapter IX identifies emotion with psyche, while Chapter I makes the identification in reverse: the denial of psychic reality and the denial of emotion go hand in hand. In Chapter X A the search for the underlying centre of emotion becomes confused with the age-old search for the soul, while Chapter X B involves the soul with the vegetative nervous system. The hyphen in the S-R theory (Chapter XII) is also such a substitute. In each case the concept of psyche or a replacement is necessary to the explanation. Emotion cannot be explained without it.

Taking the formal cause of emotion to be the psyche, the conclusions about the *efficient cause* become more intelligible. There it was said that the symbol activates the whole person. In so far as the psyche is a whole embracing both consciousness and the unconscious, both subjective and objective levels, the symbol activates emotion

273

as the whole psyche. Emotion is the psychological response to the symbol. Therefore, symbolic realization transforms the whole personality (Chapter XIV). The primary language of the soul as a whole, the primary way the soul grasps reality is as symbolic reality. An emotion is the psyche symbolized; it is like a rite, a ceremony, a magical propitiation of objective powers (Chapter XV). Each emotion has as *causa efficiens* an appropriate symbol and each emotion has as *causa formalis* an appropriate formal pattern or quality. *These two, symbol and form, correspond with each other.* Analysis of the forms of emotional behaviour shows appropriate symbols; an encounter with a symbol corresponds to a specific quality and pattern of emotional behaviour. This correspondence of symbol and form is more exact the less the emotion is coloured by subjective consciousness. The more universal the symbol, the more collective the behaviour pattern.

So too the formal cause sheds light upon the *material cause* as energy. There appeared an apparent paradox between the statement that emotion is an aspect of universal energy and the statement that emotion is the energy 'located' in the body situation. It is the psyche, as form of the body (Aristotle), which 'locates' emotion in the relatively closed field of the body situation. Emotion is in the field only as qualities or physiognomic characters; it is going on all the time everywhere, but only *in potentia*. In actuality, it is only known as it comes into existence due to psyche. *Energy only can become emotion through psyche.* (If we look at the symbolic products of the mentally ill we find the landscape without life, or the dream of only natural or cosmic phenomena often indicates a pathology in the affective sphere.) Not until the soul joins the world of objects does their emotional aspect come into being.

Several clarifications follow upon the hypothesis that the formal cause of emotion is the psyche as a complex whole. First, it becomes evident why central psychological problems are called emotional problems, or as was said: ' "Emotion" and "psychic" are terms which are frequently used interchangeably in the literature.'[1] Therefore, the development of emotion is the development of the soul, as has been stressed in all great ethical treatises and spiritual disciplines. Also, it becomes more evident why emotion is the bugbear of theoretical brain models which as analogues of separate functions do not reproduce the psyche as a complex whole.

Further, we can see why the *transference* has such a primary role in psychotherapy. Affective contact is psychic contact. Reduction of the transference to specific schemas of the mother-child relation or infantile experiences, to sociological notions of isolation or religious

[1] Malmo, R. B., 'Research: Experimental and Theoretical Aspects', in RDPM, p. 87.

notions of sin and confession are unnecessary; they confuse the fundamental issue. The primary contact with the soul of another person is emotion. This is evident to the plain man who sizes up the nature of his fellows through style and manner, physiognomy and tone of voice. These are revelations of the other person as a total pattern, reflecting his central truth. In short, emotion is wholeness and the affective contact is the first level of healing, of making whole. Therefore the patient continually provokes the emotion of the therapist, involving him in anger, in love and desire, in hope and anxiety, in order to get a whole reaction. It is only this wholeness perhaps which works a cure. Or, as Landauer says (p. 158) emotion makes us aware of ourselves as a whole. It produces organization (Chapter XVIII).

Let us not fancy that this wholeness must be a harmony, an ataraxic state confined to the specifications of the rational will. The psyche as a whole includes maladapted and inferior functions, too. It is a condition of completion and not necessarily of perfection. Thus cacophony is as appropriate to emotion as is harmony.

With this we come to a new understanding of the *order-disorder problem*. Taking emotion as the psyche as a whole, it becomes evident why emotion can be disorder, may be a danger and might have to be repressed or released. *The soul's great unified force is too great for the partial systems of the conventional set.* The pattern of organization with which the ego is identified must be large enough to withstand the psyche acting as a whole. The centre of gravity, so to speak, of the person cannot sit too high up or too onesidedly, else it is surely overthrown by the centre. (Here we can recall those terms 'abdication', 'being overwhelmed', 'Erschütterung', 'bouleversement', etc.) In order to live emotion positively, one's subjective centre must be close to the centre of oneself as a whole, close to the objective psychic levels. One must live close to emotion itself.

To put this another way, the dangerous *excess* of emotion (which is not emotion itself although Chapter VII would make this identity) is due to the difference in degree between the energetic and formal aspects of the psyche. Psyche and emotion are not the same. Emotion is the energetic aspect of psyche; psyche has a formal aspect as well. This formal aspect is not just intelligence, level of consciousness, self-control, the 'G' factor, the Rorschach 'F', flexibility, nor tension-tolerance, yet it has to do with all these descriptions. To put it simply, the formal aspect is the container of the energetic aspect. It too is the psyche as a whole, but more from the point of view of formal organization. The disorder of emotional excess is due to the improper relation of these two aspects of the psyche. Here we find the importance of education and of the early years of life (Chapters

XIII, XV and XVIII). The formal side is developed too often independently of the energetic side: grammar versus games. In therapy one must often go back to very early years to find a symbolic bridge between the energetic and formal aspects, and re-educate the patient by means of aesthetic, imaginative and social methods neglected in 'normal' education. Until the vessel is shaped, therapy of emotion may often require suppression or release of the energetic aspect for the sake of the container. Sometimes this alone can save a formless psyche from being destroyed by its emotion. Emotion is not always good nor always bad; it can either kill or cure, and it can only be 'dosed' (Chapter XVIII) in respect to the quality of the formal organization of the psyche.

F. *CAUSA FINALIS*

It is usual to distinguish between two notions of the final cause. The first is the more ancient one as given by Aristotle: 'The purpose and the good (for this is the end of all generation and change)' (*Metaphys.* 983a); 'the end, i.e. that for the sake of which a thing is; . . .' (*Metaphys.* 1013a). The second is the more modern idea of the end of a process, not as a purpose or goal, but as the conclusion or finish of an operation. Are purpose and finish irreconcilable opposites? If one holds for purpose does this mean finalism, vitalism, and a teleology with a transcendent subject who pulls the event towards the best of possible goals? Or, if one holds for finish, does this mean that the conclusion of every event is a barren mechanistic stop determined completely from behind by efficient causes?

A solution to this old riddle can be derived from Aristotle, who unites the end of a process with its purpose as follows: 'For if a thing undergoes a continuous change and there is a stage which is last, this stage is the end or "that for the sake of which" ' (*Physica* II, 194a). This last stage or outcome—whatever it might be—is what a process has achieved. *This means we take the end of every emotional process to be an achievement.* This achievement is neither a dead finish, nor a good goal. Yet, it is both at once: every result is an achievement and this achievement is the purpose of the process. Every purpose is nothing more or less than the actual result attained. The result of a process is its purpose; its purpose is its result. This solution keeps us within the phenomenological approach in that purposes are observable phenomena, i.e. results, and results are always intentional.[1]

Here it is important not to be confined by the notion of time. Not only is emotion taken as a *process* in time, but we are also speaking of

---

[1] 'Finis est prior in intentione, sed est posterior in executione'—Thomas Aquinas (*Summa Theol.*, Ia–IIae, xx, 1 ad 2).

it as a phenomenological *event*. The final cause is temporally the last stage of a process, but it is not later than emotion when this is conceived as an event. Just as we argued that what initiated a motion (the efficient cause) is not something prior to or separate from an event, so too the final cause is not later than the event. The achievement of emotion is not only the consequent of the emotional process; the achievement is the emotion itself. Emotion is achievement. The final cause taken this way is thus clearly distinct from the other causes. The final cause is not some material potentiality which works itself through to a goal, nor is it some efficient stimulus initiating a motion from the future, nor is it a formal essence which gives shape to a process as it goes along. It is a result and this result is 'that for the sake of which', the achievement of the event. It is the event itself viewed under the aspect of its issue. We need not assume along with Aristotle that the issue of an event is its good; yet because it is natural to evaluate issues and results rather than formal essences, material substrates and efficient stimuli, it is under this rubric that we become involved with the *value of emotion*.

And so we ask for the fourth time, 'why'; this time in the sense of what is the issue of emotion; what does it achieve; for the sake of what does it come about at all? The answers are the hypotheses of the final cause. They can be outlined as follows:

I. Emotion achieves *survival*:

    A. Its end is the release of energy (Chapter VI, etc.).
    B. Its end is homeostatic regulation (X A, etc.).
    C. Its end is a back action upon the stimuli (XII).

II. Emotion achieves *signification*:

    A. Its end is the qualification of all experience (IX).
    B. Its end is expression, communication and the revelation of values and truth (XV).
    C. Its end is ultimately the signification of life in terms of 'not-being' (evil, *Angst*, and sex) (XIII).

III. Emotion achieves *improvement*:

    A. Through emotion physical energy emerges into consciousness (VI).
    B. Emotion presents images and is the matrix of the new and creative (XIV and XVIII).
    C. Emotion amplifies isolated functions to a general level (VIII) and is whole-making.

The broadest concept with which we can integrate these various descriptions of the final cause is the concept of *change*. This can be described in terms of (I) biological survival as changes in the internal or external milieu, or (II) in terms of a change in the significance of experience, or (III) in terms of improvement. Neither denying intentionality to such changes nor claiming that these changes are a useless remnant of the past and a disorder refutes that the outcome of emotion is change. As said above we take the outcome to be an achievement. Thus emotion achieves change; as its result *is* change, so is its purpose *to* change. That for the sake of which emotion occurs is change. Further, *emotion is itself change*, because the final cause, like all the causes, is an aspect of the event itself. Emotion is always alteration when viewed from the point of view of the final cause.

This change has been formulated in many ways throughout Part II. Chapter XII described change as *motion*, either as locomotion between subject and object, or within the subject as quantitative increase or decrease or as qualitative alteration. Ribot says succinctly: '. . . the fundamental and irreducible fact at the root of all emotion: attraction or repulsion, desire or aversion, in short, motion or arrest of motion.'[1] Chapter VI speaks of *energetic* changes, Chapter X C of *physiological* changes, while Chapter XIV discusses emotion as a change in *representations,* Chapter XVI presents change as *conflict*, Chapter XVII as *disorder* and Chapter XVIII as new *organization*. Further, there have been accounts of this change in terms of need and disbalance and also in terms of a relatively self-activating principle (as cortex, unconscious will, spirit, etc,). There is, in short, no argument in the literature about taking emotion as change. The word itself emotion = *ex-movere* brings out its dynamic aspect. And Drever's definition (Part I) which enjoys general agreement mentions widespread changes during emotion. It is not that the theories do not describe emotion as a change in energetic, physiological, sociological, psychological sectors, rather the problem lies in evaluating this change and defining it more closely.

Therefore, just as it was necessary to define the formal cause not just as psyche but as the whole psyche, so it is necessary to conceive the final cause of emotion as that kind of change called *transformation*. And just as the closer definition of the formal cause helped distinguish emotion from other activities of the soul, so too emotion is set apart from other changes by the notion of transformation.

What we mean by 'transformation' is evident from what has gone before. From our discussion of emotion as a *symbol*, it is clear that emotion is not just a change in conscious representations, but a transformation of them in terms of symbolic reality. When we say emotion is a transformation of *energy*, we speak of the quality of the

[1] Ribot, Th., *The Psychology of the Emotions*, London, 1897, p. 91.

energy, not just a change in direction or intensity. And the discussion of emotion as the activity of the *psyche* as a whole again leads one to take it as a transformation of that whole rather than as a change of its partial functions. As transformation of the whole it becomes evident why it involves all the changes in will, perception, values, social relations, physiology, etc., described in our theories. Transformation is the wider concept; the changes aspects of it. The changes in conscious representations, in direction and intensity of energy and in the soul's partial activities are all aspects of the transformation going on. From this hypothesis that emotion achieves transformation, the other hypotheses of the final cause fall in place.

Returning to the outline of these hypotheses, let us interpret the role of emotion in *biological survival* in terms of transformation. Emotion is the adaptation syndrome; it is the organism's only full response to the demands for change life presents us with. When the organism must be transformed if it is to survive, emotion appears on the scene. The transformation goes on in many sectors at once: release of physical energy, re-ordering of homeostasis, changes in the subject-object relation. Psychologically, there is a change in *signification*. To speak accurately, change is always going on and every moment involves survival, thus emotion qualifies all experience. But such continuous adjustments are subliminal; one commonly calls only the more drastic ones emotion. In these, values and attitudes are transformed and emotion expresses this alteration. As was said in Chapter XV, emotion is always directed at an audience. There is urgent information to be communicated. This can be taken as the message of uncertainty, the revelation of a fundamental nothingness (Chapter XIII) which is contrary to survival and runs paradoxically parallel with it particularly in the most intense moment of biological life, the sexual act—if we are to believe the authors of Chapter XIII, (Sex, *Angst*, and 'not-being' are related). Emotion comes into play in emergency situations (Chapter X A), which have been described also as conflict, as 'bouleversement', as 'Umschichtung', as a total 'Erschütterung'. A person's worth disappears, consciousness is in abeyance; the whole person stands in question (Chapter XVII). Even in the great affirmation of joy one's survival is uncertain; since one is grasped and transformed partly beyond one's awareness. Emotion is an activity not of the subject's own doing. Thus it is always a *passio*, a test, a crisis situation, when adaptation through reasoning or instinct or other partial functions no longer are enough.[1] All such

---

[1] Here we fall upon a difference between emotion and instinct. Instinct conserves; emotion transforms. One might even say: instinct adapts in terms of the past; emotion in terms of the future. (Although emotion accompanies instinct, Chapter III, there is no need to reduce emotion to an instinctoid basis. On our view, rather the reverse

lesser means of survival have failed. Thus, emotion reveals the truth about the peril of ourselves and the world (Chapter XV). 'Chuang Tzu says: "The existence of things is like a galloping horse. With every motion it changes. Every second it is transformed." ' [1] Conceived biologically this truth is: transform or perish.

This would imply that emotion is an acute episode, but oddly enough chronic symptoms, long dark depressions and states of ineffable boredom or unswerving attachments to things and people, too, serve survival. Transformation goes on at many levels beyond superficial notions of crises. In this way the emergency theory of emotion seems not to cover the ground—unless we take 'emergency' in a broader way. Transform or perish can be conceived psychologically—even eschatologically. Emotion would then be a crisis of the soul and would have to do with its survival, its life or death. An emotion is relatively short-lived, as the theories often contend; but only providing the crisis (biological, psychological or eschatological) is short-lived. The chronic emotion which marks our times reveals the truth of our age. It is a time in which the partial functions of reason, will, instinct, belief have each failed to give adaptation. The emotional symptoms of our time, whether strictly described in psycho-somatic terminology or presented through the phenomena of daily life (delinquency, divorce, addictions, conversion, etc.) are all attempts of the psyche to transform in response to the crisis. Even the parathymias of schizophrenia, the misplaced emotions of hysterics and the primitive reactions of catatonic rage might be taken as having a survival value. They are witness to the crisis of the patient and attempts at transformation.

What then characterizes a successful transformation? When is an emotion a 'good' emotion? What is the 'justification of emotion'

position is maintained, since we take emotion as the primary activity of the psyche and instinct as a partial function.) Emotion performs two functions when associated with instinct. First, through emotion instinct is open to transformation and education (Chapters XIV and XVIII); second, through emotion instinct is raised to a molar event (Chapter VIII) involving the whole person. Depending upon the degree of differentiation of the *emotion* (not the sexual instinct), sexuality can range between lust murder and pyromania on the one hand to the mystical ecstasy of divine love on the other. Neither extreme is a function of sexual instinct as such, but is a result of the accompanying emotion which transforms the energy of instinct and symbolizes it. Investigators of human sexuality might well notice this difference between instinct and emotion. The orgasm in women or the age at which men's potency is maximum as well as the other questions charted by these gentlemen will never be determined by their studies of instinct mechanisms alone. It is always emotion that decides these things since in human sexuality only pathologies show an isolated instinct not amplified and transformed by emotion. (See further on the relation of instinct and emotion—other than McDougall as presented in Chapter III above—J. C. Whitehorn, 'Concerning Emotion as Impulsion and Instinct as Orientation', *Am. J. Psychiat.*, 1932.)

[1] Chung-yuan Chang, 'Creativity as Process in Taoism', *Eranos Jahrbuch* XXV, Zurich, 1957, p. 403.

as one symposium asks.[1] We can approach this question conversely: 'When is emotion not "good"?' Here the answers have been several: some would insist all emotion is disorder, an *action manquée*; some would hold that only negative emotions (hatred, despair, anger, say) are not good, are never justifiable. Others would put the point that only repressed and unconscious emotion is not good. While in Chapter XVIII where emotion was taken most positively, intense emotions (Leeper) or those which do not fit in with self-actualization (Goldstein) could be classed as not 'good'.

In order to give our answer to this question of value—by far the prickliest fruit on the giant cactus of emotion theory—we must first make some distinctions. First, not all that passes for emotion is genuine. There are substitutes: deep feelings, vigorous willing, drive and instinct behaviour, tumults of sensation. These conditions are not symbolic, energetic activities of the whole psyche as described above. Nor are they transformations as described here. (Such states are always incomplete compared with emotion. They lack either an element of meaningful consciousness, or the gross physiological demonstrations, or the disordered irrationality, or the spontaneous alteration of representations, etc.) Second, there is a difference between emotion abortive in itself and abortive emotion due to a disorder in the causes. For example, there might be a deficiency in the formal cause should the psychic level not be adequate to the excess of energy. Or there can be anomalies in the field of energy distribution. And perhaps the efficient cause is either not a symbol (an electrical charge, a drug, a glandular product) or the symbolic functioning of the patient is disordered. The source of the failed emotion under these conditions is not in the emotion but in the causes: formal, material, efficient.

Now we are left with the original question: what characterizes a successful transformation, a 'good' emotion? The position we took in regard to the final cause—a purpose is nothing more or less than the achieved result—obliges us to take emotion in and for itself as *always having achieved its purpose*. It must therefore be a successful transformation always and *always 'good'*. However, if we separate the result of emotion from the emotional process itself, then the question of value turns upon the value of the aftermath. Does the transformation bear fruit? Does it lead to a work of art or a nervous breakdown? Does it kill or cure? Practically, this means that the value of emotion can be determined by an examination of its expressed result. *It is not emotion that is good or bad, but its expression.*

[1]'Symposium: The Justification of Emotions' (Mary Warnock and A. C. Ewing), *The Aristotelian Society*, Suppl. Vol. XXXI, London, 1957.

The expression of emotion of course involves other factors which are not emotion, particularly the formal aspect of the psyche (its quality and organization as touched upon above). And the evaluation of emotional expression goes beyond theory of emotion; it opens into theories of art, of disease, of social morality and ethics, etc. Nevertheless, from the point of view which separates a process from its result, a successful transformation must be judged by positive after-effects. In order to achieve successful emotions it becomes necessary to acquire ability in emotional expression. Methods for this were sketched all through Part II and they cover even the emotions of fear, hatred and greed, the expression of which can be highly differentiated and successful. Direct expression—even of genuine, of 'good' emotion—is often just what makes emotion abortive. It is often too violent and too peculiar for our standards of collective morality. Nevertheless, emotion itself remains 'good', so that one is required to use the methods of indirect expression. 'Symbolic circuition', 'symbolic realization', 'active imagination' (Chapter XIV) are often first necessary before emotion can be lived directly in daily life (Chapters XV and XVIII).

Judging emotional expression is always risky. If we keep in mind that the survival or adaptation value of emotion can be taken in many ways, e.g. in terms of biological, sociological, psychological and eschatological reality, an emotion, abortive in one frame of reference, may be successful in another. Further complicating the judging of 'good' emotion is the notion of adaptation. Do we mean adaptation for the individual or for the collective (either as biological species, social group, or collective psyche)? Let us use self-hatred leading to suicide as example. It may be an abortive transformation for the individual from the standpoint of biological and eschatological reality; yet it may be a successful transformation, a 'good' emotion, in that it corresponds to the individual's psychological reality. It may be his individual death, and yet be survival for the social group (suicide rather than murder). Emotion always has some survival value and reveals some truth about reality, but this truth is symbolic, not merely sociological or biological. We cannot therefore condemn an emotion without giving it full hearing, without trying to grasp the transformation as symbolic. The peculiar emotional behaviour of our time may perhaps be an adaptation to reality and have survival value, if not only for the individual, perhaps also for the collective psyche of the species. How often are neuroses—abortive emotion from many points of view—also creative adaptations. The 'emotional' behaviour of the schizophrenic and the 'teddy-boy' with the 'cosh' may—either through a purgatory suffering of the individual or by confronting the species with the unexplored peculiarities of its own psyche—

perhaps be contributing to survival no less valuably than the 'un-emotional' behaviour of the engineer dumping radio-active wastes in the seas. Emotion is an achievement of the whole soul whose full dimensions include many unknowns. It is, as said before, a symbolic phenomenon and a reflection of objective psychic constellations. It is *transpersonal* and best respected as such. Too often the therapist with too narrow a view of emotion sees it as an abortive transformation and rushes in with relief. One could expect Job's friends or the companions of Jesus in Gethsemane today to step forward with a tranquillizer. In short, emotion, no matter how bizarre, must be taken in awful earnest before diagnosing it abortive.

The third achievement of emotion as given in the outline is *improvement*. This improvement can be taken as an energetic transformation of the physical into the psychological (Chapter VI), as a creative transformation of the old into the new (Chapter XVIII), and as a molar transformation of the part into the whole (Chapter VIII). These improvements, as well as others in the realm of therapy and education, have been already stressed in Chapter II. Here it might be well to point out that emotion is an improvement which does not depend on its consequences. It may or may not build a work of art or develop new images or free energy. *It is not these after-effects which make emotion an improvement. Emotion is itself an improvement.* To speak strictly: my state of being during emotion is an improvement over my state of being without emotion, regardless of what happens afterwards. How are we to understand this fundamental question of emotion as an improvement?

Here we can recall that the main hypotheses put forward throughout this work, of which the notions of change and motion discussed above form aspects, conceive emotion as a *relation*. Be it between subject and object, man and world, two kinds of willing, instinct and imagination, conscious and unconscious or sections of a divided psyche, different cerebral or physiological systems, etc., emotion is the '*Zwischenfunktion*' that relates. In the light of this we can say: my state of being is improved during emotion because in emotion I exist in a paradoxical relation. I am not *only*, but *both*. My will is frustrated; there is conflict, disorder and unconsciousness. I have fallen into my ancestral past and into my flesh. Yet in this fall I am re-united with the world, with my body, with the objective psyche and with a will and reason beyond my own doing. I am improved because I live what I am: inheritor of my ancestor's sins, prisoner of my flesh and victim of forces greater than my will. I am complete. Also, I live in the bonds of this very moment, the time just exactly as it is. This concrete precision of my existence, painful and ugly as it can be at times, is the improvement of being 'right', *echt* or *eigentlich*, of being

Integration

in Tao. This improvement is survival, adaptation and signification all together.

From the point of view of the ego, this fall—described in many theories as the 'downward discharge' of emotion—signifies not improvement, but uncertainty. Or, as was said in Chapter XVIII: emotional behaviour is not security behaviour. Thus, this fall is usually too much of a risk; instead, emotion is damped down, let loose or avoided at all costs even to the point of agonizing psychosomatic symptoms, all conditions due, as we have already suggested, to the related problems of *excess* and *development*. Different ways of developing emotion have been discussed. In addition to mentioning again 'active imagination' (Chapter XIV), we might point to the education of emotion through changes in values and meanings (Chapter XV) and the living of emotion consciously in daily life (Chapter XVIII). Individuals who have developed their emotion by means of these arts, or others like love, adventure, meditation or those other disciplines usually called the Arts, tend to cultivate emotional behaviour. They recognize that only emotion can provide complete adaptation because it is the psyche's method of renewal, *par excellence*. It is an encounter with spirit (Chapter XIX). This means choosing a life, not *au dessus de la mêlée* but a life of descent into the flesh. As Freud,[1] James,[2] and Watson[3] each point out, an essential fact of emotion is that it terminates in the subject's own body. Whether one likes this or not, the fact remains as psychosomatic symptoms demonstrate. Therefore, the very first step in the development of emotion is going with the downward discharge. One chooses the gross demonstrations of the body which by this choice become less autonomous and are given the dignity of consciousness. This is living emotion in terms of a final cause given in Chapter XVIII: to love one's own body.[4]

The prolongation of the therapeutic situation beyond the cure of symptoms and the problems of social adjustment can be seen in the light of emotional development. An analysis—and we mean in particular that sort which involves an active confrontation of analyst and analysand, two human beings, with risk and love and meditation

[1] Freud, S., 'The Unconscious' (1915), *Coll. Papers*, IV, London, 1949, p. 111 fn. ('Das Unbewusste', *Gesammelte Schriften*, V, Wien/Leipzig/Zürich, 1925, p. 494).
[2] James, W., 'The Emotions', Chapter XXV in *The Principles of Psychology* (Dover Edition), 1950, p. 442.
[3] Watson, J. B., *Psychology from the Standpoint of a Behaviourist*, Philadelphia and London, 3rd edn. 1929, p. 227.
[4] The paradox of the descent into emotion is nicely imaged in the Kundalini Yoga where the emotional centre (*Manipura*) just below the diaphragm is both a seething cauldron, place of Rudra the 'howler', and means 'filled-with-jewels'. A fall into the flesh is at the same time a discovery of spiritual riches, as we pointed out in Chapter XIX.

and openness to the elaboration of symbolic images—has become a last refuge of traditional teaching of individuals in our culture. To meet this need for emotional cultivation, psychotherapy has expanded beyond its origins in physical medicine and has moved toward religious, and even if need be oriental, methods of psychic development.

Lack of emotional development—whether described topologically as distance from the centre, or energetically as the inert potential of the conventional set, or formally in terms of an uncouth quality of the psyche—yields emotional excess. Emotion can be abortive also because of this excess, an excess in this case due to the absence of consciousness. Ego-consciousness, after struggling to suppress emotion, suddenly abdicates in its favour (Chapter XVII). Instead of living emotionally, there is only a blind acting out. This kind of enantiodromia will never develop emotion since it is only unconscious (unadapted) behaviour. The two systems are not lived simultaneously; one has replaced the other. It is not a symbolic event because the conscious aspect is missing, or only recovered later in an *esprit de l'escalier*. This kind of emotion fails to fulfil our theory; it is not complete emotion—even if named 'emotion' by many psychologists who one must suppose know only it and not the real thing. As a partial activity of the psyche, an activity without consciousness, it is an *emotion manquée* and belongs rightly among the semi-pathological states described by Janet (Chapter XVI). Abortive emotion of this kind occurs, as the attitudes betrayed in theory after theory have shown, for *one main reason: consciousness is unable to accept emotion and live it.* (This denial is of course also bound up with rejection of any final cause for emotion. We refuse to admit: first, any good in it; second, any purpose for it; and third, even any end or stop to it—it is 'always going on'.) This refusal to meet the challenge of emotion, this *mauvaise foi* of consciousness is fundamental to our 'age of anxiety'. It is characteristic of—even instrumental in—what has been called 'the contemporary failure of nerve'. We do not face emotion in honesty and live it consciously. Instead emotion hangs as a negative background shadowing our age with anxiety and erupting in violence. A 'therapy' of this condition depends altogether upon a change in the attitude of consciousness towards emotion—a change for which this work attempts to provide a ground. If there is anything novel in this synthesis of final causes it is this: *emotion is always to be valued more highly than the conscious system alone.* This tends to run counter to the main stream of thinking about emotion in the psychology, philosophy, physiology and therapy of today.

285

G. CODA

Having the four hypotheses of the four causes of emotion, the integration asked for in the first chapter takes place as follows: Emotion is 'symbol', 'energy', 'psyche' and 'transformation' as described above. *Each emotion has: its own pattern of behaviour and quality of experience which is always a total attitude of the whole psyche* (causa formalis); *its own distribution and intensity of energy in the field of the human body situation* (causa materialis); *its own symbolic stimulus which is partly conscious and partly not presented to consciousness* (causa efficiens); *its own achieved transformation which has some survival value and is some improvement compared with non-emotional states* (causa finalis). These four causes correspond with each other. The quality and pattern of an emotion is only that quality and pattern given by a specific symbol which in turn corresponds with the specific organization and intensity of energy and a specific kind of transformation. What makes an emotion 'joy' and not 'disgust' or 'shame' always depends upon the specific constellation of the four causes. The causes correspond to each other because, in fact, each is emotion itself in one of its aspects. As de La Chambre[1] in the seventeenth century and Duchenne[2] in the nineteenth asserted, each emotion has its own peculiar characteristics of expression which accord with the purposeful result being achieved. Although using different language, modern studies so well represented in Dunbar's massive compendium (EBC) show that different constellations of factors—energy balance, psychological attitudes, symbolic situations, symptomatic behaviour results—correspond with different emotions. More exact coordination of the factors, that is, the analysis of an emotion, awaits deeper understanding of the *causa efficiens* and *causa formalis* in particular. Practically also our theory suggests that the more collective the *causa efficiens* (the symbol), the more typical the pattern of behaviour and the more statistically average the energy organization. Thus, studies on the more primitive emotions like fear and rage lend themselves better to experimental methods. Our theory also suggests why the concept of emotion has become central to the problems of our time. If emotion is the meeting place of physical energy and the soul and if it also has to do with symbols and the transformation of the person, then the contemporary dissolution of symbols and the problems of transformation of modern man will be reflected there (Chapter XIX). Further, this theory accounts on a general level for psychosomatic symptoms, which can be mani-

---

[1] de la Chambre, M. C., *Les Caractères des passions*, Amsterdam, 1658, I, 12.

[2] Duchenne, G. B., *Mécanisme de la physiognomie humaine, ou Analyse électro-physiologique d'expression des passions*, Paris, 1862, Eng. summary by E. B. Kaplan, *Physiology of Motion* (by Duchenne), Philadelphia, 1949.

festations in the realm of physical energy of the transformations of the soul, including those transformations involving the soul's most metaphysical and religious symbols.—With these suggestions and intuitions we come to the end. This is a coda and a coda is 'a passage added after the natural completion of a movement, so as to form a more definite and satisfactory conclusion' (OED). To fulfil this, then, we can condense our result: *emotion is that transformation of the energy of the conventional set which is achieved by the whole psyche and which is initiated by a symbol.*

Also here, it is appropriate to pick up again the major and minor themes of this work: *theory* and *therapy*. They were sounded in the first chapter where the task was set: 'Can a unified theory of emotion be developed which might provide a basis for psychotherapy and find agreement within systematic psychology?' Whereas the first concern of our work appeared to be the major theme of theory and methods of explanation, it grows evident as we come to the end that the minor theme of therapy has become dominant. From one point of view, therapeutic methods are the consequences of theoretical explanations; from another point of view, therapy is 'that for the sake of which' we have a theory at all. However we put it, *explanatory and therapeutic psychology in regard to emotion are enmeshed with each other* as we have sought to point out in chapter after chapter. Partial theories and partial therapies go together, e.g. emotion conceived as a thalamic function entails therapeutic methods in terms of the thalamus. We have tried to expose the fundamental failures of partial explanations, and steadfastly we have refused to make the same error of using simple events to account for complex ones. Therefore, we have never defined emotion, the very concept in question, nor differentiated it absolutely from affect, *passion, orexis, Sindsbevaegelse, Gemütsbewegung, Stimmung,* etc.[1] Any definition would whittle down the complexity to fit some ready-made frame. And so the frame we have used of 'symbol', 'energy', 'psyche' and 'transformation' is composed of concepts even more general—yes, and more difficult perhaps—than the concept 'emotion'. The formula given above to satisfy the form of a coda is *not a definition but a condensation*, the meaning of which depends wholly upon the amplification of its terms as found through the work.

To repeat, explanatory and therapeutic psychology in regard to emotion are enmeshed with each other. We offer that a unified theory of emotion is both a systematic explanation and a therapeutic method. The theory we have set out is both a systematic explanation

---

[1] See KB, pp. 1–3, for historical differentiation of some of these terms; also FE 37, p. 123; M. Steinitzer, *Die menschlichen und tierischen Gemütsbewegungen als Gegenstand der Wissenschaft,* Munich, 1889, pp. 17–26; as well as any philosophical dictionary.

which integrates the great range of viewpoints of modern psychology and includes also, we suggest, a method of psychotherapy of the kind stressed, namely, *development*. As was pointed out in the first chapter, the method has been one of amplification, the circumambulation from all sides for the sake of enlargement of consciousness. This has been attempted, first, through a differentiated amplification by means of the eighteen groups of hypotheses and, second, by an integrated amplification by means of the four causes. Our method has attempted to explain in the sense of '*rendre manifeste ce qui est enveloppé et caché*',[1] to make clear (*erklären*) or to enlighten (*erhellen*), to unfold (*expliquer*), even if not to make plain or lay out flat.

Our method, therefore, is a 'therapy' in that going through the work—that continual confrontation with the 'why' of emotion—is an enlargement of comprehension. It is a process of enlightenment which can result in an acceptance, an affirmation even, of emotion, which is precisely what, as said often and again, is required for its development. The prolonged encounter with the problem of emotion is already—by admitting it as a problem—an attempt on the part of consciousness to come to terms with it, which is the first step towards the development of any problem. Or, to put it another way, the circumambulation of this phenomenon has altered our relation to it. It has been an emotional event itself and affects consciousness. Our theory, then, not only gives ground for the therapy of development but is based on an explanatory method which perhaps has started this development itself.

The development of emotion through an affirmation by consciousness, as last phrase of the coda, is the most personal statement of the work. Neither can a long and careful rational exposition of this position, nor can any amount of exhortation bring this about. Behind the difficulty of affirmation lies the healthy, natural tendency to avoid the numinous and demonic, that dark unruly horse of the Phaedrus myth, violent yet harnessed to the chariot in which we sit and which we try to manage. What to do about this horse has occupied the great philosophers and religious teachers for thousands of years. Many alternatives have been formulated. The ancients spoke of *mediopatheia, apatheia, ataraxia* and *catharsis*. Some Church fathers suggested governing, while sectarians have offered on the one hand a radical, disciplined annihilation of the horse, or on the other, an enthusiastic loss of identity in favour of the animal in Dionysian orgy. More recently, methods of 'abreaction', 'acting out', or mechanical and chemical therapy have been put forward. All of these we have refused in favour of the notion of development. But by development we do not mean a progressive climb away from the dark beast so as

[1] Smith, F. V., *The Explanation of Human Behaviour*, London, 1951, p. 28.

to escape it. Nor do we mean a dropping of the reins in favour of the whip such as the charioteer does in a scene of such blood and cruelty (*Phaedrus*, 254), that it serves to indicate how subtly the dark horse can creep under the human skin of the charioteer who believes himself superior. No, this is not the way; but Plato himself gives us another image—the reins. We are reined to the horse, it to us. This is emotional existence, driving and being driven, the true image of *homo patiens*. Here we come close to the image of the centaur which Benoit[1] proposes as the Zen image for solving emotional states. These passionate mythological monsters, one of whom was the wise instructor of such culture heroes as Achilles, Hercules and Aesculapius, represent a humanization of emotional driving power. Centaurs were said to be able to capture wild bulls which expresses the idea that wilder emotion can be tamed by conscious emotion, or as was said before in Chapter XIV, 'only through emotion can emotion be cured'. And it was a centaur, mythology tells us, who taught mankind something of the arts of music and medicine—as if to say the origins of healing our emotional malaise are to be found in the union of mind with flesh, of wisdom with passion.

Therefore, Nietzsche,[2] though he too in writing of emotion uses the metaphor of the horse and reins, leads us astray when he advises using the reins without pleasure, coolly, detachedly. This only furthers the split between horseman and horse and reveals Nietzsche's contempt for *homo patiens*, which he too in the end was forced to become. Such advice is a pathological denial of the reality of what reins are: ties, attachments, the very bonds and binds (*peirata*[3]) of fate. Development means a qualitative process of constant relationship approximating to the nature of the centaur, whereby through the harness of reins and chains 'I become the horse and the horse me'.

We use the symbol of the Phaedrus myth because we have come to the end of rational explanation. The phenomenon of emotion is always partly outside consciousness. We can never know ultimately what emotion is, what it achieves or what sets it going. It remains a symbolic event; emotion is a 'gift' said William James.[4] But not, as he said, a gift either of flesh or spirit, but a gift of both flesh and spirit. Thus its danger for a gift can be a curse or a blessing, or a blessing in disguise. It can never be altogether understood because the psyche as a whole is not grasped by consciousness alone. Emotion is always therefore a risk. To be known it must be lived. Perhaps this is why no matter how thoroughly amplified, the problem of emotion, theory and therapy, remains perennial and its solution ineffable.

[1] Benoit, H., *The Supreme Doctrine*, London, 1955, pp. 117–34; 146–60.
[2] Nietzsche, F., *Der Wille zur Macht*, ¶ 928.   [3] OET, Part III, Chapter II.
[4] James, W., *The Varieties of Religious Experience*, London, 1906, p. 151.

ABBREVIATIONS

ANCL   *Ante-Nicene Christian Library, Translations of the Writings of the Fathers down to A.D. 325* (ed. by A. Roberts and J. Donaldson), 24 vols., Edinburgh, 1867–72.

EBC   *Emotions and Bodily Changes:* F. Dunbar, Columbia Univ., N.Y., 1954 (4th edn.).

ECM   *Emotions and Clinical Medicine:* S. Cobb, N.Y., 1950.

EGP   *Early Greek Philosophy:* J. Burnet, London, 1948 (4th edn.).

EM   *Emotions and Memory:* D. Rapaport, N.Y., 1950 (2nd edn.).

ERE   *Encyclopaedia of Religion and Ethics* (ed. by J. Hastings), Edinburgh, 1908.

FE 28   *Feelings and Emotions—The Wittenberg Symposium* (ed. by M. Reymert), Clark Univ., 1928.

FE 37   *Feeling and Emotion: A History of Theories;* H. M. Gardiner, R. C. Metcalf and J. G. Beebe-Center, N.Y., 1937.

FE 50   *Feelings and Emotions—The Mooseheart Symposium* (ed. by M. Reymert), N.Y., 1950.

KB   *Kritische Darstellung der Geschichte des Affektbegriffes (Von Descartes bis zur Gegenwart)*; K. Bernecker (Dissertation), Berlin, 1915.

OED   *Oxford English Dictionary.*

OET   *The Origins of European Thought, about the Body, the Mind, the Soul, the World, Time and Fate;* R. B. Onians, Cambridge, 1954 (2nd edn.).

RDPM *Recent Developments in Psychosomatic Medicine* (ed. by E. D. Wittkower and R. A. Cleghorn), London, 1954.

SS   *In Search of the Soul, and the Mechanism of Thought, Emotion, and Conduct;* B. Hollander, 2 vols., London, n.d.

GENERAL BIBLIOGRAPHICAL INDEX

Numbers in square brackets refer to the page in this book where the reference is mentioned.

Abelard, *Ethica, Scito Te Ipsum*. [132, 138]

Abély, P., 'Etude clinique', *Les Facteurs Vasculaires et Endocriniens de l'Affectivité* (A. M. P. Abély, A. Assailly et B. Lainé), Paris, 1948. [7]

Adler, A., 'Feelings and emotions from the standpoint of individual psychology', FE 28. [185–6]

Adrian, E. D., 'The conception of nervous and mental energy', *Brit. J. Psychol.*, 1923–4. [80]

Akhilananda, Swami, *Hindu Psychology*, London, 1948. [182]

Albertus Magnus, *De Mirabilibus Mundi*. [62, 264]

Alexander, F., Book Review of *Psychosomatic Diagnosis*, by F. Dunbar, in *Psychosom. Med.*, 1945. [71]

—— 'The logic of emotions', *Int. J. Psycho-Anal.*, 1935. [56]

—— *Psychosomatic Medicine, Its Principles and Applications*, N.Y., 1950. [20]

—— 'Three fundamental dynamic principles of the mental apparatus and of the behavior of living organisms', *Dialectica*, 1951. [67]

Allen, G., *Physiological Aesthetics*, London, 1877. [117]

Allendy, R., *Le Symbolisme des Nombres*, Paris, 1948. [248]

Allison, H. W., and Allison, S. G., 'Personality changes following transorbital lobotomy', *J. Abn. Soc. Psychol.*, 1954. [3, 176]

Allport, F. H., *Social Psychology*, Cambridge, U.S.A., 1924. [127]

—— *Theories of Perception and the Concept of Structure*, N.Y. and London, 1955. [199]

Allport, G. W., *Becoming* (The Terry Lectures), Yale Univ., 1955. [138, 219]

—— *Personality* (1951, London reprinting of 1937 U.S.A. edition). [42, 148, 195]

Angier, R. P., 'The conflict theory of emotion', *Am. J. Psychol.*, 1927 (Washburn Commemorative Volume). [201–2]

Anton-Stephens, D., 'Preliminary observations on the psychiatric uses of chlorpromazine', *J. Ment. Sci.*, 1954. [4]

Aristotle (*Collected Works*, ed. by W. D. Ross, Oxford), *Metaphysica*. [19–20, 27, 246–7, 249, 266–7, 276]

—— (*Collected Works*, ed. by W. D. Ross, Oxford), *Physica*. [19–20, 153, 200, 247, 276]

Arnheim, R., 'Emotion and feeling in psychology and art', *Confin. Psychiat.*, 1958. [32, 224]

Arnold, M. B., 'An excitatory theory of emotion', FE 50. [111–12]

Augustine, *De Civitate Dei*. [117, 131, 180]
—— *De Trinitate*. [160]
Aveling, F., 'Emotion, conation and will', FE 28. [166]
Ax, A., 'The physiological differentiation between fear and anger in humans', *Psychosom. Med.*, 1953. [51]
Babkin, B., 'The conditioning of emotions', FE 50. [147]
Bard, P., 'The neuro-humoral basis of emotional reactions', in *The Foundations of Experimental Psychology* (ed. C. Murchison), Clark Univ., U.S.A., 1929. [102]
Barnett, S. A., 'The "expression of the emotions" ', *New Biology*, 22 (Penguin Book), 1957.
Bartlett, F. C., 'Feeling, imaging and thinking', *Brit. J. Psychol.*, 1925-6. [178, 199]
Beck, S. J., 'Emotional experience as a necessary constituent in knowing', FE 50. [87, 166, 190, 219]
Beebe-Center, J. G., 'Feeling and emotion', in *Theoretical Foundations of Psychology* (ed. by H. Helsen), N.Y., 1951. [6, 15, 18, 34, 36, 82, 147, 244]
Bekhterev, V. M., 'Emotion as somato-mimetic reflexes', FE 28. [48, 145]
Bell, C., *Art*, London, 1914. [223]
Belouino, P., *Les Passions dans leurs Rapports avec la Religion*, Paris, 1873. [160]
Benassi, P., 'Sulle attuali concezioni delle emozioni', *Riv. sper. freniat*, 1957.
Benoit, H., *The Supreme Doctrine*, London, 1955. [79, 289]
Bentley, M., 'Is "emotion" more than a chapter heading?' FE 28. [7]
Bergson, H., *Creative Evolution*, London, 1928. [213]
—— *The Two Sources of Morality and Religion*, N.Y., 1956. [225-26, 229]
Berkeley, G., *Alciphron, or The Minute Philosopher*, London, 1732. [199]
Berman, L., *The Glands Regulating Personality*, N.Y., 1930. [120]
Bernard, T., *Hatha Yoga* (Ph.D. Thesis), Col. Univ., N.Y., 1944. [129]
Bernecker, K., *Kritische Darstellung der Geschichte des Affektbegriffes*, Berlin, 1915 (Dissertation). [131, 159, 211, 287]
Bertrand-Barraud, D., *Les Valeurs Affectives*, Paris, 1924. [192]
Best, C. H., and Taylor, N. B., *The Physiological Basis of Medical Practice*, Baltimore, 1943. [113]
Bichat, F. X., 'Recherches physiologiques sur la vie et la mort', in *Anatomie Générale*, nouv. ed., Paris, 1818. [115]
Bindra, D., 'Organization in emotional and motivated behaviour', *Canad. J. Psychol.*, 1955. [212]
Binswanger, L., *Grundformen und Erkenntnis menschlichen Daseins*, 2nd edn., Zürich, 1953. [160, 162]
Bitter, W., *Meditation in Religion und Psychotherapie*, Stuttgart, 1958. [181]
Blatz, W., 'The cardiac, respiratory and electrical phenomena involved in the emotion of fear', *J. Exper. Psychol.*, 1925. [131]
Bleuler, E., *Affectivity, Suggestibility, Paranoia*, Utica, N.Y., 1912. [88]
—— 'Das autistische Denken', *Jhb. f. Psychoanal. Psychopath. Forsch.*, 1912. [175]

Byrne, O., *The Evolution of the Theory and Research on Emotions* (unpubl. M.A. Thesis), Columbia Univ., N.Y., 1927. [68]

Cameron, N., *The Psychology of Behavior Disorders*, Boston, 1947. [116]

Cannon, W. B., *Bodily Changes in Pain, Hunger, Fear and Rage* (2nd edn.), Boston, 1929 (1953 printing). [102]

—— 'The James-Lange theory of emotions: A critical examination and an alternative theory', *Am. J. Psychol.*, 1927 (Washburn Commemorative Volume). [101]

—— 'Neural organization for emotional expression', FE 28. [101]

—— *The Wisdom of the Body*, N.Y., 1932. [102]

—— 'Voodoo Death', *Psychosom. Med.*, 1957. [228]

Carp (ed.), *The Affective Contact* (Report from International Congress for Psychotherapeutics), Amsterdam, 1952. [3, 274–5]

Carr, H., 'The differentia of an emotion', FE 28. [208]

Carus, C. G., *Vorlesungen über Psychologie*, Leipzig, 1831. [211]

Cason, H., 'An interacting-pattern theory of the affectivities', *Psychol. Rev.*, 1933. [78, 244]

Cassirer, E., 'Language as an expression of emotion', in *The Philosophy of Symbolic Forms*, Vol. I, Yale Univ., 1953. [196]

Cellérier, L., 'La vie affective secondaire', *Rev. Phil.*, 1927. [45]

de la Chambre, M. C., *Les Caractères des Passions*, Amsterdam, 1658. [150, 286]

Chang, Chung-yuan, 'Creativity as process in Taoism', *Eranos Jahrbuch*, *XXV*, Zürich, 1957. [280]

Chenu, M. D., 'Les catégories affectives dans la langue de l'école', *Le Cœur*, Paris, 1950. [189]

Choisy, M., 'Recherches expérimentales des émotions', *Arch. di Psicol. Neurol. e Psichiat.*, 1953. [133, 183]

Claparède, E., 'Feelings and emotions', FE 28. [5, 50–1, 196]

Cobb, S., *Emotions and Clinical Medicine*, N.Y., 1950. [7, 14, 40, 157, 176, 235, 243]

Collingwood, R. G., *The Principles of Art*, Oxford, 1938. [5, 62, 189, 196, 226]

de Condillac, E. B., *Traité des Sensations*, Paris, 1754. [155]

Cooke, W., *Mind and the Emotions in Relation to Health, Disease and Religion*, London, 1852. [182]

Costello, C., 'The effects of pre-frontal leucotomy upon visual imagery and the ability to perform complex operations', *J. Ment. Sci.*, 1956. [175]

Crichton, A., *An Inquiry into the Nature and Origin of Mental Derangement*, 2 vols., London, 1798. [117]

Crile, G. W., *The Origin and Nature of the Emotions*, Philadelphia, 1915. [156–7]

De Crinis, *Der Affekt und seine körperlichen Grundlagen*, Leipzig, 1944. [3, 119–20]

Darrow, C., 'Emotion as functional decortication', *Psychol. Rev.*, 1935. [110]

Darwin, C., *The Expression of the Emotions in Man and Animals*, (1872), London, 1904. [126, 130, 156, 196]

Das, B., *The Science of the Emotions*, Madras, 1924. [160]

Dejean, R., *L'Emotion*, Paris, 1933. [187]

Dembo, T., 'Der Aerger als dynamisches Problem', *Psychol. Forsch.*, 1931. [140]

Denison, J. H., *Emotion as the Basis of Civilization*, N.Y. and London, 1928. [5]

Descartes, R., *The Philosophical Works of Descartes*, Vol. I, Dover Edition, U.S.A., 1955. [7, 40]

Descuret, J. B. F., *La Médecine des Passions*, 3rd edn., Paris, 1860. [210–12]

Dewey, J., 'The theory of emotion', *Psychol. Rev.*, 1894, 1895. [201]

—— 'Theory of valuation', *Inter. Enc. of Unified Science*, 2, 4, Chicago, 1939. [189]

Dibblee, G. B., *Instinct and Intuition*, London, 1929. [195]

Dictionnaire encyclopédique du Bouddhisme (Hôbôgirin) ed by S. Lévi, J. Takakusu and P. Demiéville, Tokyo, 1929. [210]

Donovan, S., 'The festal origin of human speech', *Mind* (O.S.), 16–17 [196]

Dorfman, W., 'Endocrines and emotions', *N.Y. State J. Med.*, 1954. [120]

Doust, J. W. L., and Schneider, R. A., 'Studies in the physiology of awareness: an oximetrically monitored controlled stress test', *Canad. J. Psychol.*, 1955. [235–6]

—— ——'Studies in the physiology of awareness: the effect of rhythmic sensory bombardment on emotions, blood oxygen saturation and the levels of consciousness', *J. Ment. Sci.*, 1952. [235–36]

Drever, J., *A Dictionary of Psychology* (Penguin Reference Books), London, 1952. [8, 278]

—— *Instinct in Man*, Cambridge, 1917. [192–3, 203–4]

Ducas, A., *Discours sur les Passions de l'Amour de Pascal*, Algiers, 1953. [232]

Duchenne, G. B., *Mécanisme de la Physionomie Humaine, ou Analyse Electro-Physiologique de l'Expression des Passions*, Paris, 1862, (Eng. summary in E. B. Kaplan, *Physiology of Motion* (by Duchenne), Philadelphia, 1949). [196, 286]

Duffy, E., 'Emotion: An example of the need for reorientation in psychology', *Psychol. Rev.*, 1934. [15, 32]

—— 'An explanation of "emotional" phenomena without the use of the concept "emotion" ', *J. General Psychol.*, 1941. [32]

—— 'Leeper's "motivational theory of emotion" ', *Psychol. Rev.*, 1948. [32]

Dugas, L., 'Les passions', *Nouveau Traité de Psychologie* (ed. G. Dumas), Vol. 6, Paris, 1938. [196]

Dumas, G., 'Introduction à l'étude de l'expression des émotions', *Rev. Philos*, 1926. [195, 197]

—— *Nouveau Traité de Psychologie*, II, 3, III, 2, Paris, 1932–3. [155]

Dunbar, F., *Emotions and Bodily Changes* (4th edn.), Columbia Univ., 1954. [3, 117, 120, 122, 286]

—— *Psychosomatic Diagnosis*, N.Y., 1943. [48–9, 70–1]

Dunlap, K., 'Emotion as a dynamic background', FE 28. [35, 117–18]

Duprat, G. L., 'La psycho-physiologie des passions dans la philosophie anciene', *Arch. f. d. Gesch. der Phil.*, XI, 1905. [125, 234]

Elmgren, J., 'Emotions and sentiments in recent psychology', FE 50. [7, 41]

Empson, W., *Seven Types of Ambiguity* (2nd edn.), London, 1949. [21]

English, H. B., and English, A. C., *A Comprehensive Dictionary of Psychological and Psychoanalytical Terms*, N.Y., London and Toronto, 1958. [6, 243]

Entralgo, P. L., *Mind and Body*, London, 1955. [211, 238, 286]

Eriugena, J. S., *De divisione naturae*. [248, 259]

Ewing, A. C., 'The justification of emotions', *The Aristotelian Society, Suppl.*, Vol. XXXI, London, 1957. [131, 281]

Fabing, H. D., 'The dimensions of neurology' (Pres. Address), *Am. Acad. of Neurol.*, 1955. [123]

—— 'Toads, mushrooms and schizophrenia', *Harper's Magazine*, 214, N.Y., May 1957. [124]

Farmer, E., and Chambers, E. G., 'Concerning the use of the psychogalvanic reflex in psychological experiments', *Brit. J. Psychol.*, 1924–5. [83]

Fearing, F., 'Group behavior and the concept of emotion', FE 50. [190]

Federn, P., *Ego Psychology and the Psychoses*, London, 1953. [58]

Fenichel, O., 'The ego and the affects', *Psychoanal. Rev.*, 1941. [56]

Féré, Ch., *The Pathology of Emotions*, London, 1899. [114, 228]

Ferrari, G., 'Psicologia dei moribundi', *Riv. di Psicol.*, 1920. [130]

Finley, K. H., 'Emotional physiology and its influence on thought content', *J. Nerv. Ment. Dis.*, 1953. [128–9]

Flemyng, M., *The Nature of the Nervous Fluid, or Animal Spirits, Demonstrated*, London, 1751. [75–6]

Flugel, J. C., 'The death instinct, homeostasis and allied concepts', *Studies in Feeling and Desire*, London, 1955. [67]

Forti, E., *L'Emotion, la volonté et le courage*, Paris, 1952. [214]

Fouillée, A., *L'Evolutionisme des idées-forces* (5th edn.), Paris, 1911. [172]

Frank, P., *Modern Science and Its Philosophy*, Harvard Univ. Press, 1949. [14]

v. Franz, M.-L., 'Die Aktive Imagination in der Psychologie von C. G. Jung', in W. Bitter (ed.), *Meditation in Religion und Psychotherapie*, Stuttgart, 1958. [181]

Freeman, W., 'Frontal lobotomy 1936–1956; a follow-up study of 3000 patients from one to twenty years', *Am. J. Psychiat.*, 1957. [176]

Freeman, W., and Watts, J. W., *Psychosurgery*, Oxford and Springfield, Ill., 2nd edn., 1950. [176]

Freud S., 'Analysis of a phobia in a five-year-old boy' (1909), *Coll. Papers*, Vol. III. [162]

—— *Delusion and Dream*, London, 1921. [56]

—— *A General Introduction to Psychoanalysis*, N.Y., 1953 (Riviere translation). [76, 169–70]

—— *Inhibitions, Symptoms and Anxiety*, 1926 (Internat. Psychoanal. Library, No. 28). [162]

—— *The Interpretation of Dreams*, London, 1954. [55]

Freud, S., 'The "uncanny" ', *Coll. Papers*, IV, London, 1919. [162]
—— 'The unconscious' (1915), *Coll. Papers*, IV, London, 1949. [54–5, 284
Frink, H. W., *Morbid Fears and Compulsions*, London, 1921. [204]
Gardiner, H. M., Metcalf, R. C., and Beebe-Center, J. G., *Feeling and Emotion:A History of Theories*, N.Y., 1937. [112, 150, 161, 174, 180, 198]
Gastaut, H., 'The brain stem and cerebral electrogenesis in relation to consciousness', *Brain Mechanisms and Consciousness, A Symposium* (ed. by J. F. Delafresnaye), Oxford, 1954. [84]
Geiger, M., 'Fragment über den Begriff des Unbewussten und die psychische Realität', *Jbch. f. Phil. u. phänomen. Forsch.*, 1921. [96, 143]
Geikie-Cobb, J., *The Glands of Destiny* (3rd edn.), London, 1947. [120–21]
Gellhorn, E., *Physiological Foundations of Neurology and Psychiatry*, Univ. of Minn., U.S.A., 1952. [112]
Gemelli, A., 'Orienting concepts in the study of affective states, Part II', *J. Nerv. Ment. Dis.*, 1949. [130, 169–73]
George, F. H., 'Machines and the brain', *Science*, 127 (1958). [213]
Gerard, R. W., Discussion following 'The central mechanism of the emotions', by Spiegel, Wycis *et al.*, *Am. J. Psychiat.*, 1951. [94]
Gesell, A., 'Emotion from the standpoint of a developmental morphology', FE 50. [130, 155–6]
Gilbert, A. R., 'Recent German theories of stratification of personality', *J. Psychol.*, 1951. [97, 246]
Gilson, E., *History of Christian Philosophy in the Middle Ages*, London, 1955. [161]
Glover, E., 'The psycho-analysis of affects', *Int. J. Psycho-Anal.*, 1939. [56–7]
Gold, H., 'How to evaluate a new drug', *Am. J. Med.*, 1954. [123]
Goldberger, E., 'Simple method of producing dreamlike visual images in the waking state', *Psychosom. Med.*, 1957. [181]
Goldstein, K., 'On emotions: considerations from the organismic point of view', *J. Psychol.*, 1951. [221, 226–27]
Gooddy, W., 'Cerebral representation', *Brain*, 1956. [113]
Gordon, K., 'Imagination and emotion', *J. Psychol.*, 1937. [225]
Grace, W. J., and Graham, D. T., 'Relationship of specific attitudes and emotions to certain bodily diseases', *Psychosom. Med.*, 1952. [51]
Gray, J. S., 'An objective theory of emotion', *Psychol. Rev.*, 1935. [120–21]
Gregory of Nyssa, 'On the Making of Man', *Select Works and Letters* (Library of Nicene and Post-Nicene Fathers of the Christian Church, Vol. V), Oxford and N.Y., 1893. [114, 161–4]
—— 'The Great Catechism' (same volume). [161]
—— 'On virginity' (same volume). [162]
Grimberg, L., *Emotion and Delinquency*, London, 1928. [5, 7]
Grinker, R. R., 'Discussion on symposium on neurohumoral factors in emotion', *Arch. Neurol. Psychiat.*, 1955. [113]
Grossart, Fr., 'Zur Kritik der herrschenden Gefühlstheorien', *Arch. f. d. Gesamte Psychol.*, 1930; 'Gefühl und Strebung', *idem.*, 1931. [6, 18, 54]

Hocart, A. M., 'Ritual and Emotion', *The Life-Giving Myth*, London, 1952. [224]

Hoisington, L. B., 'Pleasantness and unpleasantness as modes of bodily experience ', FE 28. [94–5]

Hollander, B., *In Search of the Soul*, London, N.D. [75, 114, 172, 234]

Horiou Toki, M., 'Si-do-in-dzou, Gestes de l'officiant', *Ann. Musée Guimet, Bibl. d'Études*, Paris, 1899. [163]

Horney, K., *Neurosis and Human Growth*, London, 1951. [150, 210]

Housman, A. E., *The Name and Nature of Poetry*, Cambridge, 1933. [222–3]

Howard, D. T., 'A functional theory of the emotions', FE 28. [208]

Hull, C., *Principles of Behavior*, N.Y., 1943. [32]

Hunt, W. A., 'Recent developments in the field of emotion', *Psychol. Bull.*, 1941.

Hunt, J. McV. *et al.*, 'Situational cues distinguishing anger, fear and sorrow', *Am. J. Psychol.*, 1958. [147]

Hunter, W. S., 'The nature of instinct and its modifications', *Psychosom. Med.*, 1942. [116]

Husserl, E., *Ideas*, London and N.Y., 1931. [10]

Huxley, A., *The Doors of Perception*, London, 1954. [124]

Irons, D., 'Nature of Emotion', *Phil. Rev.*, 1897.

Jacobi, J., *Complex, Archetype, Symbol*, London and N.Y., 1959. [173]

—— *The Psychology of Jung* (5th edn.), London, 1951. [20]

Jacobson, E., *Progressive Relaxation*, Univ. of Chicago, 1929. [128]

Jacobson, E., a MS., 1951 (quoted by D. Rapaport, *Int. J. Psycho-Anal.*, 1953). [57]

James, W., *The Principles of Psychology* (1890), (Dover Edition), N.Y., 1950. [40, 49–50, 284]

—— *The Varieties of Religious Experience*, London, 1906. [231, 289]

Janet, P., *Automatisme psychologique* (3rd edn.), 1889. [46, 202, 285]

—— *L'Etat mental des hystériques* (3rd edn.), Paris, 1931. [202–3, 285]

—— 'Fear of action as an essential element in the sentiment of melancholia', FE 28. [203]

—— *Principles of Psychotherapy*, London, 1925. [203]

Jaspers, K., *Allgemeine Psychopathologie* (4th edn.), Berlin and Heidelberg, 1946. [243]

Jeans, Sir James, *Physics and Philosophy*, Cambridge, 1942. [96]

Jeness, A., 'The recognition of facial expressions of emotion', *Psychol. Bull.*, 1932. [195]

Jonas, H., 'Motility and emotion', *Actes de XIème Congrès International de Philosophie*, VII (Bruxelles, 1953), Amsterdam and Louvain. [150–1]

Jores, A., 'Hormone und Psyche', *Wien. Klin. Wchnschr.*, 1954. [121]

Jorgensen, C., 'A theory of the elements in the emotions', FE 28, [40]

Jung, C. G., *Ueber die Psychologie der Dementia praecox*, Halle, 1907 (*Coll. Works*, III). [59–60]

—— *Psychological Types*, London, 1923 (*Coll. Works*, VI). [15, 18, 60, 167, 229, 269]

Jung, C. G., 'Spirit and Life', *Contributions to Analytical Psychology*, London, 1928 (*Coll. Works*, VIII). [61]

—— *The Integration of the Personality*, London, 1940. [61]

—— *Symbolik des Geistes*, Zürich, 1948 ('A Psychological Approach to the Dogma of the Trinity', *Coll. Works*, XI). [248]

—— *Gestaltungen des Unbewussten*, Zürich, 1950 ('Concerning Mandala Symbolism', *Coll. Works*, IX). [248]

—— *Aion*, Zürich, 1951 (*Coll. Works*, IX). [248]

—— *Psychology and Alchemy*, London, 1953 (*Coll. Works*, XII). [248]

—— 'The Phenomenology of the Spirit in Fairy Tales', *Spirit and Nature*, *Papers from the Eranos Yearbooks*, N.Y. and London, 1954 (*Coll. Works*, IX). [234]

—— 'The Spirit of Psychology', same volume (*Coll. Works*, VIII). [64–5, 172–4]

—— *Von den Wurzeln des Bewusstseins*, Zürich, 1954. [248]

—— *Symbols of Transformation*, London, 1956 (*Coll. Works*, V). [77]

—— *The Transcendent Function* (1916), privately printed, Zürich, 1957 (*Coll. Works*, VIII). [181]

—— 'The Psychological Aspects of the Kore' (*Coll. Works*, IX). [181]

—— 'Psychological Aspects of the Mother Archetype' (*Coll. Works*, IX). [206]

Jung, C. G., and Pauli, W., 'Synchronicity: An acausal connecting principle', *The Interpretation of Nature and the Psyche*, London, 1955. [61–2]

Jung, R., 'Symposion ü.d. Zwischenhirn', *Hel. Physiol. et Pharmacol. Acta* 8, Suppl. 6, 1950. [106]

Kafka, G., 'Ueber Uraffekte', *Acta Psychologica*, 7, 1950. [149]

Kaiser, J. R., 'The psychology of thrill', *Ped. Sem.* 27, 1920. [159]

Kalinowsky, L. B., and Hoch, P. H., *Shock Treatments and other Somatic Procedures in Psychiatry*, N.Y., 1946. [74]

Kant, I., *Anthropologie* (Cassirer edn.), Berlin, 1923. [66, 77, 197, 214]

Kantor, J. R., *Principles of Psychology*, N.Y., 1924. [208]

Karnosh, L., 'Neurology and human emotions', *J. Am. Med. Assoc.*, 1951. [7]

Karsten, A., 'Psychische Sättigung', *Psych. Forsch.*, 1928. [140]

Katz, D., *Gestalt Psychology*, London, 1951. [139]

Keller, W., *Psychologie und Philosophie des Wollens*, München and Basel, 1954. [132]

Kennard, M. A., 'Automatic interrelation with the somatic nervous system', *Psychosom. Med.*, 1947. [127]

—— 'The electroencephalogram in psychological disorders—a review', *Psychosom. Med.*, 1953. [84]

Kierkegaard, S., *The Concept of Dread*, Princeton, 1946. [162–4]

King, C. D., *The Psychology of Consciousness*, London, 1932. [47]

Klages, L., *Grundlegung der Wissenschaft vom Ausdruck* (7th edn.), Bonn, 1950. [82–3, 196]

Klopfer, B., and Ainsworth, M., *et al.*, *Developments in the Rorschach Technique*, Vol. I, N.Y. and London, n.d. [72]

Klüver, H., 'Functional differences between the occipital and temporal lobes', *Cerebral Mechanisms in Behavior* (ed. by L. Jeffress), N.Y. and London, 1951. [193–4]

Knapp, P. H., 'Conscious and unconscious affects: A preliminary approach to concepts and methods of study', in *Research in Affects* (Psychiatric Research Reports, 8, 1957). [85, 199, 225, 272]

Koffka, K., *Principles of Gestalt Psychology*, London, 1935. [35–6, 48, 139–40)

Köhler, W., *Gestalt Psychology*, London, 1930 (and N.Y. 1947 edn.). [139]

—— *Die physischen Gestalten in Ruhe und im stationären Zustand*, Erlangen, 1924. [52]

Krapf, E. E., 'Ueber Kälte- und Wärmeerlebnisse in der Uebertragung', in *Entfaltung der Psychoanalyse* (ed. A. Mitscherlich), Stuttgart, 1956. [78]

Kraus, F., *Allgemeine und spezielle Pathologie der Person*, 2 vols., Leipzig, 1919–26. [110]

Kretschmer, W. E., Jr., 'Meditation in der Psychologie und Psychiatrie der Gegenwart', *Zschft. f. Rel. u. Geistesgesch.*, 1958. [181]

—— 'Die meditativen Verfahren in der Psychotherapie', *Zschft. f. Psychotherapie u. med. Psychol.*, 1951. [181]

Kris, E., *Psychoanalytic Explorations in Art*, N.Y., 1952. [224, 238]

Krueger, F., 'The essence of feeling', FE 28. [93–4]

Kubie, L. S., 'The central representation of the symbolic process in relation to psychosomatic disorders', RDPM. [108]

—— 'Influence of symbolic processes on the role of instincts in human behavior', *Psychosom. Med.*, 1956. [108, 183]

Kühn, H., 'Die Bedeutung des Fühlens für den Erlebnisaufbau', *Der Nervenartz*, 1947. [90]

Kurtz, P., 'An approach to psychodynamic appraisal', *J. Nerv. Ment. Dis.*, 1953. [111]

Lacey, J., Bateman, B., and Van Lehn, R., 'Autonomic response specificity', *Psychosom. Med.*, 1953. [156]

Lacroze, R., *L'Angoisse et l'Emotion*, Paris, 1938. [163–4]

Lactantius, *De Ira Dei*. [117]

Lagerborg, R., *Des Gefühlsproblem*, Leipzig, 1905. [117]

Laignel-Lavastine, M., *The Concentric Method in the Diagnosis of Psychoneurotics*, London, 1931. [46, 243]

Landauer, K., 'Affects, passions and temperament', *Int. J. Psycho-Anal.*, 1938. [56, 158, 221]

Landis, C., 'An attempt to measure emotional traits in juvenile delinquency', *Studies in the Dynamics of Behavior* (ed. by K. Lashley), Univ. of Chic., 1932. [12–13, 272]

—— 'Emotion', *Psychology*, Boring, Langfeld and Weld, N.Y., 1935. [36, 135–6, 244]

—— 'The interpretation of facial expression in emotion', *J. General Psychol.*, 1929. [136, 196]

Landis, C., and Hunt, W., *The Startle Pattern*, N.Y., 1939. [154]

Landolt, H., 'Elektroenzephalographische Untersuchungen bei nicht katatonen Schizophrenien', *Schweiz. Zschft. f. Psychol. u. ihre Anwendungen*, 1957. [88–9]

—— 'Ueber Verstimmungen, Dämmerzustände und Schizophrene Zustandsbilder bei Epilepsie', *Schweiz. Arch. f. Neurol. u. Psychiat.*, 1955. [88–9]

Lange, C., 'Om Sindsbevaegelser', Köbenhavn, 1885, in *The Classical Psychologists*, London, 1912, and in German translation by H. Kurella, Leipzig, 1887. [116, 122, 125–6]

Langfeld, H. S., 'The role of feeling and emotion in aesthetics', FE 28. [223]

—— 'Feeling and emotion in art', FE 50. [224]

Langworthy, O. R., 'Newer concepts of the central control of emotions: A Review', *Am. J. Psychiat.*, 1955.

Lasagna, L., von Felsinger, J., and Beecher, H., 'Drug induced mood changes in man, I and II', *J.A.M.A.*, 1957. [123]

Lavin, A., *et al.*, 'Centrifugal arousal in the olfactory bulb', *Science*, 129 (1959). [235]

Laycock, T., *A Treatise on the Nervous Diseases of Women*, London, 1840. [78]

Leeper, R. W., 'A motivational theory of emotion to replace "emotion as a disorganized response" ', *Psychol. Rev.*, 1948. [207, 217–18]

Lehmann, A., *Die Hauptgesetze des menschlichen Gefühlslebens* (2nd edn.), Leipzig, 1914. [175, 223, 243]

Lersch, P., *Aufbau der Person*, München, 1952. [91–2]

Lévy-Bruhl, L., *Les Fonctions mentales dans les sociétés inférieures* (2nd edn.), Paris, 1912. [172]

Lewin, B. D., *The Psychoanalysis of Elation*, London, 1951. [97]

Lewin, K., *A Dynamic Theory of Personality*, N.Y., 1935. [140–1]

—— *Principles of Topological Psychology*, N.Y., 1936. [90–1, 140]

Lhermitte, J., 'Le cœur dans ses rapports avec les états affectifs', *Le Cœur, Etudes Carmélitaines*, chez Desclées de Brouwer, 1950. [98]

Liddell, H. S., 'Conditioning and the emotions', in *Twentieth Century Bestiary (First Book of Animals)*, N.Y., 1955. [145–6]

Lindsley, D. B., 'Emotion and the electroencephalogram', FE 50. [104]

—— 'Emotion', *Handbook of Experimental Psychology* (ed. by Stevens), N.Y. and London, 1951. [103–5, 244]

Lindworsky, J., 'Orientierende Untersuchungen über höhere Gefühle', *Arch. f. d. ges. Psychol.*, 1928. [70–1]

Lipps, T., *Leitfaden der Psychologie*, Leipzig (3rd edn.), 1909. [94–5]

London, I., 'Theory of emotions in Soviet dialectic psychology', FE 50. [119, 136]

López Esnaurrízar, M., 'Las emociones y el simpático', *Medicina México*, 1953. [119, 122]

Lotze, R. H., *Medizinische Psychologie*, Leipzig, 1852. [115, 117]

Lund, F. H., *Emotions*, N.Y., 1939. [135]

Luria, A. R., *The Nature of Human Conflicts, or Emotion, Conflict and Will*, N.Y., 1932. [180–1, 202]

Maass, J. G. F., *Versuch ueber die Gefühle, bes. ueber die Affekten,* Halle and Leipzig, 1811–12. [92]

—— '*Versuch ueber die Leidenschaften*', Halle and Leipzig, 1805–07. [92, 180]

MacCurdy, J. T., *The Psychology of Emotion,* London, 1925. [135, 171–3, 235]

MacLean, P. D., 'The limbic system ("visceral brain") in relation to central gray and reticulum of the brain stem: Evidence of inter-dependence in emotional processes', *Psychosom. Med.,* 1955. [105–7]

—— 'Psychosomatic disease and the "visceral brain" ', *Psychosom. Med.,* 1949. [107–8]

—— 'Studies on limbic system ("visceral brain") and their bearing on psychosomatic problems', RDPM. [79, 107, 235]

MacLeod, A. W., Wittkower, E. D., and Margolin, S. G., 'Basic concepts of psychosomatic medicine', RDPM. [72, 141]

MacMurray, J., *Reason and Emotion,* London, 1935. [191, 200, 238]

Maine de Biran, F. P. G., 'Essai sur les fondemends de la psychologie' (1812), *Œuvres Inédites,* Paris, 1859. [131]

Malebranche, N., *De la Recherche de la Vérité* (Garnier ed.), 1674. [221]

Mall, G., *Konstitution und Affekt,* Leipzig, 1936. [156]

Malmo, R. B., 'Research: experimental and theoretical aspects', RDPM. [36, 114, 274]

Malmud, R. S., 'Poetry and the emotions', *J. Abn. Soc. Psych.,* 1927–8. [47]

Malraux, A., *The Creative Act,* N.Y., 1949 (*La Création Artistique,* 1948). [222]

Mangan, G., 'A Review of Published Research on the Relationship of Some Personality Variables to ESP Scoring Level', *Parapsychological Monographs,* 1, N.Y., 1958. [5]

Marañón, G., 'The psychology of gesture', *J. Nerv. Ment. Dis.,* 1950. [197–8]

Margetts, E. L., 'Historical notes on psychosomatic medicine', RDPM. [3]

Marston, W. M., 'Analysis of emotions', *Encyclopedia Britannica* (14th edn.), 1929. [6, 18]

—— *Emotions of Normal People,* London, 1928. [68–9]

Maslow, A., 'The instinctoid nature of basic needs', *J. of Personality,* 1953–4. [211]

Masserman, J. H., 'A biodynamic psychoanalytic approach to the problems of feeling and emotion', FE 50. [6, 33, 35]

—— *Principles of Dynamic Psychiatry,* Philadelphia, 1946. [47, 210]

Massignon, L., 'L'idée de l'esprit dans l'Islam', *Eranos Jahrbuch XIII,* Zürich, 1946. [233, 235]

Mayer, C. F., 'Metaphysical trends in modern pathology', *Bull. Hist. Med.,* 1952. [142]

McDougall, W., 'Organization of the affective life', *Acta Psychologica,* 1937. [38]

—— *An Outline of Psychology* (12th edn.), London, 1948. [45, 172, 46]

McFie, J., Piercy, M. F., and Zangwill, O., 'The Rorschach Test in obsessional neurosis with special reference to the effects of pre-frontal leucotomy', *Brit. J. Med. Psychol.*, 1951. [175]

McGill, V., *Emotions and Reason*, Springfield, Ill., 1954. [190, 207]

McGinnies, E., 'Emotionality and perceptual defense', *Psychol. Rev.*, 1949. [218]

McKellar, P., *A Textbook of Human Psychology*, London, 1952. [218]

McKinney, J., 'What shall we choose to call emotion', *J. Nerv. Ment. Dis.*, 1930. [68]

Meier, C. A., 'Moderne Physik—Moderne Psychologie', in *Die Kulturelle Bedeutung der Komplexen Psychologie*, Berlin, 1935. [96]

Meinong, A., 'Ueber emotionale Präsentation', *Wien. Sitzungsberichte*, 183, 1917. [192]

Merry, J., 'Excitatory group psychotherapy', *J. Ment. Sci.*, 1953. [72–3]

Mesmer, F. A., *Mémoire sur la découverte du magnétisme animal*, Genève, 1779. Eng. transl. G. Frankau, *Mesmerism*, London, 1948. [73]

Messer, A., *Psychologie* (5th edn.), Leipzig, 1934. [81]

Metzger, W., *Gesetze des Sehens*, Frankfurt a/M, 1953. [53]

Meyer, M. F., 'That whale among the fishes—the theory of emotions', *Psychol. Rev.*, 1933. [32]

Meyer, A., 'Discontent', *Collected Papers of Adolf Meyer, IV*, Baltimore, 1952. [157]

Meynert, T., *Sammlung von populär-wissenschaftlichen Vorträgen*, Vienna and Leipzig, 1892. [117]

Michotte, A. E., 'The emotions regarded as functional connections', FE 50. [150]

Minkowski, E., 'L'Affectivité', *L'Evolution Psychiatrique*, 1947. [149]

Mittelman, B., and Wolff, H. G., 'Affective states and skin temperature', *Psychosom. Med.*, 1943, p. 243. [78]

du Moulin, P., *A Treatise on Peace of Soul and Content of Mind* (trans. by J. Scrope), Salisbury, 1765. [187]

Mühl, A., 'Problems in general medicine from the emotional standpoint', *Psychoanal. Rev.*, 1929.

Naccarati, S., 'Hormones and emotions', *Med. Rec.*, 1921. [121]

Nahm, M. C., 'The philosophical implications of some theories of emotion', *Phil. of Sci.*, 1939. [177–8]

Nemesius of Emesa, 'De natura hominis', 16 (Library of Christian Classics IV), London, 1955. [114, 209, 212–13]

Neumann, E., 'Der schöpferische Mensch und die "grosse Erfahrung" ', *Eranos Jahrbuch* XXV, Zürich, 1957. [225]

—— *The Origins and History of Consciousness*, London, 1954. [64]

Nielsen, J., and Sedgwick, R., 'Instincts and emotions in an anencephalic monster', *J. Nerv. Ment. Dis.*, 1949. [113]

Niemeyer, L. H. C., *Commentatio de Commercio inter animi pathemata*, Göttingen, 1795. [227]

Nietzsche, F., *Der Wille zur Macht* (Kroner edn.), Leipzig, 1912. [92, 227, 289]

de Nogales Quevedo, C., *Psiquismo y Secreciones Internas: Emoción Nosógena*, Barcelona, 1950. [187, 198]

Nony, C., 'The biological and social significance of the expression of the emotions', *Brit. J. Psychol.*, 1922–3. [197]

Nogué, J., 'Le symbolisme spatial de la qualité', *Rev. Phil.*, 1926. [97]

Novey, S., 'A clinical view of affect theory in psycho-analysis', *Int. J. Psycho-Anal.*, 1959. [56]

Nunberg, H., *Allgemeine Neurosenlehre*, Bern, 1932. [56]

Nuttin, J., 'Intimacy and shame in the dynamic structure of personality', FE 50. [136]

Ogden, C. K., and Richards, I. A., *The Meaning of Meaning*, 1923, London (7th edn.), 1945. [189]

Onians, R. B., *The Origins of European Thought about the Body, the Mind, the Soul, the World, Time and Fate*, Cambridge, 1954. [76–7, 98–9, 172, 175, 232–35, 289]

Orwell, G., *Nineteen Eighty-Four*, London, 1949 (Penguin Books 1954). [15]

Otto, R., *The Idea of the Holy*, Oxford, 1923. [194]

Oxford English Dictionary. [8, 43, 267, 287]

Papez, J. W., 'A proposed mechanism of emotion', *Arch. Neurol. Psychiat.*, 1937. [103]

Pascal, *Pensées*. [189]

Pasquarelli, B., and Bull, N., 'Experimental investigations of the body-mind continuum in affective states', *J. Nerv. Ment. Dis.*, 1951. [130]

Paulhan, F., *The Laws of Feeling*, London, 1930. [204, 215]

Pauli, W., 'The influence of archetypal ideas on the scientific theories of Kepler', *The Interpretation of Nature and the Psyche*, London, 1955. [96, 248]

Petrie, A., *Personality and the Frontal Lobes*, London, 1952. [176]

Phillips, M., *The Education of the Emotions through Sentiment Development*, London, 1937. [200]

Pieron, H., 'Emotion in animals and man', FE 28. [81]

Pillsbury, W. B., 'The utility of emotions', FE 28. [45]

Pinel, P., *Traité médico-philosophique sur l'aliénation mentale*, Paris, 1801. [117]

Plato, *Phaedrus; Parmenides; Laws*. [132, 164, 201, 209, 233, 289]

Plessner, H., *Lachen und Weinen* (2nd edn.), Bern, 1950. [215]

Plotinus, *Enneads*. [174, 210]

Plutarch, *Moralia*, 'Of common conceptions, against the Stoics', ed. by W. Goodwin, London, 1870, Vol. IV. [36]

Plutchik, R., 'Some problems for a theory of emotion', *Psychosom. Med.*, 1955. [15, 42]

Pope, A., *An Essay on Man*. [205]

Portman, A., 'Die Bedeutung der Bilder in der lebendigen Energiewandlung', *Eranos Jahrbuch* XXI, Zürich, 1953. [174]

Poynter, F. N. L. (ed.), *The History and Philosophy of Knowledge of the Brain and its Functions*, Oxford, 1958. [75]

Precker, J. A., 'Toward a theoretical brain-model', *J. of Personality*, 1953–54. [33]

Prescott, D. A., *Emotion and the Educative Process*, Washington, 1938. [137, 219]

Price, H. H., *Thinking and Experience*, London, 1953. [188]

—— 'Haunting and the "psychic ether"', *Tomorrow*, 5, 1957. [63]

Prince, M., 'Can emotion be regarded as energy?' FE 28. [67–8, 264]

Rapaport, D., *Emotions and Memory* (2nd edn.), N.Y., 1950. [58, 175]

—— 'On the psycho-analytic theory of affects', *Int. J. Psycho-Anal.*, 1953. [58–9]

Razran, G., 'Soviet psychology since 1950', *Science* 126 (1957). [136]

Read, H., *Education through Art*, London, 1943. [220]

—— 'Poetic consciousness and creative experience', *Eranos Jahrbuch*, XXV, Zürich, 1957. [224]

Reich, W., *Character Analysis* (3rd edn.), N.Y., 1949. [73–4, 150]

Reichenbach, H., *The Rise of Scientific Philosophy*, Univ. of Calif., 1951. [16, 189, 247]

Reid, L. A., 'Instinct, emotion and the higher life', *Brit. J. Psychol.*, 1923. [191–2, 225]

Reid, J. R., 'Introduction' to *Emotions and Clinical Medicine* by S. Cobb, N.Y., 1950. [245]

Reymert, M. (ed.), *Feelings and Emotions—The Moosheart Symposium*, N.Y., 1950. [98]

—— (ed.), *Feelings and Emotions—The Wittenberg Symposium*, Clark Univ., 1928. [24]

Rhine, J. B., and Pratt, J. G., *Parapsychology*, Springfield, Ill., 1957. [63]

Ribot, Th., *Essay on the Creative Imagination*, London, 1906. [222]

—— *The Psychology of the Emotions*, London, 1897. [49, 172, 196, 243, 278]

—— *La psychologie des sentiments* (3rd edn.), Paris, 1899. [49, 243]

Richards, I. A., *Speculative Instruments*, London, 1955. [189]

Richmond, J., and Lustman, S., 'Autonomic function in the neonate: 1. Implication for psychosomatic theory', *Psychosom. Med.*, 1955. [156]

Richter, C. P., 'On the phenomenon of sudden death in animals and man', *Psychosom. Med.*, 1957. [228]

Rignano, E., *Biological Memory*, London, 1926. [168]

—— *De l'origine et de la nature mnémonique des tendances affectives*, Bologna, 1911. [168]

—— *The Psychology of Reasoning*, London, 1923. [221]

Rivers, W. H. R., *Conflict and Dream*, London, 1923. [45]

—— *Instinct and the Unconscious*, Cambridge, 1920. [45]

Rof Carballo, J., 'Fisiopatologia de la emoción', *Medicina Clinica*, Barcelona, 1950. [109, 159]

Rohracher, H., *Einführung in die Psychologie* (4th edn.), Wien and Innsbruck, 1951. [60]

Rome, H. P., 'The dynamics of emotions', *Minn. Med.*, 1953. [159]

de Ropp, R. S., *Drugs and the Mind*, N.Y., 1957. [123]

Rosenzweig, N., 'The Affect System: Foresight and Fantasy', *J. Nerv. Ment. Dis.*, 1958. [188]

Rothacker, E., *Die Schichten der Persönlichkeit* (4th edn.), Bonn, 1948. [79]

Ruckmick, C. A., *The Psychology of Feeling and Emotion*, N.Y. and London, 1936. [39–40, 157–8]

Rush, B., *Medical Inquiries and Observations upon the Diseases of the Mind*, Philadelphia, 1812. [123]

Russell, B., *The Analysis of Mind*, London, 1921. [167–8]

Ryle, G., *The Concept of Mind*, London, 1949. [35, 249]

Sabshin, M., and Ramot, J., 'Pharmacotherapeutic evaluations and the psychiatric setting', *Arch. Neurol. Psychiat.*, 1956. [123]

Sargant, W., and Slater, E., *An Introduction to the Physical Methods of Treatment in Psychiatry*, (2nd edn.), Edinburgh, 1948. [72]

—— 'On chemical tranquillizers', *Brit. Med. J.*, 1956. [122]

Sartre, J. P., *Esquisse d'une théorie des émotions* (3rd edn.), Paris, 1948, (*The Emotions: Outline of a Theory*, N.Y., 1948). [9, 11, 186—7]

Sarwer-Foner, G. J., 'The transference and nonspecific drug effects in the use of the tranquilizing drugs, and their influence on affect', *Research in Affects* (Psychiatric Research Reports 8, 1957). [123–4]

Saul, L. J., *Emotional Maturity*, Philadelphia, 1947. [217]

—— *Bases of Human Behavior*, Philadelphia, 1951. [39, 195]

Saul, L., Davis, H., and Davis, P., 'Psychologic correlations with the encephalogram', *Psychosom. Med.*, 1949. [84]

Scheidemantel, F. C. G., *Die Leidenschaften als Heilmittel betrachtet*, Leipzig, 1787. [227]

Scheler, M., 'Der Formalismus in der Ethik and die materiale Wertethik', *Jhrbch. f. Phil. u. phänomen. Forsch.*, Halle, 1916–22. [192]

—— *Zur Phänomenologie und Theorie der Sympathiegefühle*, Halle, 1913 (*The Nature of Sympathy*, London, 1954). [11]

Schilder, P., 'Studies concerning the psychology and symptomatology of general paresis', in *Organization and Pathology of Thought* (ed. D. Rapaport), N.Y., 1951. [195]

Schiller, F., *On the Aesthetic Education of Man*, London, 1954. [220]

Schlosberg, H., 'Three dimensions of emotions', *Psychol. Rev.*, 1954. [83, 85]

Schneider, A., 'Die Psychologie Alberts des Grossen', *Beiträge z. Gesch. d. Phil. d. Mittelalters*, IV, 5 and 6, Münster, 1903. [75, 114, 119]

Schopenhauer, A., 'Animalischer Magnetismus und Magie', *Ueber den Willen in der Natur* (Coll. Works, Frauenstädt and Hübscher Edition, Leipzig, 1938). [62, 182]

—— *Ueber die vierfache Wurzel des Satzes vom zureichenden Grunde* (*On the Fourfold Root of the Principle of Sufficient Reason*, London, 1889). [246–47]

Schou, H. I., *Some Investigations into the Physiology of Emotions*, Copenhagen and London, 1937. [102–3]

Schrödinger, E., 'The spirit of science', in *Spirit and Nature, Papers from the Eranos Yearbooks*, N.Y. and London, 1954. [260]

Schultz-Hencke, H., *Der Gehemmte Mensch*, Leipzig, 1940. [94, 201]

Schultz, J. H., *Das Autogene Training* (3 Aufl.), Leipzig, 1937. [129]

Sechehaye, M. A., *Symbolic Realization*, N.Y., 1951. [182]

Selye, H., *Stress*, Montreal, 1950. [141]

Semon, R., *Die Mneme* (3rd edn.), Leipzig, 1911. [168]

Senaut, J. F., *The Use of the Passions*, London, 1649. [1, 159–60]

Sergi, G., 'Ueber den Sitz und die psychiche Grundlage der Affekte', *Zschft. f. Psychol. u. Physiol. d. Sinnesorg.*, 1897. [99, 116]

Seydl, E., 'Alkuins Psychologie', *Jhbch. f. Phil. u. spek. Theol.*, Paderborn, 1911. [119]

Shand, A. F., *The Foundations of Character* (2nd edn.), London, 1920. [5, 38, 160]

—— 'Character and the emotions', *Mind*, N.S., V, 1896. [43]

Sherrington, Sir Charles, *The Integrative Action of the Nervous System* (1947 edn.), Cambridge, 1952. [87, 127, 149]

—— *Man on His Nature* (2nd edn.), N.Y., 1953. [76–7, 233]

Shute, C., *The Psychology of Aristotle*, N.Y., 1941. [19]

Silberer, H., 'Bericht über eine Methode gewisse symbolische Halluzinationen Erscheinungen hervorzurufen und zu beobachten', *Jhrb. f. Psychoanal. Psychopath. Forsch.*, 1909. (Eng. trans. in *Organization and Pathology of Thought* (ed. D. Rapaport)), N.Y., 1951. [181]

Sinnot, E. W., *The Biology of the Spirit*, London, 1956. [233]

Smith, A., and Kinder, E. F., 'Changes in psychological test performances of brain-operated schizophrenics after 8 years', *Science*, 129 (1959). [176]

Smith, F. V., *The Explanation of Human Behaviour*, London, 1951. [288]

Smith, N. Kemp, 'Fear: Its nature and diverse uses', *Philos.*, 1957. [227]

Smith, W. Whately, *The Measurement of Emotion*, London, 1922. [7, 83, 203]

Solomon, M., 'The mechanism of the emotions', *Brit. J. Med. Psychol.*, 1927. [111]

Spearman, A., *Psychology Down the Ages*, Vols. I and II, London, 1937. [130, 131, 152]

Spencer, H., *The Principles of Psychology*, London, 1855. [117]

Spiegel, E., and Wycis, H. *et al.*, 'The central mechanism of the emotions', *Am. J. Psychiat.*, 1951. [113]

Spies, T. D., in *Newsweek* (Internat. ed.), XLIX, 24, June 1957. [129]

Spinoza, *Ethica*. [33, 106, 117, 160, 180]

Stanley, H. M., *Studies in the Evolutionary Psychology of Feeling*, London, 1895. [168]

Stein, L., 'What is a symbol supposed to be?' *J. Analyt. Psychol.*, 1957. [173]

Steinitzer, M., *Die Menschlichen und Tierischen Gemütsbewegungen als Gegenstand der Wissenschaft*, Münich, 1889. [287]

Stern, W., *Allgemeine Psychologie*, Haag, 1935. [88]

—— ' "Ernstspiel" and the affective life', FE, 28. [97]

Stieler, G., 'Die Emotionen', *Arch. f. d. Ges. Psychol.*, 1925. [116–17]

Störring, G., *Psychologie des menschlichen Gefühlslebens*, Bonn, 1916.

Stout, G. F., *A Manual of Psychology* (5th edn.), London, 1938. [5, 39, 243]

Strasser, S., *Das Gemüt*, Utrecht, Antwerpen and Freiburg, 1956. [97, 214–215]

Stratton, G. M., 'The function of emotion as shown particularly in excitement', *Psychol. Rev.*, 1928. [218]

Sullivan, H. S., *Clinical Studies in Psychiatry*, N.Y., 1956. [43]

—— *The Interpersonal Theory of Psychiatry*, London, 1955. [46]

Summers, M., *The Physical Phenomena of Mysticism*, London, 1950. [235]

Suttie, I., *The Origins of Love and Hate*, London, 1935. [159]

Suzuki, D. T., 'The awakening of a new consciousness in Zen', *Eranos Jahrbuch XXIII*, Zürich, 1955. [220]

Tertullian, 'De Anima', ANCL XV. [106, 114–15, 209, 212–13]

——'De Testimonio Animae Liber Adversus Gentes', *Opera . . . Omnia*, Paris, 1616 (ANCL, XI). [10]

Terzian, H., and Dalle Ore, G., 'Syndrome of Klüver and Bucy reproduced in man by bilateral removal of the temporal lobe', *Neurology*, 1955. [194]

Thalbitzer, S., *Emotion and Insanity*, London, 1926. [81–2]

Thomas Aquinas, *De Trinitate* (Philosophical Texts, ed. by T. Gilby, Oxford, 1951). [178]

—— *Summa Theologica* (Philosophical Texts, ed. by T. Gilby, Oxford, 1951). [106, 178, 276]

Thorndike, E. L., *Mental and Social Measurements*, N.Y., 1913. [84]

Thouless, R. H., 'The affective function of language', FE 50. [189]

Thurstone, L. L., *The Vectors of the Mind*, Univ. of Chicago, 1935. [41]

The Times (London), July 17, 1957. [123]

Tissot, S. A., *Traité des nerfs et de leurs maladies*, Lausanne, 1789. [227]

Titchener, E. B., 'An historical note on the James-Lange theory of emotion', *Am. J. Psychol.*, 1914. [115]

Tolman, E. C., 'A behavioristic account of the emotions' (reprinted from the *Psychol. Rev.*, 1923) in *Collected Papers in Psychology*, Univ. of Calif., 1951. [145]

Tow, P. MacD., *Personality Changes Following Frontal Leucotomy*, Oxford, 1955. [97, 176–7]

Troland, L. T., 'A system for explaining affective phenomena', *J. Abn. Psychol.*, 1920. [82]

Tucker, A. (Ed. Search), *The Light of Nature Pursued*, Vol. II, London, 1768. [155]

Tuke, D. H., *Illustrations of the Influence of the Mind upon the Body*, London, 1872. [114, 127]

Tuttle, H. S., 'Emotion as substitute response', *J. General Psychol.*, 1940. [205]

Tyrell, G., *Apparitions*, London, 1953. [63]

Ubeda Purkiss, Fr. M., 'Desarrollo histórico de las doctrinas sobre las emociones', *La Ciencia Tomista* 248, 1953; 250, 1954. [115]

Veith, I., 'Non-western concepts of psychic function', in *The History and Philosophy of Knowledge of The Brain and its Functions*, ed. by F. N. L. Poynter, Oxford, 1958. [98]

Verworn, M., *Kausale und Konditionale Weltanschauung* (3rd edn.), Jena, 1928. [20]

Walde, A., *Lateinisches Etymologisches Wörterbuch* (3rd edn.), Heidelberg, 1938–40. [43]

—— *Vergleichendes Wörterbuch der Indogermanischen Sprachen*, Berlin and Leipzig, 1928. [99]

Wallace, E., *Outlines of the Philosophy of Aristotle* (3rd edn.), Cambridge, 1887. [21]

Waller, A. D., 'Concerning emotive phenomena', *Proc. Royal Soc.*, Series B, 1920. [83–84]

Wallon, H., *L'Evolution psychologique de l'enfant*, Paris, 1950. [154]

Warnock, M., 'The justification of emotions' (Symposium), *The Aristotelian Society, Suppl. Vol. XXXI*, 1957. [84, 281]

Warren, H. C., *Dictionary of Psychology and Cognate Sciences*, 1934. [6]

Washburn, M., 'Emotion and thought: A motor theory of their relations', FE 28. [127–8]

Watson, J. B., *Psychology from the Standpoint of a Behaviorist*, Philadelphia and London (3rd edn., 1929, first edn. 1919). [128, 145, 146–7, 284]

Webb, W. B., 'A motivational theory of emotions', *Psychol. Rev.*, 1948. [144]

Weber, A. O., and Rapaport, D., 'Teleology and the emotions', *Phil. of Sci.*, 1941. [200]

Wechsler, D., 'Further comment on the psychological significance of the galvanic experiment', *Brit. J. Psychol.*, 1925–6. [83]

Weiss, A. P., 'Feeling and emotion as forms of behaviour', FE 28. [144–5]

Wenger, M., 'Emotion as visceral action: an extension of Lange's theory', FE 50. [118]

White, W. A., 'The frustration theory of consciousness', *Psychoanal. Rev.*, 1929. [78]

Whitehead, A. N., *Modes of Thought*, Cambridge, U.S.A., 1938. [69–70, 193–4, 215]

Whitehorn, J., 'Physiological changes in emotional states' in the *Inter-Relationship of Body and Mind*, Baltimore, 1939. [97]

—— 'Concerning emotion as impulsion and instinct as orientation', *Am. J. Psychiat.*, 1932. [280]

Wiener, N., *The Human Use of Human Beings, Cybernetics and Society* (2nd edn.), N.Y., 1954. [120, 199, 219]

Wikler, A., 'A critical analysis of some current concepts in psychiatry', *Psychosom. Med.*, 1952. [243, 257]

Wilde, O., *The Picture of Dorian Gray*, London, 1891. [216]

Wilhelm, R., and Jung, C. G., *The Secret of the Golden Flower*, London, 1931. [75, 153]

Wili, W., 'The history of the spirit in antiquity', *Spirit and Nature, Papers from the Eranos Yearbooks*, N.Y. and London, 1954. [232]

Williams, D., 'The structure of emotions reflected in epileptic experiences', *Brain*, 1956. [41]

Williams, R. J., 'Some implications of physiological individuality', FE 50. [156]

Wittkower, E., 'Studies on the influence of emotions on the functions of the organs', *J. Ment. Sci.*, 1935. [6]

Wolf, A., *Spinoza's Short Treatise*, London, 1910. [249]

Wolff, C., *The Psychology of Gesture*, London, 1945. [207, 215–16]

Woodger, J. H., *Physics, Psychology and Medicine*, Cambridge, 1956. [3, 11, 23, 189, 241]

Woodworth and Marquis, *Psychology* (20th edn.), London, 1949. [243]

Wordsworth, W., *Lyrical Ballads with other Poems*, Vol. I (2nd edn. London, 1800. [223]

Wreschner, A., *Das Gefühl*, Leipzig, 1931. [159]

Wright, T., *The Passions of the Minde in Generall*, London, 1604. [196]

Wundt, W., *Lectures on Human and Animal Psychology*, London and N.Y., 1894. [168, 175]

Yakovlev, P. I., 'Motility, Behavior and the Brain: Stereodynamic organization and neural co-ordinates of behavior', *J. Nerv. Ment. Dis.*, 1948. [222]

Young, P. T., *Emotion in Man and Animal*, N.Y., 1943. [196, 205, 208, 219, 229, 243]

Zeller, E., *The Stoics, Epicureans and Sceptics*, London, 1892. [112, 135, 174]

Zilboorg, G., *A History of Medical Psychology*, N.Y., 1941.

—— 'The emotional problem and the therapeutic role of insight', *Yearbook of Psychoanalysis*, Vol. IX, N.Y., 1953. [3, 219]

Zinkin, J., Book Review in *J. Nerv. Ment. Dis.*, 1954. [6]

SUBJECT INDEX

313

fluid, 75–6

fluid model of the soul, 71–77, 197, 204

forces, emotional, 41–3, 260

form, 267n.

Freud, S., 3, 54–7, 65, 70, 110, 142, 159, 160, 179, 284; on *Angst*, 162; on inherited memory, 168–70; on unconscious emotions, 54–6

function, and structure, 101–3, 106, 113

fury, 85; *see also* anger

'Geist', 215, 232, 237

Gemüt, 92, 98

genesis, emotion and, 154–65

genetic endownment, 252, 255

Gestalt psychology, 48, 139–40, 210, 256

gesture, 197, 207

gifts, emotions as, 96, 231–2, 289

glands, 120, 145, 155, 252

God: absence of emotion in, 117, 126; and evil, 161, 164; image of, as curative, 181–2; and disorder, 209; e. leading to God, 92, 192, 195, 238

gut(s), 234, 252; *see also* visceral

haruspicy, 234n.

heart, 98–9, 153

heat, 77–9, 206

hedonism, 67, 74

Hemmung, 201

heredity, 156, *see also* genetic endowment

'higher' and 'lower', 115–16, 125

historical method, 17, 18

homeostasis, 67, 102, 118, 120, 263

hormones, 120–2

horse: as image, 79; Plato's myth of, 201, 209, 212, 280, 288–9

humour, 254; wit, 179

hypnosis, 130

hypothalamus, 213n.

hypothesis: choice of, 23; fundamental, 29

ib, 99

ideas and emotions, *see* representations, values

idées-forces, 172

images: and emotion, 175 ff.; unconscious, 171; *see also* memory images

imagination: active, 181, 282, 284; impoverishment of, 176–8

imperfection, and evil, 210

improvement, 277, 283–4

inertia, 206, 260, 263

inhibition, cortical, 110–11, 252

initiation ceremonies, 220

inner and outer, 90, 94–6, 254

insight, emotional, 3, 219

inspiration, 232–3, 237, 238

instinct, 49, 169–70, 171, 173–4; and emotion, difference, 279–80n.

integration, problem of, 18, 23

intensity, 258; affective, 82; i. mobilization, 32

intention, 137–8, 215

intra-systemic sign, emotion as, 198

introspection, 34, 37, 95

intuition, 229n., 235n., 270n.

inwardness, of emotion, 91 ff., 271

irrationality, 191, 209

irritation, 67, 76, 85

isomorphism, 47, 71, 48–53, 121, 262, 271–3; simple, 51–2; sophisticated, 52–3

James, William, 49–50, 51, 52, 231, 284n., 289

Jung, C. G., 3, 15n., 18, 20, 39, 59–65, 77n., 167n., 172–3, 174, 206, 229n., 232, 234n., 235, 238, 248, 269n.

knowing, as emotional experience, 220

Kundalini yoga, 98, 284n.

laughter, 254

learning: emotion and, 219–21, 255; *see also* knowledge

leucotomy, 116, 175–6

libido, 76–7, 160; damming up of, 204

life: emotion as essence of, 97–8, 151, 262, 273; stages of, 153, 255, 256

limbic lobe, 105–6

linguistic analysis, 5

liquid, 76–7n.

liver, 98, 234

lobectomy, 193–4

lobotomy, prefrontal, 3, 176

location: physiological, 100–34; psychological, 90–9

locomotion, motion and, 152

love, 159–60, 194, 261

magic, 62–3, 186, 274